120-00

BURREN

PEDIATRIC CARDIOLOGY
For Practitioners

Second Edition

Pediatric Cardiology for Practitioners

Second Edition

Myung K. Park, M.D.

Professor of Pediatrics
Head, Division of Cardiology
University of Texas Health Science Center
San Antonio, Texas

YEAR BOOK MEDICAL PUBLISHERS, INC.
Chicago • London • Boca Raton

3 4 5 6 7 8 9 0 CC 92 91 90

Library of Congress Cataloging-in-Publication Data

Park, Myung K. (Myung Kun), 1934–
  Pediatric cardiology for practitioners.

  Includes bibliographies and index.
  1. Pediatric cardiology. I. Title. [DNLM: 1. Heart
Defects, Congenital. 2. Heart Diseases—in infancy &
childhood.   WS 290 P235p]
RJ421.P37   1988   618.92'12   88-144
ISBN 0-8151-6617-6

Sponsoring Editor: Nancy E. Chorpenning
Associate Managing Editor, Manuscript Services: Deborah Thorp
Production Project Manager: Gayle Paprocki
Proofroom Supervisor: Shirley E. Taylor

To my wife, Issun, and our boys Douglas, Christopher, and Warren.

Foreword to the First Edition

I was very honored by Dr. Park's request that I review his manuscript and write a foreword. Having carefully read it, I am even more pleased to be able to write a foreword with unqualified praise and to recommend this book to my colleagues in pediatrics and family medicine. I think that it is so well organized and logical that serious students and even pediatric cardiologists in training will find it useful.

One of the more obvious difficulties encountered by a busy house officer or a practitioner is that most textbooks are organized to be useful to the individual who already knows the diagnosis. This "Catch-22" is resolved by Dr. Park's presentation, which permits scanning and rapid identification of the problem area, and then stepwise progresses to the clinical diagnosis, the medical management of the problem, and the general potential of surgical assistance.

This book is both concise and thorough, a relatively rare combination in the medical literature. It spares the practitioner the great detail usually found in a cardiology textbook on esoteric details of the echocardiogram, catheterization, angiocardiogram, and surgical procedures. The presentations are practical, giving drug dosages, intervals, and precautions. Although he presents alternative views where appropriate, Dr. Park is courageous in presenting his own recommendations, which are well thought out and, above all, logical.

It is easy for me to see the impact of Dr. Park's career in this excellent book. He had a thorough general pediatric training, followed by several years in pediatric cardiology and cardiovascular physiology in this country. After some years in academic pediatric cardiology in Canada, he returned to this country and served as a family practitioner in a small community in the state of Washington. He learned well the problems of practicing in an area where consultants were not convenient for the practitioner, nor was it easy to transport a patient quickly to a major center. He returned to a research fellowship in pharmacology, and consequently knows more about the dynamics of cardiovascular drugs than anyone I can think of in the field of pediatric cardiology. For the past several years he has actively taught and practiced pediatric cardiology in a university setting and learned the process of transmitting the information and the skills that he has acquired in his career. This book reflects all of these experiences, and the balance between science and practical considerations is reflected in every page, with the particular clarity of a natural teacher.

I am proud of my earlier association with Dr. Park, and particularly proud of his present contribution to pediatric cardiology.

Warren G. Guntheroth, M.D.
Professor of Pediatrics
Head, Division of Pediatric Cardiology
University of Washington
  School of Medicine
Seattle, Washington

Preface to the First Edition

Since I started teaching pediatric cardiology, I felt that there was a need for a book that was written primarily for noncardiologists, such as medical students, house staff, and practitioners. Although many excellent pediatric cardiology textbooks are available, they are not very helpful to the noncardiologist, since they are filled with many details that are beyond the need or comprehension of practitioners. In addition, these books are not very effective in teaching practitioners how to approach children with potential cardiac problems; they are usually helpful only when the diagnosis is known. This book is intended to meet the need of noncardiologist practitioners for improving their skills in arriving at clinical diagnosis of cardiac problems, using basic tools available in their offices and community hospitals. This book will also serve as a quick reference in the area of pediatric cardiology. Although echocardiograms, cardiac catheterization, and angiocardiograms provide more definite information about the problem, these tools are not discussed at length in this book, since they are not routinely available to practitioners, and their use requires special skills.

In writing a small, yet comprehensive book, occasional oversimplification was unavoidable. Major emphasis was placed on the effective utilization of basic tools: history taking, physical examination, ECGs, and chest roentgenograms. Significance of abnormal findings in each of these areas is discussed, with differential diagnosis whenever applicable. A section is provided for pathophysiology for in-depth understanding of clinical manifestations of cardiac problems. Accurate but succinct discussion of congenital and acquired cardiac conditions is presented for quick reference. Indications, timing, procedures, risks, and complications for surgical treatment of cardiac conditions are also briefly discussed for each condition. Common cardiac arrhythmias are presented, with brief discussion of description, causes, significance, and management of each arrhythmia. A special section addresses cardiac problems of the neonate; another is devoted to special problems, such as congestive heart failure, systemic hypertension, pulmonary hypertension, chest pain or syncope, etc.

I would like to thank my teachers and my colleagues, past and present, who directly and indirectly influenced me and taught me how to teach pediatric cardiology, and those students and house staff who gave me valuable suggestions during the early stages of this book. My special thanks are due Dr. Warren G. Guntheroth, who encouraged me to write this book, read the entire manuscript, and gave me many helpful suggestions. I gratefully acknowledge Mrs. Linda Barragan for the expert secretarial assistance, Mr. Ronald Reif for careful proofreading, and the Department of Educational Resources, University of Texas Health Science Center at San Antonio, for their superb art and photographic works, especially Mrs. Deborah Felan for her excellent art work.

Finally, it is impossible to express adequately my debt to my brother, Young Kun, and my sister Po Kun, who provided me with powerful stimulus, encouragement, and hearty support throughout my schooling and who maintained confidence in me. Most of all, I am deeply indebted to my lovely wife and our wonderful boys, who accepted with understanding the inconvenience associated with my long preoccupation with this book.

Myung K. Park, M.D.

Preface to the Second Edition

Since the publication of the first edition of this book, significant changes have taken place in many areas of pediatric cardiology, thus making a new edition necessary. Major changes addressed in the second edition include the addition of the section, "Special Tools in Evaluation of Cardiac Patients," and an updating of surgical management. Considerable revisions have been made in most chapters. A brief chapter, "Hyperlipidemia in Childhood," has been added.

Although purposefully omitted in the first edition, echocardiography has gained such popularity that most pediatricians and family practitioners are exposed to this test, and an introductory knowledge is thought to be helpful; only basic views of two-dimensional and M-mode echocardiogram are illustrated. Other subjects in this edition include exercise tolerance test, ambulatory ECG monitoring, cardiac catheterization and angiocardiography, and therapeutic use of cardiac catheters.

In updating surgical management, it was sometimes difficult to suggest the procedure of choice, optimal age, and mortality of operation, as they vary greatly from center to center and are expected to continue to change with time. Attempts were made to give wide ranges of values for optimal age and mortality rate of operations. Readers are cautioned to consider local situations before making any recommendations to the patient.

I am most grateful to Dr. Warren G. Guntheroth for his valuable suggestions in many areas. I also wish to thank Mrs. Myra Weaver, P.A.-C., for her editing and suggestions, and Mrs. Linda Barragan for her assistance with typing. Grateful acknowledgment is made to Mr. Dieter F. Karkut and Mrs. Deborah Felan of the Department of Educational Resources, University of Texas Health Science Center at San Antonio for their unselfish, professional support with photography and art work. I owe the most to my wife and our boys, to whom this book is dedicated; without their support, understanding, and sacrifice, this work would not have been possible.

Myung K. Park, M.D.

Frequently Used Abbreviations

AR	Aortic regurgitation
AS	Aortic stenosis
ASD	Atrial septal defect
CHD	Congenital heart disease or defect
CHF	Congestive heart failure
COA	Coarctation of the aorta
ECD	Endocardial cushion defect
ECHO	Echocardiography or echocardiographic
HOCM	Hypertrophic obstructive cardiomyopathy
IHSS	Idiopathic hypertrophic subaortic stenosis
IVC	Inferior vena cava
LA	Left atrium or left atrial
LAD	Left axis deviation
LAH	Left atrial hypertrophy
LBBB	Left bundle branch block
LICS	Left intercostal space
LLSB	Lower left sternal border
LPA	Left pulmonary artery
LPLs	Left precordial leads
LRSB	Lower right sternal border
LSB	Left sternal border
LV	Left ventricle or left ventricular
LVH	Left ventricular hypertrophy
MLSB	Mid-left sternal border
MPA	Main pulmonary artery
MR	Mitral regurgitation
MRSB	Mid-right sternal border
MS	Mitral stenosis
MVPS	Mitral valve prolapse syndrome
PA	Pulmonary artery or posteroanterior
PAC	Premature atrial contraction
PAPVR	Partial anomalous pulmonary venous return
PAT	Paroxysmal atrial tachycardia
PBF	Pulmonary blood flow
PDA	Patent ductus arteriosus
PR	Pulmonary regurgitation
PS	Pulmonary stenosis
PV	Pulmonary vein or pulmonary venous
PVC	Premature ventricular contraction
PVM	Pulmonary vascular markings
PVOD	Pulmonary vascular obstructive disease
PVR	Pulmonary vascular resistance

RA   Right atrium or right atrial
RAD   Right axis deviation
RAH   Right atrial hypertrophy
RBBB   Right bundle branch block
RICS   Right intercostal space
RPA   Right pulmonary artery
RPLs   Right precordial leads
RV   Right ventricle or right ventricular
RVH   Right ventricular hypertrophy
S1   First heart sound
S2   Second heart sound
S3   Third heart sound
S4   Fourth heart sound
SEM   Systolic ejection murmur
SVC   Superior vena cava
SVR   Systemic vascular resistance
TAPVR   Total anomalous pulmonary venous return
TGA   Transposition of the great arteries
TOF   Tetralogy of Fallot
TR   Tricuspid regurgitation
TS   Tricuspid stenosis
ULSB   Upper left sternal border
URSB   Upper right sternal border
VSD   Ventricular septal defect
WPW   Wolff-Parkinson-White

Contents

PART I

Basic Tools in Routine Evaluation of Cardiac Patients

Initial cardiac evaluation of a child in an office practice is usually accomplished by (a) history taking, (b) physical examination that includes inspection, palpation, and auscultation, (c) electrocardiogram, and (d) chest roentgenogram.

The weight of the information gained from these different techniques varies with the type and severity of the disease. For example, if a mother has a history of having had German measles early in pregnancy, congenital heart defect and other malformations are almost always present (rubella syndrome), of which patent ductus arteriosus (PDA) and peripheral pulmonary artery stenosis are the two most common cardiovascular defects. One should be looking for these defects when examining the child. Auscultation may be the single most important source of information for the diagnosis of acyanotic heart disease such as ventricular septal defect (VSD) or PDA, whereas auscultation is rarely diagnostic in cyanotic congenital heart disease (CHD) such as transposition of the great arteries (TGA) in which the heart murmur is often absent. Careful palpation of the peripheral pulses is more important than auscultation in the detection of coarctation of the aorta (COA). Measurement of blood pressure is the most important diagnostic tool in the detection of hypertension. The ECG and chest x-ray films have strengths and weaknesses in their ability to assess the severity of heart disease. The ECG is very good at detecting hypertrophy and, therefore, conditions of pressure overload, but it is less reliable at detecting dilatation from volume overload. The chest x-ray films are most reliable in establishing volume overload but poor in demonstrating hypertrophy without dilatation.

In the next five chapters, an in-depth discussion of basic tools will be presented, followed by flow diagrams which aid in arriving at a correct diagnosis of pediatric cardiac problems.

1 / History Taking

As in evaluation of any other system, history taking is a basic step in cardiac evaluation. Maternal history during pregnancy is often helpful in the diagnosis of congenital heart disease (CHD), as certain prenatal events are known to be teratogenic. Past history including the immediate postnatal period provides more direct information relevant to the cardiac evaluation. Family history is also helpful in relating a cardiac problem to other medical problems that may be prevalent in the family. Table 1-1 lists more important aspects of history taking in a child with a potential cardiac problem. Each of the items will be discussed in some detail.

I. GESTATIONAL AND NATAL HISTORY

Infections, medications, and excessive smoking or alcohol intake may cause CHD, especially if they take place very early in pregnancy.

A. **Infections:** Maternal rubella infection during the first trimester of pregnancy commonly results in multiple anomalies, including cardiac defects. Infections by cytomegalovirus, herpesvirus, and coxsackievirus B are highly suspected to be teratogenic if they occur in the early part of pregnancy. Infections by these viruses later in pregnancy may cause myocarditis.

B. **Medications including alcohol and smoking:** Several medications are highly suspected teratogens. Amphetamines have been associated with VSD, PDA, atrial septal defect (ASD), and TGA. Other medications suspected to cause congenital heart disease include anticonvulsants (hydantoin has been associated with pulmonary stenosis [PS], aortic stenosis [AS], COA, or PDA, and trimethadione with TGA, tetralogy of Fallot [TOF], or hypoplastic left heart syndrome), progesterone/estrogen (VSD, TOF, TGA), and alcohol (fetal alcohol syndrome in which VSD, PDA, ASD, and TOF are common). Although cigarette smoking has not been proved to be teratogenic, it causes an intrauterine growth retardation.

C. **Maternal conditions:** There is a high incidence of cardiomyopathy in infants of diabetic mothers. In addition, these babies have a higher incidence of structural heart defects (e.g., TGA, VSD, PDA). Maternal lupus erythematosus or collagen disease has been associated with a high incidence of congenital heart block in the offspring. The incidence of CHD increases to 3%–4% if the mother has CHD, even postoperative.

D. **Birth weight:** Often, birth weight provides important information as to the nature of the cardiac problem. If an infant is small for gestational age, this may indicate intrauterine infections. Rubella syndrome is a typical example. Infants with high birth weight, often seen in the offspring of diabetic mothers, have a higher incidence of cardiac anomalies. Infants with TGA often have a birth weight greater than average; of course, these infants are cyanotic.

3

TABLE 1–1.

Selected Aspects of History Taking

Gestational and natal history
   a. Infection, medications, excessive smoking or alcohol
     intake during pregnancy
   b. Birth weight
Postnatal (or past) history
   a. Weight gain and development, including feeding pattern
   b. Cyanosis, "cyanotic spells," and squatting
   c. Tachypnea, dyspnea, puffy eyelids
   d. Frequency of respiratory infection
   e. Exercise tolerance
   f. Heart murmur
   g. Chest pain
   h. Joint symptoms
   i. Neurologic symptoms
   j. Medications
Family history
   a. Hereditary disease
   b. Congenital heart disease
   c. Rheumatic fever
   d. Sudden unexpected death
   e. Diabetes mellitus, arteriosclerotic heart disease,
     hypertension, etc.

II. POSTNATAL HISTORY

A. Weight gain and development, including feeding pattern: Weight gain and general development may be delayed in infants and children with congestive heart failure (CHF) or severe cyanosis. Weight is affected more significantly than height. If weight is severely affected, suspect a more general dysmorphic condition. Poor feeding of recent onset may be an early sign of CHF in infants, especially if the poor feeding is due to fatigue and dyspnea.

B. Cyanosis, "cyanotic spells," and squatting: If the parents think that their child is cyanotic, ask about the onset of cyanosis (in the nursery or shortly after coming home?), its severity, permanent or paroxysmal nature, or whether the cyanosis becomes worse after feeding.

A true "cyanotic spell" is seen most frequently in infants with tetralogy of Fallot (TOF) and requires immediate attention. Ask about the time of its appearance (in the morning on waking up or following feeding, etc.), duration of the spell, and frequency of the spells. Most important, ask whether the infant was breathing *fast* and *deep* during the spell, or was holding his breath. This helps to differentiate between a true cyanotic spell and a breath-holding spell.

Ask whether the child squats when he is tired or if the child has a favorite position (such as knee-chest position) when he is tired. A history of squatting is strongly suggestive of cyanotic heart disease, particularly TOF.

C. Tachypnea, dyspnea, and puffy eyelids: These are signs of congestive heart failure. Left heart failure produces tachypnea with/without dyspnea. Tachypnea becomes worse with feeding, eventually resulting in poor feeding and poor weight gain. A sleeping respiratory rate of more than 40/min is noteworthy, and a rate of more than 60/min is definitely abnormal, even in a newborn infant.

Wheezing or persistent cough at night may be an early sign of CHF. Puffy eyelids and sacral edema are signs of systemic venous congestion. The ankle edema commonly seen in adults is not seen in infants.

D. **Frequency of respiratory infections:** Congenital heart defects with a large left-to-right shunt (and increased pulmonary blood flow) predispose to lower respiratory tract infections. Frequent upper respiratory tract infections are not related to CHD, although children with a vascular ring may sound as if they have a chronic upper respiratory tract infection.

E. **Exercise tolerance:** Decreased exercise tolerance may be caused by large left-to-right shunt lesions, cyanotic defects, valvular stenosis or regurgitation, or arrhythmias. Obese children may be inactive and may have decreased exercise tolerance in the absence of heart disease. An excellent assessment of exercise tolerance may be obtained by asking the following questions: Does he keep up with other children? How many blocks can he walk or run? How many flights of stairs can he climb without fatigue? Does the weather or the time of day influence his exercise tolerance?

In infants who do not walk or run, an estimate of exercise tolerance may be gained by history of feeding pattern (see above). The parents often volunteer to say that the child takes naps; however, many normal children nap regularly.

F. **Heart murmur:** If the presence of a heart murmur is the chief complaint, obtain information about the time of its first appearance and the circumstances of its discovery. The heart murmur heard within a few hours of birth usually indicates a stenotic lesion (AS or PS) or small left-to-right shunt lesions (VSD or PDA). The murmur of large left-to-right shunt lesions, such as VSD or PDA, may be delayed because of slow regression of pulmonary vascular resistance (PVR). The onset of the murmur in the case of a stenotic lesion is not affected by the PVR, and the murmur is usually heard shortly after birth. A heart murmur that is first noted on a routine examination of a healthy-looking child is more likely to be innocent, especially if the same physician has been following up the child's progress. The presence of a febrile illness is often associated with the discovery of the heart murmur.

G. **Chest pain:** If chest pain is the chief complaint, ask whether it is activity-related. (Do you have chest pain only when you are active or does it come even when you watch television?) Also ask about the duration (in seconds, minutes, or hours), nature of the pain (stabbing, squeezing), and radiation to other parts of the body (neck, left shoulder, or left arm). Ask whether the pain was accompanied by syncope or palpitation. Does deep breathing improve or worsen the pain? (Cardiac origin, except for pericarditis, will not be affected by respiration.) Also ask the parents if there has been a recent cardiac death in the family. Three most common cardiac conditions that may cause chest pain are aortic stenosis (usually associated with activity), pulmonary vascular obstructive disease (PVOD), and mitral valve prolapse syndrome (not necessarily associated with activity, but there may be a history of palpitation). Other less common cardiac conditions that can cause chest pain include severe pulmonary stenosis, pericarditis of various etiology, and Kawasaki's disease (in which stenosis or aneurysm of coronary arteries is common). The majority of children with complaints of chest pain do not have a cardiac condition (see chap. 31 for further discussion).

H. **Joint symptoms:** When joint pain is the chief complaint, ask about the number of joints involved, duration of the symptom, and migratory or stationary nature of the pain. Ask if there has been a recent sore throat; if so, ask whether a throat culture was taken. Has the child had rashes suggestive of scarlet fever? Can (or could) he walk on his feet? If so, it is not likely a rheumatic joint. Pain in rheumatic joints is so severe that children refuse to walk. Ask whether rubbing the joint alleviates the pain. If it does, it is not likely a rheumatic joint. It is important to ask about aspirin or other analgesics administered (dose, number, and timing), since even small doses of salicylates may suppress the full manifestation of joint symptoms of rheumatic fever or may abolish joint pain completely. Also ask whether the joint was swollen, red, hot, or tender. Ask about abdominal pain, chest pain (pericarditis), and nosebleeds, which may be seen in rheumatic fever (see chap. 20).

I. Neurologic symptoms: History of stroke suggests embolization or thrombosis secondary to cyanotic CHD with polycythemia or infective endocarditis. History of headache may be a manifestation of cerebral hypoxia with cyanotic heart disease, severe polycythemia, or brain abscess in cyanotic children. Although it is claimed in adults, hypertension with/without COA is a rare cause of headache in children. Choreic movement strongly suggests rheumatic fever. History of syncope may suggest arrhythmias, particularly ventricular arrhythmias, and may be seen in long QT syndrome (Jervell and Lange-Nielsen syndrome, Romano-Ward syndrome) and mitral valve prolapse syndrome. Syncope related to exercise may be due to severe AS. It should be pointed out, however, that vasodepressor syncope without underlying cardiac disease is the most common syncope in children.

J. Medications: Note name, dosage, timing, and duration of both cardiac and noncardiac medications. Medications may be responsible for chief complaints or certain physical findings. Tachycardia and palpitation may be caused by cold medications or antiasthmatic drugs such as aminophylline and related drugs.

III. FAMILY HISTORY

A. Hereditary disease: Some hereditary diseases may be associated with certain forms of congenital heart diseases. For example, Marfan's syndrome is frequently associated with aortic aneurysm or with aortic and/or mitral insufficiency. Pulmonary stenosis (secondary to dysplastic pulmonary valve) is common in Noonan's syndrome. Lentiginous skin lesion (leopard syndrome) is often associated with PS and cardiomyopathy. Common hereditary diseases in which heart disease is a frequent finding are listed in Table 1–2.

B. Congenital heart disease: The incidence of CHD in the general population is about 1%, or, more precisely, 8 of 1,000 live births, not including PDA in premature infants.

The incidence of CHD increases with the number of the family members who have a defect. When there is one affected first-order relative (one parent or one sibling), the incidence increases by three-fold (to about 3%). If there are two affected first-order relatives (both parents, one parent and one sibling, or two siblings), the incidence increases to 9% (three-fold increase over one affected first-order relative). If there are three affected first-order relatives, the incidence may be as high as 50%. In general, lesions with higher incidence (such as VSD) tend to have a higher risk for recurrence, and lesions with lower incidence (for example, persistent truncus arteriosus) have a lower risk for recurrence.

TABLE 1–2.

Hereditary Diseases in Which Congenital Heart Disease is a Frequent Finding

Hereditary Disease	Mode of Inheritance	Common Cardiac Disease	Important Features
Apert's syndrome	AD	VSD, TOF	Irregular craniosynostosis with peculiar head and facial appearance Syndactyly of digits and toes
Crouzon's disease (craniofacial dysostosis)	AD	PDA, COA	Ptosis with shallow orbits Craniosynostosis, maxillary hypoplasia
Ehlers-Danlos syndrome	AD	Aneurysm of aorta and carotids	Hyperextensive joints, hyperelasticity, fragility and bruisability of skin
Ellis-van Creveld syndrome (chondroectodermal dysplasia)	AR	Single atrium	Neonatal teeth, short distal limbs, polydactyly, nail hypoplasia
Friedreich's ataxia	AR	Cardiomyopathy	Late onset ataxia, skeletal deformities
Glycogen storage disease II (Pompe's)	AR	Cardiomyopathy	Large tongue and flabby muscles, cardiomegaly; ECG: LVH and short PR; normal FBS and GTT
Holt-Oram syndrome (cardiac-limb)	AD	ASD, VSD	Defects or absence of thumb or radius
Hypertrophic obstructive cardiomyopathy (HOCM)	AD	Hypertrophic obstructive subaortic stenosis	
Leopard syndrome	AD	PS, long PR interval, cardiomyopathy	Lentiginous skin lesion, ECG abnormalities, Ocular hypertelorism, Pulmonary stenosis, Abnormal genitalia, Retarded growth, Deafness
Long QT syndrome: Jervell and Lange- Nielsen Romano-Ward	AR AD	Long QT interval, ventricular tachyarrhythmias	Congenital deafness (not in Romano-Ward), syncope due to ventricular arrhythmias. Family history of sudden death
Marfan's syndrome	AD	Aortic aneurysm, aortic regurgitation and/or mitral regurgitation	Arachnodactyly, subluxation of lens
Mitral valve prolapse syndrome (primary)	AD	Mitral regurgitation, dysrhythmias	Thoracic skeletal anomalies (80%)

(Continued.)

TABLE 1–2. *(cont.)*.

Hereditary Disease	Mode of Inheritance	Common Cardiac Disease	Important Features
Mucopolysaccharidosis		Aortic regurg./	Coarse features, large tongue,
Hurler's (type I)	AR	mitral regurg.,	depressed nasal bridge, kyphosis,
Hunter's (type II)	XR	coronary artery	retarded growth, hepatomegaly,
Morquio's (type IV)	AR	disease	corneal opacity (not in Hunter's),
			mental retardation
Muscular dystrophy (Duchenne's type)	XR	Cardiomyopathy	Waddling gait, "pseudohypertrophy" of calf muscle
Neurofibromatosis (von Recklinghausen's disease)	AD	PS, COA, pheochromocytoma	Café-au-lait spots, acoustic neuroma, variety of bone lesions
Noonan's syndrome	AD	PS (dystrophic pulmonary valve)	Similar to Turner's syndrome but may occur in phenotypic male and without chromosomal abnormality
Osler-Weber-Rendu syndrome	AD	Pulmonary AV fistulas	Hepatic involvement; telangiectases, hemangiomas or fibrosis
Tuberous sclerosis	AD	Rhabdomyoma	Adenoma sebaceum (2–5 years of age), convulsion, mental defect
Williams's syndrome (supravalvular aortic stenosis)	AD	Supravalvular aortic stenosis, PA stenosis	Mental retardation, peculiar "elfin" facies, hypercalcemia of infancy?

AD = autosomal dominance; AR = autosomal recessive; XR = sex-linked recessive; FBS = fasting blood sugar; GTT = glucose tolerance test.

C. Rheumatic fever: Rheumatic fever frequently occurs in more than one member of the family, and there is a higher incidence of rheumatic fever among relatives of rheumatic children. Although knowledge of genetic factors in rheumatic fever is incomplete, it is generally agreed that there is an inherited susceptibility (possibly through a single autosomal recessive gene) to rheumatic fever.

2 / Physical Examination

As is true with an examination of any child, the order and extent of physical examination of infants and children with potential cardiac problems should be individualized. The more innocuous procedures, such as inspection, should be done first, and the more frightening or uncomfortable parts should be delayed until the latter part of the examination.

Supine is the preferred position for examination of the patient in any age group. However, older infants and young children, 1–3 years of age, may be examined initially while sitting on their mothers' laps if they refuse to lie down.

The growth chart should reflect height and weight in terms of absolute values as well as in percentiles. Accurate plotting (and following the growth curve) is an essential part of initial (and follow-up) evaluation.

I. INSPECTION

Much information can be gained by simple inspection without disturbing a sleeping infant or frightening a child with a stethoscope. Inspect the following: (1) general appearance and nutritional state; (2) any obvious syndrome or chromosomal abnormalities; (3) color, i.e., cyanosis, pallor, or jaundice; (4) clubbing; (5) respiratory rate, dyspnea, and retraction; (6) sweat on the forehead; and (7) the chest.

A. **General appearance and nutritional state**

Note whether the child is in any distress, well-nourished or undernourished, happy or cranky.

B. **Syndromes or chromosomal abnormalities**

Note any obvious syndromes or chromosomal abnormalities that suggest certain specific congenital heart defects. For example, about 50% of children with Down's syndrome have congenital heart disease, and the two most common defects are endocardial cushion defect (ECD) and VSD. A girl with Turner's syndrome may have COA, and a child with a missing thumb or deformities of a forearm may have an ASD or a VSD (Holt-Oram syndrome or cardiac-limb syndrome). Table 2–1 shows cardiac defects associated with common chromosomal abnormalities. See Table 1–2 for cardiac anomalies in some hereditary diseases.

C. **Color**

Note if the child is cyanotic, pale, or jaundiced. If there is cyanosis, note its degree and distribution (throughout the body or on the lower or upper half of the body). Mild cyanosis is difficult to detect. The arterial saturation is usually 85% or lower before cyanosis is detectable in patients with normal hemoglobin. Cyanosis is more readily appreciated in natural light than in artificial light. Cyanosis of the lips may be misleading, particularly in children who have deep pigmentation. Check other areas, such as the tongue, buccal mucosa, nail beds, or conjunctiva as well. Not all children with cyanosis have cyanotic CHD; it may be an effect of respiratory diseases or CNS disorders. Cyanosis associated

9

TABLE 2–1.

Congenital Heart Defects in Selected Chromosomal Aberrations

Conditions	Incidence of CHD, %	Common Defects in Decreasing Order of Frequency
5p− (Cri du chat syndrome)	25	VSD, PDA, ASD
Trisomy 13	90	VDS, PDA, dextrocardia
Trisomy 18	99	VSD, PDA, PS
Trisomy 21 (Down's syndrome)	50	ECD, VSD
Turner's syndrome (XO)	35	COA, AS, ASD
Klinefelter's variant (XXXXY)	15	PDA, ASD

AS = aortic stenosis; ASD = atrial septal defect; CHD = congenital heart disease; COA = coarctation of aorta; ECD = endocardial cushion defect; PDA = patent ductus arteriosus; PS = pulmonary stenosis; VSD = ventricular septal defect.

with arterial desaturation is called central cyanosis, and that associated with normal arterial saturation is called peripheral cyanosis. Peripheral cyanosis may be seen in exposure to cold, congestive heart failure (CHF) (due to sluggish peripheral blood flow), or polycythemia. Cyanosis, even of a mild degree, in a newborn infant requires thorough investigation, including arterial blood gas determination. Also check cyanosis against the hematocrit (polycythemic infants may be cyanotic without arterial desaturation).

Pallor may be seen in infants with vasoconstriction from congestive heart failure or circulatory shock or in infants with severe anemia. Newborn infants with severe CHF and those infants with congenital hypothyroidism may have prolonged physiologic jaundice (PDA and PS are common findings in congenital hypothyroidism). Hepatic disease with jaundice may cause arterial desaturation due to pulmonary arteriovenous fistula (arteriohepatic dysplasia).

D. Clubbing

Long-standing arterial desaturation (usually more than 6 months), even that too mild to be detected by inexperienced persons, results in clubbing of the fingernails and toenails. When fully developed, clubbing consists of a widening and thickening of the end of the fingers and toes, accompanied by convex fingernails and loss of angle between nail and nail bed (Fig 2–1). Reddening and shininess of the terminal phalanges are seen in the early stage of clubbing. It appears earliest and most marked in the thumb. Clubbing may also be associated with (a) lung disease (abscess), (b) cirrhosis of the liver, and (c) subacute bacterial endocarditis, as well as occurring in normal persons (familial clubbing).

E. Respiratory rate, dyspnea, and retraction

Note the respiratory rate on every infant and child. Count for a whole minute if the infant breathes irregularly. Respiratory rate will be faster in children who are crying, upset, eating, or febrile. The most reliable respiratory rate is that taken during sleep. After finishing a bottle of formula, an infant may breathe faster than normal for 5–10 minutes. A respiratory rate of more than 40/min is unusual and more than 60/min is definitely abnormal at any age, including the newborn period. Tachypnea, along with tachycardia, is the earliest sign of left ventricular failure. Note if the child has dyspnea or retraction, a sign of a more severe degree of left heart failure.

F. Sweat on the forehead

Infants with CHF often have a cold sweat on the forehead. This is an expression of sympathetic overactivity as a compensatory mechanism for the decreased cardiac output.

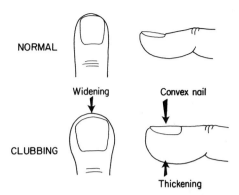

NORMAL

Widening

Convex nail

CLUBBING

Thickening

FIG 2–1.
Diagrammatic illustration of normal and clubbed fingers.

G. Inspection of the chest

Precordial bulge with or without actively visible cardiac activity suggests *chronic* cardiac enlargement. Acute dilatation of the heart does not cause precordial bulge. Pigeon chest in which the sternum protrudes on the midline is usually not due to cardiomegaly.

Pectus excavatum rarely, if ever, causes cardiac embarrassment. It may be a cause of pulmonary systolic ejection murmur (SEM) or a large cardiac silhouette on a posteroanterior (PA) view of chest roentgenogram, compensating for the diminished anteroposterior (AP) diameter of the chest.

Harrison's groove, a line of depression in the bottom of the rib cage along the attachment of the diaphragm, indicates poor lung compliance of long duration, such as that seen in large left-to-right shunt lesions.

II. PALPATION

Palpation should include the peripheral pulses and the precordium for thrill, the point of maximal impulse (PMI), and hyperactivity. Although ordinarily palpation is the next step after inspection, auscultation may be more fruitful on a sleeping infant who might awaken and become uncooperative.

I. Peripheral Pulses

A. Count the pulse rate and note any irregularities in the rate and volume. Normal pulse rate varies with age and the status of the patient. The younger the patient, the faster the pulse rate. Increased pulse rate may indicate excitement, fever, CHF, or arrhythmia. Bradycardia may mean heart block, digitalis toxicity, etc. Irregularity of the pulse suggests arrhythmias, but sinus arrhythmia (an acceleration with inspiration) is normal.

B. Compare the right and left arm and an arm and a leg for volume of the pulse. Every patient should have palpable pedal pulses, either dorsalis pedis, tibialis posterior, or both. It is often easier to feel pedal pulses than the femoral pulses, particularly on sleeping infants. Attempts at palpating a femoral pulse often wake up a sleeping infant or upset a toddler. If one feels a good pedal pulse, COA is effectively ruled out, particularly if the blood pressure in the arm is normal.

Weak leg pulses and strong arm pulses suggest COA. The right brachial pulse stronger than the left brachial pulse is associated with (a) COA proximal to or near the origin of the left subclavian artery or (b) supravalvular aortic stenosis.

C. Bounding pulses are found in aortic run-off lesions such as PDA, aortic insufficiency, large systemic arteriovenous fistula, or, rarely, persistent truncus arteriosus. Pulses are bounding in premature infants because of the lack of subcutaneous tissue and because many have a PDA.

D. Weak, thready pulses are found in cardiac failure or circulatory shock or in the leg of a patient with COA. Systemic-pulmonary artery shunt (either classic Blalock-Taussig or modified Gore-Tex shunt) or the subclavian flap angioplasty for repair of COA may cause absent or weak pulse in the arm affected by surgery.

E. Pulsus paradoxus (paradoxical pulse) is suspected when there is marked variation in the volume of arterial pulses with respiratory cycle. The term "pulsus paradoxus" does *not* indicate a phase reversal; it is an exaggeration of normal reduction of systolic pressure during inspiration. Accurate evaluation requires sphygmomanometry (Fig 2–2). This condition may be associated with cardiac tamponade secondary to pericardial effusion or constrictive pericarditis, or severe respiratory difficulties seen with asthma or pneumonia. It is also seen in patients who are on respirators with high pressure settings, but then the blood pressure will increase with inflation.

The presence of pulses paradoxus is confirmed by the use of sphygmomanometer as follows:

a. Raise the cuff pressure about 20 mm Hg above systolic pressure.

b. Lower the pressure slowly until one hears Korotkoff sound I for some but not all cardiac cycles and note the reading (line A on Fig 2–2).

c. Lower the pressure further until one hears systolic sounds for all cardiac cycles and note the reading (line B on Fig 2–2).

d. If the difference between readings A and B is greater than 10 mm Hg, pulsus paradoxus is present.

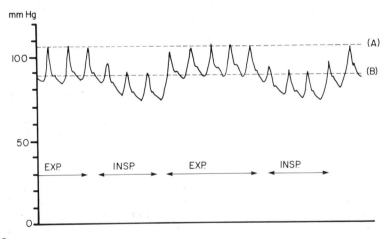

FIG 2–2.
Diagrammatic drawing of pulsus paradoxus. Note the reduction of systolic pressure of more than 10 mm Hg during inspiration.

II. Chest

Palpate the following: (A) apical impulse, (B) point of maximal impulse (PMI), (C) hyperactivity of the precordium, and (D) palpable thrill.

A. Apical impulse.—Palpation of apical impulse is usually superior to percussion in detection of cardiomegaly. Note its location and diffuseness. Percussion in infants and children is inaccurate and adds little. The apical impulse is normally at the 5th intercostal space (5ICS) in the midclavicular line after the age of 7 years. Before this age, the apical impulse is in the 4ICS just to the left of the midclavicular line. Apical impulse displaced laterally and/or downward suggests cardiac enlargement.

B. Point of maximal impulse (PMI).—The PMI is helpful in determining whether the right or left ventricle is dominant. With right ventricular dominance, the impulse is maximal at the lower left sternal border (LLSB); with left ventricular dominance, the impulse is maximal at the apex. If the impulse is more diffuse and slow-rising, it is called a "heave"; if it is well-localized and sharp-rising, it is called a "tap." Heaves are more often associated with volume overload and taps with pressure overload. Normal newborns and infants have more right ventricular dominance, and therefore more right ventricular impulse, than older children.

C. Hyperactive precordium.—The presence of a hyperactive precordium is a characteristic of heart disease with increased volume overwork such as that seen in CHD with large left-to-right shunts (PDA, VSD, etc.) or in heart disease with severe valvular regurgitation (aortic regurgitation, mitral regurgitation, etc.)

D. Thrill.—Palpation for thrill is often of real diagnostic value. A thrill on the chest is felt better with the palm of the hand than with the tips of fingers. However, one has to use the fingers to feel a thrill in the suprasternal notch and over the carotid arteries.

    a. Thrill in the upper left sternal border (ULSB) originates from the pulmonary valve or pulmonary artery and therefore is present in PS, PA stenosis, or, rarely, PDA.

    b. Thrill in the upper right sternal border (URSB) is usually of aortic origin and is seen in aortic stenosis (AS).

    c. Thrill in the LLSB is characteristic of VSD.

    d. Thrill in the suprasternal notch (SSN) suggests AS, but may be found in PS, PDA, or COA.

    e. The presence of a thrill over the carotid artery or arteries accompanied by a thrill in the SSN is suggestive of diseases of the aorta or aortic valve (COA, AS, etc.). An isolated thrill in one of the carotid arteries (without thrill in the SSN) may be an isolated carotid bruit.

    f. Thrill in the intercostal space is found in older children with severe COA with extensive intercostal collaterals.

III. BLOOD PRESSURE MEASUREMENT

Every child should have blood pressure (BP) measurement as part of the physical examination whenever possible. However, there are numerous problems associated with indirect BP measurement in infants and children. Unacceptably wide ranges of normal BP values have been reported in the literature. Among large epidemiologic studies, differences in the 95th percentile systolic BP are as large as 30 mm Hg for certain age groups. A new set of normal BP data recommended by the NIH Task Force on Blood Pressure Control in Children (1987) is considerably lower than those reported by the Task Force in 1977, causing further confusion, and the methodology used in both recommendations is subject to criticism.

One must select the correct size of the BP cuff. Cuffs that are too narrow will overestimate the true BP, and cuffs too wide will underestimate the true pressure. It is wrong to select the cuff based solely on the length of the arm, because many children with thick arms may become "iatrogenically" hypertensive. The width of the inflatable part of the cuff (bladder) should be 125%–155% of the diameter (or 40%–50% of the circumference) of the limb (either arm or leg) on which BP is to be determined (Fig 2–3). This is the standard recommended by the American Heart Association for the adult, and the same recommendation should apply for children. Cuff size determined this way compensates for variation in thickness of the arm, which is the most important factor determining the compression of the underlying artery and, thereby, the accuracy of auscultatory pressure. In addition, the air bladder should be long enough to completely or nearly completely encircle the limb.

The same selection criterion applies for the leg pressure determination. Even with a considerably wider cuff selected for the thigh, the systolic pressure in the thigh will be 10–20 mm Hg higher than that obtained in the arm. This is not because the pressure in the femoral artery is higher than that in the brachial artery, but it is a result of the lack of a well-designed cuff for the thigh. The systolic pressure in the thigh obtained with sphygmomanometry using appropriate cuffs should be at least equal to that in the arm; if it is lower, coarctation of the aorta is likely. Thigh BP determinations are mandatory in a child with hypertension in the arm. The presence of a femoral pulse does not rule out a coarctation.

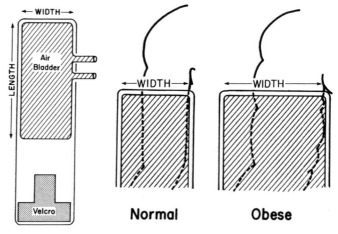

FIG 2–3.
Diagram showing a method of selecting an appropriate-sized blood pressure cuff. The selection is based on the thickness rather than the length of the arm. The end of the cuff is at the top, and the cuff width is then compared with the diameter of the arm. The width of the inflatable part of the cuff (bladder, *cross-hatched areas*) should be 125%–155% of the diameter (or 40%–50% of the circumference) of the arm.

Some confusion still exists as to which should be taken as the diastolic signal—the point of muffling (phase IV) or the point of disappearance (phase V) of the Korotkoff sounds. In general, the point of muffling is closer to the true diastolic pressure than the point of disappearance in children. When the points of muffling and of disappearance are more than 6 mm Hg apart, both values should be noted; for example, 110/75–50 mm Hg, where 110 mm Hg is systolic pressure (the phase I of Korotkoff sound), 75 mm Hg is the point of muffling, and 50 mm Hg is the point of disappearance. When the points of muffling and of disappearance are less than 6 mm Hg apart, record phase V as the diastolic pressure.

Although there is no single reliable set of normative BP values, a working guide of normal BP values is needed until more reliable data become available. Table 2–2 shows BP values adapted from the NIH Task Force (1987). It appears that after 13 years of age, boys' BP values are higher than those of girls.

Recently, accuracy of indirect BP measurement by an oscillometric method (Dinamap) has repeatedly been demonstrated. The cuff width 40%–50% of the circumference (or 125%–155% of the diameter) of the arm is also appropriate for the Dinamap method. The oscillometric method is not only accurate but also provides other advantages over the auscultatory method: it eliminates observer-related variations, it can be successfully used in infants and small children, it eliminates controversies over the diastolic signals, and it provides mean pressure and heart rate. Unpublished data on normal BP values by the Dinamap method are presented in Table 2–3 for newborns and children up to 5 years of age.

TABLE 2–2.
A Working Guide to Normal Blood Pressure*

Age	Mean Values, mm Hg (Systolic/ Diastolic)	90th Percentile, mm Hg (Systolic/ Diastolic)	95th Percentile, mm Hg (Systolic/ Diastolic)
1–7 days†	72/—	86/—	96/—
1–4 wk†	84/—	100/—	104/—
1–12 mo.	94/52	105/68	110/70
1–5 yr	94/56	108/68	114/70
6–10 yr	98/62	114/74	118/78
11–13 yr	106/66	120/78	124/82
14–18 yr	(B) 116/68‡	(B) 130/82	(B) 136/86
	(G) 108/66‡	(G) 122/80	(G) 126/82

*Modified from the NIH Task Force (1987): Report of the Second Task Force on Blood Pressure Control in Children—1987. *Pediatrics* 1987; 79:1–25.
†Obtained by Doppler flow detector; therefore, no diastolic pressures are given.
‡B = boys; G = girls.

TABLE 2–3.
Normal Blood Pressure Values [Systolic/Diastolic(Mean)] by Dinamap Monitor

Age	Mean Values, mm Hg	90th Percentiles, mm Hg	95th Percentiles, mm Hg
1–3 days	64/41 (50)	75/49 (59)	78/52 (62)
1 mo–2 yr	95/58 (72)	106/68 (83)	110/71 (86)
2–5 yr	101/57 (74)	112/66 (82)	115/68 (85)

IV. AUSCULTATION

Auscultation of the heart requires more skill but at the same time provides more valuable information than do other methods of examining the heart. Remember that the bell-type chest piece is better suited for detecting low-frequency events, whereas the diaphragm selectively picks up the high frequency events. When the bell is firmly pressed against the chest wall, it acts like the diaphragm by filtering out low-frequency sounds or murmurs and picks up high-frequency events. One should not limit examination to the four traditional auscultatory areas; the entire precordium as well as the sides and the back of the chest should be explored with the stethoscope. Attention should be given systematically to the following aspects:

a. Heart rate and regularity: Heart rate and regularity should be noted on every child. Extremely fast or slow heart rates or irregularity in the rhythm should be evaluated by an ECG and a long rhythm strip. This aspect will be discussed under arrhythmias (see chap. 23).

b. Heart sounds: Intensity and quality of the heart sounds, especially the second heart sound, should be evaluated. Also note abnormalities of the first heart sound and the third heart sound and the presence of gallop rhythm or the fourth sound.

c. Systolic and diastolic sounds: Systolic and diastolic sounds, such as ejection click in early systole and midsystolic click, provide important clues to the diagnosis. Opening snap should be noted, but it is extremely rare in pediatrics.

d. Heart murmurs: Heart murmurs should be evaluated in terms of intensity, timing (systolic or diastolic), location, transmission, and quality.

I. Heart Sounds

The heart sound should be identified and analyzed prior to the analysis of heart murmurs.

A. **First heart sound (S1).**—The first heart sound is associated with closure of the mitral and tricuspid valves, and it is best heard at the apex or LLSB. Splitting of the S1 may be found in normal children, but is infrequent. Abnormally wide splitting of S1 may be found in RBBB or Ebstein's anomaly. Splitting of S1 should be differentiated from:

a. Ejection click, which is more easily audible at the ULSB in pulmonary stenosis; in bicuspid aortic valves, the click may be louder at the LLSB or apex than at the URSB.

b. A fourth sound (S4), which is rare in children.

B. **Second heart sound (S2).**—The second heart sound in the ULSB (or pulmonary area) is of critical importance in pediatric cardiology. The S2 must be evaluated in terms of: (a) the degree of splitting of S2 and (b) the relative intensity of P2 (in relation to the intensity of A2). Although best heard with a diaphragm, both components are readily audible with the bell as well. Abnormalities of splitting of the S2 and the intensity of the P2 are summarized in Table 2–4.

a. Splitting of the S2:
In every normal child, with the exception of occasional newborn infants, two components of the S2 should be audible in the ULSB (or pulmonary

TABLE 2–4.

Summary of Abnormal S2

Abnormal splitting
  1. Widely split and fixed S2
      a. Volume overload (ASD, PAPVR)
      b. Pressure overload (PS)
      c. Electrical delay (RBBB)
      d. Early aortic closure (MR)
      e. Occasional normal child
  2. Narrowly split S2
      a. Pulmonary hypertension
      b. Aortic stenosis
      c. Occasional normal child
  3. Single S2
      a. Pulmonary hypertension
      b. One semilunar valve (pulmonary atresia, aortic
         atresia, persistent truncus arteriosus)
      c. P2 not audible (TGA, TOF, severe PS)
      d. Severe AS
      e. Occasional normal child
  4. Paradoxically split S2
      a. Severe AS
      b. LBBB, WPW syndrome (type B)
Abnormal intensity of P2
  1. Increased P2 (pulmonary hypertension)
  2. Decreased P2 (severe PS, TOF, tricuspid stenosis)

valve area): the first is the aortic closure (A2), and the second is the pulmonary closure (P2).

1) Normal splitting of the S2:

The degree of splitting of the S2 varies with respiration, increasing with inspiration and decreasing or becoming single with expiration (Fig 2–4). What causes this normal respiratory variation in splitting of the S2? Although there is a new theory based on the vascular impedance of systemic and pulmonary circuits, the traditional explanation relates these events to closure of the aortic and pulmonary valves. During inspiration, because of a greater negative pressure in the thoracic cavity, there is an increase in systemic venous return to the right

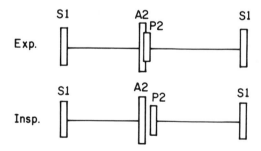

FIG 2–4.
Diagram showing relative intensity of A2 and P2 and the respiratory variation in the degree of splitting of the second heart sound at the ULSB (pulmonary area).

side of the heart. This increased volume of blood in the RV prolongs the duration of RV ejection time, delaying the closure of the pulmonary valve, which in turn widens the splitting of the S2. The absence of splitting (or single S2) or widely split S2 usually indicates an abnormality.

2) Abnormal splitting of the S2:
Abnormal splitting may be in the form of (a) wide splitting, (b) narrow splitting, (c) single S2, or, rarely, (d) paradoxical splitting of the S2.

a) A widely split and fixed S2 is found in conditions that prolong the RV ejection time or that shorten the LV ejection. It is, therefore, found in:

(1) ASD or PAPVR (conditions in which the amount of blood ejected by the RV is increased; volume overload).

(2) Pulmonary stenosis (the valve stenosis prolongs the RV ejection time; pressure overload).

(3) RBBB (a delay in electrical activation of the RV).

(4) Mitral regurgitation (a decreased forward output seen in this condition shortens the LV ejection time).

(5) Occasional normal child, including "prolonged hangout time" seen in children with dilated MPA ("idiopathic dilatation of the pulmonary artery"). In dilated MPA, the increased capacity of the artery produces less recoil to close the pulmonary valves, delaying closure.

b) A narrowly split S2 is found in conditions with early closure of the pulmonary valve (pulmonary hypertension), with a delay in aortic closure (AS), or occasional normal child.

c) A single S2 is found when (a) only one semilunar valve is present (aortic or pulmonary atresia, persistent truncus arteriosus), (b) P2 is not audible (TGA, TOF, severe PS), (c) aortic closure is delayed (severe AS), (d) P2 occurs early (severe pulmonary hypertension), or (e) occasional normal child.

d) Paradoxically split S2 is found when the aortic closure (A2) follows the pulmonary closure (P2), and, therefore, is seen in conditions in which LV ejection is greatly delayed: severe AS, LBBB, or sometimes type B Wolff-Parkinson-White (WPW) syndrome.

b. Intensity of the P2:
The *relative* intensity of P2 compared with A2 must be assessed on every child. In the pulmonary area, A2 is usually louder than P2 (see Fig 2–4). Note that A2 is *not* the S2 at the aortic area; it is the aortic component of the S2 at the pulmonary area, or ULSB. Judgment as to normal intensity of P2 is based on experience, and there is no substitute for listening to many normal children.

Abnormal intensity of P2 may suggest pathology. Increased intensity of P2 (in comparison to A2) is found in pulmonary hypertension. Decreased intensity of P2 is found in conditions with decreased diastolic pressure of the pulmonary artery (severe PS, TOF, tricuspid atresia, etc.).

C. **Third heart sound (S3).**—The third heart sound is a somewhat low-frequency sound in early diastole and is related to rapid filling of the ventricle (Fig 2–5). It is best heard at the apex or LLSB. It is commonly heard in normal children and young adults. A loud S3 is abnormal and is audible in conditions with dilated ventricles and decreased compliance; e.g., large shunt VSD, CHF. When tachycardia is present, it forms a "Kentucky" gallop.

D. **Fourth heart sound (S4) or atrial sound.**—The fourth heart sound is a relatively low-frequency sound of late diastole (presystole) and is rare in infants and children (see Fig 2–5). When present, it is always pathologic and is seen in conditions with decreased ventricular compliance or CHF. With tachycardia, it forms a "Tennessee" gallop.

E. **Gallop rhythm.**—Generally implies pathology and results from the combination of a loud S3 or S4 and tachycardia. It is commonly present in CHF. A summation gallop represents tachycardia and superimposed S3 and S4.

II. Systolic and Diastolic Sounds

A. Ejection click (or ejection sound) follows the first sound very closely and occurs at the time of onset of ventricular ejection. Therefore, it sounds like splitting of the S1. However, it is most audible at the base (either side of the upper sternal border), whereas split S1 is most audible at the LLSB (note exceptions with aortic click below). If one hears what sounds like a split S1 at the upper sternal border, it may be an ejection click (Fig 2–6).

The pulmonary click is heard at the 2LICS and 3LICS and changes in intensity with respiration, being louder on expiration. The aortic click is best heard at the 2RICS, but may be louder at the apex or mid-left sternal border (MLSB). It usually does not change its intensity with respiration.

The ejection click is most often associated with:

a. Stenosis of semilunar valves (PS or AS).

b. Dilated great arteries seen in systemic or pulmonary hypertension, idiopathic dilatation of the PA, TOF (in which the aorta is dilated), and persistent truncus arteriosus.

B. Midsystolic click with or without late systolic murmur is heard at the apex in mitral valve prolapse syndrome (see Fig 2–6 and chap. 21).

C. Diastolic opening snap is rare in children and is audible at the apex or LLSB. It occurs somewhat earlier than the S3 during diastole and originates from a stenosis of the atrioventricular (AV) valve, such as mitral stenosis (see Fig 2–6).

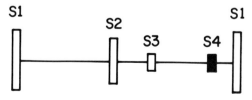

FIG 2–5.
Diagram showing the relative relationship of the heart sounds. *Filled bar* shows an abnormal sound.

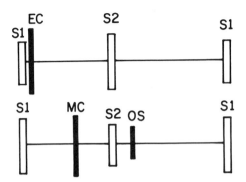

FIG 2–6.
Diagram showing the relative position of ejection click *(EC)*, midsystolic click *(MC)*, and diastolic opening snap *(OS)*. *Filled bars* show abnormal sounds.

III. Extracardiac Sounds

  A. Pericardial friction rub is a grating to-and-fro sound produced by friction of the heart against the pericardium. It usually indicates pericarditis. Intensity of the rub varies with the phase of the cardiac cycle (rather than the respiratory cycle). It may become louder when the patient leans forward. Large accumulation of fluid (pericardial effusion) may result in disappearance of the rub.

  B. Pericardial knock is an adventitious sound associated with chronic (constrictive) pericarditis and is rare in children.

IV. Heart Murmur

  Each heart murmur must be analyzed in terms of intensity (grade 1–6), timing (systolic or diastolic), location, transmission, and quality (musical, vibratory, blowing, etc.).

  1. Intensity of the murmur is customarily graded from 1 to 6.
     Grade 1: barely audible.
     Grade 2: soft but easily audible.
     Grade 3: moderately loud but not accompanied by a thrill.
     Grade 4: louder and associated with a thrill.
     Grade 5: audible with the stethoscope barely on the chest.
     Grade 6: audible with the stethoscope off the chest.

     The difference between grades 2 and 3 or grades 5 and 6 may be somewhat subjective. The intensity of the murmur may be influenced by the status of cardiac output. Thus, any factor that increases the cardiac output—i.e., fever, anemia, anxiety, or exercise—will intensify any existing murmur or may even produce one that is not audible at basal conditions.

  2. Classification of heart murmurs:
     Based on the timing of the heart murmur in relation to the S1 and S2, the heart murmur is classified into three types:

       1) Systolic murmur (ejection type and regurgitant type)

       2) Diastolic murmur (early diastolic, middiastolic, and presystolic)

       3) Continuous murmur.

For each type of murmur, the location, transmission, and quality of the murmur will be discussed when applicable.

A. Systolic murmurs

    a. Types of systolic murmurs:
The majority of heart murmurs are systolic in timing, occurring between the S1 and S2. A systolic murmur is usually classified as one of two types, depending on the timing of the *onset* of the heart murmur in relation to the S1—ejection or regurgitant.

      1) Ejection murmur (stenotic, diamond-shaped, crescendo-decrescendo): There is an interval between the S1 and the onset of the murmur. These murmurs are generally crescendo-decrescendo or "diamond-shaped" in contour (Fig 2–7,A) and usually end before the S2. The murmur may be short or long. All systolic murmurs that are not regurgitant (see below) may be classified as ejection-type murmurs. These murmurs are caused by flow of blood through stenotic or deformed semilunar valves or increased flow through normal semilunar valves, and are therefore found at the 2LICS or 2RICS. One source of confusion may be a soft S1 followed by an ejection click; only the latter may be heard. Consequently, the murmur appears to start immediately after "S1." However, this situation usually occurs at the 2LICS or 2RICS, where systolic regurgitant murmurs do not occur.

      2) Regurgitant systolic murmur: These murmurs begin *with* the first heart sound (S1) (no gap between the S1 and the murmur) and usually, but not invariably, last throughout systole (pansystolic or holosystolic).

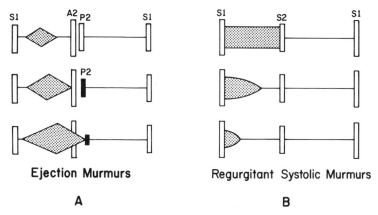

Ejection Murmurs   **Regurgitant Systolic Murmurs**

        A   **B**

FIG 2–7.
Diagram of ejection and regurgitant systolic murmurs. Classification of systolic murmurs is based primarily on the relationship of the S1 to the onset of the murmur. Both types of systolic murmurs may be long or short. **A,** short ejection-type systolic murmur with its apex of the "diamond" in the early part of systole is seen with mild stenosis of semilunar valves *(top)*. With increasing severity of obstruction to flow, the murmur becomes longer, and its apex moves toward the S2 *(middle)*. In severe PS, the murmur may go beyond the A2 *(bottom)*. **B,** regurgitant systolic murmur in children is most often due to VSD and is usually holosystolic, extending all the way to the S2 *(top)*. However, the regurgitation murmur may end in middle or early systole (not holosystolic) in some children, especially those with small shunt *(middle and bottom)*. Regardless of the length of the murmur, all regurgitant systolic murmurs are pathologic.

Therefore, analysis of the presence or absence of a gap between the S1 and the onset of the systolic murmur is of utmost importance; it is not concerned with the length or the termination of the murmur in relation to the S2 (Fig 2–7,B). Regurgitant systolic murmurs are caused by flow of blood from a chamber that is at a higher pressure throughout systole than the receiving chamber, and they are associated with *only* three conditions: ventricular septal defect, mitral regurgitation, and tricuspid regurgitation. It should be noted that none of these ordinarily occurs at the base (2LICS or 2RICS). One exception to the early onset of regurgitant systolic murmur is the late systolic murmur at the apex, following a midsystolic click in mitral valve prolapse syndrome (see chap. 21).

b. Location of the systolic murmurs:
In addition to the type of murmur (i.e., ejection vs. regurgitant), the location of the maximal intensity of the murmur is of great importance in making a clinical diagnosis of the origin of the heart murmur. For example, a regurgitant murmur heard maximally at the LLSB is characteristic of VSD. An ejection systolic murmur maximally audible at the 2LICS is usually pulmonary in origin. Also, location of the heart murmur often helps to clarify the situation in which differentiation between an ejection murmur and a regurgitant murmur is not easy. For example, a long pulmonary stenosis murmur may sound like a regurgitant murmur of VSD, but the maximal intensity at the ULSB makes it less likely to be due to a VSD (although rare, subarterial infundibular [or supracristal] VSD murmur may be maximal at the ULSB). This important topic will be discussed below in detail with Tables 2–5 through 2–8 and Figure 2–8.

c. Transmission of systolic murmurs:
The transmission of systolic murmurs from the site of maximal intensity may be helpful in determining the origin of the murmur. For example, an apical systolic murmur that transmits well to the left axilla and lower back is characteristic of mitral regurgitation, whereas one that radiates to the URSB and the neck is more likely to be of aortic valve origin. A systolic ejection murmur at the base that transmits well to the neck is more likely to be aortic in origin, and one that transmits well to the back is more likely to be of pulmonary valve or pulmonary artery origin.

d. Quality of systolic murmurs:
The quality of a murmur may be extremely helpful in the diagnosis of heart disease. Systolic murmurs of mitral regurgitation or VSD have a uniform, high-pitched quality often described as blowing. Ejection systolic murmurs of AS or PS have a rough, grating quality. A common innocent murmur in children, which is best audible between the LLSB and apex, has a characteristic vibratory or humming quality.

B. **Differential diagnosis of systolic murmurs at various locations:**
a. Upper left sternal border (ULSB) (or pulmonary area):
Systolic murmurs best heard in the ULSB are usually ejection type and may be due to one of the following:

1) Pulmonary valve stenosis (PS).

2) Atrial septal defect (ASD).

3) Innocent pulmonary flow murmur of newborn.

4) Innocent pulmonary flow murmur of older children.

5) Pulmonary artery stenosis.

6) Aortic stenosis (AS).

7) Tetralogy of Fallot (TOF).

8) Coarctation of the aorta (COA).

9) Patent ductus arteriosus (PDA) with pulmonary hypertension. (A continuous murmur of PDA is ordinarily loudest in the left infraclavicular area.)

10) Total anomalous pulmonary venous return (TAPVR).

11) Partial anomalous pulmonary venous return (PAPVR).

Conditions 1 through 4 are more common than the rest of the list. Characteristic physical findings, ECG, and x-ray findings that are helpful in differential diagnosis of these conditions are listed in Table 2–5.

b. Upper right sternal border (URSB) (or aortic area):
The systolic murmurs at the URSB are also ejection type and are caused by the narrowing of the aortic valve or its neighboring structures. The intensity of this ejection murmur varies from grade 2 to 5/6, and the murmur transmits well to the neck, rather than to the back, with thrill over the carotid arteries. The ejection murmur of AS may be heard equally well at the "pulmonary area" as well as the apex. However, the murmur of pulmonary stenosis does not transmit well to the URSB and the neck. The ECG may show LVH with/without "strain," depending on the severity of the obstruction.

The systolic murmurs in the URSB are caused by:

1) Aortic valve stenosis (AS).

2) Subvalvular aortic stenosis (subaortic stenosis).

3) Supravalvular aortic stenosis.

Characteristic physical, ECG, and x-ray findings that are helpful in differential diagnosis of these conditions are presented in Table 2–6.

c. Lower left sternal border (LLSB):
Systolic murmurs that are maximally audible at this location may be either of the regurgitant or ejection type and may be due to one of the following conditions:

1) Ventricular septal defect (VSD) (small muscular VSD may be heard best between the LLSB and apex).

2) Vibratory (or musical) innocent murmur (Still's murmur).

3) Hypertrophic obstructive cardiomyopathy (formerly known as idiopathic hypertrophic subaortic stenosis [IHSS]).

4) Tricuspid regurgitation.

5) Tetralogy of Fallot (TOF).

Characteristic physical, ECG, and x-ray findings which are helpful in differential diagnosis of these conditions are presented in Table 2–7.

TABLE 2–5.

Differential Diagnosis of Systolic Murmurs at the Upper Left Sternal Border (Pulmonary Area)

Condition	Important Physical Findings	Chest X-rays	ECG Findings
Pulmonary valve stenosis	SEM, grade 2–5/6, *Thrill (±) S2 may be split widely when mild *Ejection click (±) at 2LICS Transmit to the back	*Prominent MPA (poststenotic dilatation) Normal PVM	Normal if mild, RAD *RVH RAH if severe
Atrial septal defect	SEM, grade 2–3/6 *Widely split and fixed S2	*Incr. PVM *RAE & RVE	RAD RVH *RBBB (rsR')
Pulmonary flow murmur of newborn	SEM, grade 1–2/6 No thrill *Good transmission to the back and axillae Newborns	Normal	Normal
Pulmonary flow murmur of older children	SEM, grade 2–3/6 No thrill Poor transmission Ejection click (±)	Normal Occasional pectus excavatum or straight back	Normal
Pulmonary artery stenosis	SEM, grade 2–3/6 Occasional continuous murmur P2 may be loud *Transmits well to the back and both lung fields	Prominent hilar vessels (±)	RVH or normal
Aortic stenosis	SEM, grade 2–5/6 *Also audible in 2RICS *Thrill (±) at 2RICS and SSN *Ejection click at apex, 3LICS, or 2RICS (±) Paradox, split S2 if severe	Absence of prominent MPA Dilated aorta	Normal or LVH
Tetralogy of Fallot	*Long SEM, grade 2–4/6, louder at MLSB Thrill (±) Loud, single S2 (=A2) Cyanosis, clubbing	*Decr. PVM *Normal heart size Boot-shaped heart Right aortic arch (25%)	RAD *RVH or CVH RAH (±)
Coarctation of aorta	SEM, grade 1–3/6 *Loudest at left interscapular area (back) *Weak or absent femorals Hypertension in arms Freq. assoc. AS, bicuspid aortic valve, or MR	*Classic "3" sign on plain film or "E" sign on barium esophagogram Rib notching (±)	LVH in children RBBB (or RVH) in infants
Patent ductus arteriosus	*Continuous murmur, at left infraclavicular area	*Incr. PVM *LAE, LVE	Normal, LVH, or CVH

TABLE 2–5. *(cont.)*.

Condition	Important Physical Findings	Chest X-rays	ECG Findings
	Occasional crescendic systolic only Grade 2–4/6 Thrill (±) Bounding pulses		
Total anomalous pulmonary venous return (TAPVR)	SEM, grade 2–3/6 Widely split and fixed S2 (±) *Quadruple or quintuple rhythm *Diastolic rumble at LLSB *Mild cyanosis (↓ Po_2) and clubbing (±)	*Incr. PVM RAE & RVE Prominent MPA "Snowman" sign	RAD RAH *RVH
Partial anomalous pulmonary venous return (PAPVR)	Physical findings similar to those of ASD *S2 may not be fixed unless associated with ASD	*Incr. PVM *RAE & RVE "Scimitar" sign (±)	Same as in ASD

AS = aortic stenosis; Decr. = decreased; Incr. = increased; CVH = combined ventricular hypertrophy; 2LICS = second left intercostal space; LLSB = lower left sternal border; MLSB = mid-left sternal border; LVE = left ventricular enlargement; LVH = left ventricular hypertrophy; MPA = main pulmonary artery; MR = mitral regurgitation; PVM = pulmonary vascular markings; RAD = right-axis deviation; RAE = right atrial enlargement; RAH = right atrial hypertrophy; RBBB = right bundle branch block; RVE = right ventricular enlargement; RVH = right ventricular hypertrophy; SEM = systolic ejection murmur; SSN = suprasternal notch.
Asterisks (*) in this and following tables indicate findings that are particularly characteristic of the condition.

TABLE 2–6.

Differential Diagnosis of Systolic Murmurs at the URSB (Aortic Area)

Condition	Important Physical Findings	Chest X-rays	ECG Findings

Aortic valve stenosis	SEM, grade 2–5/6, at 2RICS, may be loudest
	  at 3LICS
	*Thrill (±), URSB, SSN & carotid arteries
	*Ejection click
	*Transmits well to neck
	S2 may be single
		Mild LVE (±)
		Prominent
		  ascending
		  aorta or
		  aortic knob
			Normal or LVH
			  w/wo "strain"

Subaortic stenosis	SEM, grade 2–4/6 *AR murmur almost always present in discrete stenosis No ejection click	Usually normal	Normal or LVH

Supravalvular aortic stenosis	SEM, grade 2–3/6
	Thrill (±)
	No ejection click
	*Pulse & BP may be greater in R than L arm
	*Peculiar facies and mental retardation
	Murmur may transmit well to the back (PA
	  stenosis)
		Unremarkable	Normal, LVH
			  or CVH

AR = aortic regurgitation; CVH = combined ventricular hypertrophy; LVE = left ventricular enlargement; LVH = left ventricular hypertrophy; 3RICS = third right intercostal space; SEM = systolic ejection murmur; SSN = suprasternal notch; URSB = upper right sternal border.
Asterisks (*) indicate findings that are more characteristic of the condition.

TABLE 2-7.

Differential Diagnosis of Systolic Murmurs at the LLSB

Condition	Important Physical Findings	Chest X-rays	ECG Findings
Ventricular septal defect (VSD)	*Regurgitant systolic, grade 2–5/6 May not be holosystolic Well-localized at LLSB *Thrill often present P2 may be loud	*Incr. PVM *LAE & LVE (cardiomegaly)	Normal LVH or CVH
Endocardial cushion defect, complete	Similar to findings of VSD *Diastolic rumble at LLSB *Gallop rhythm common in infants	Similar to large VSD	*Superior QRS axis LVH or CVH
Vibratory innocent murmur (Still's)	SEM, grade 2–3/6 *Musical or vibratory with midsystolic accentuation *Max. between LLSB & apex	Normal	Normal
Hypertrophic obstructive cardiomyopathy (HOCM or IHSS)	SEM, grade 2–4/6 Medium-pitched Max. LLSB or apex Thrill (±) *Sharp upstroke of brachial pulses May have MR murmur	Normal or globular LVE	LVH Abnormally deep Q waves in V5 and V6
Tricuspid regurgitation	*Regurgitant systolic, grade 2–3/6 *Triple or quadruple rhythm (in Ebstein's) Mild cyanosis (±) Hepatomegaly with pulsatile liver and neck vein distention when severe	Normal PVM RAE if severe	RBBB, RAH & 1° AV block in Ebstein's
Tetralogy of Fallot	See Table 2–5 Murmurs can be louder at ULSB		

CVH = combined ventricular hypertrophy; LAE = left atrial enlargement; LLSB = lower left sternal border; LVE = left ventricular enlargement; LVH = left ventricular hypertrophy; MR = mitral regurgitation; PVM = pulmonary vascular markings; RAE = right atrial enlargement; RAH = right atrial hypertrophy; RBBB = right bundle branch block; SEM = systolic ejection murmur.
Asterisks (*) indicate findings that are more characteristic of the condition.

---

d. The apical area:

Systolic murmurs that are maximally audible at the apex may be either of the regurgitant or ejection type and are due to one of the following conditions:

1) Mitral regurgitation.

2) Mitral valve prolapse syndrome (MVPS).

3) Aortic stenosis (AS).

4) Hypertrophic obstructive cardiomyopathy (HOCM or IHSS).

5) Vibratory innocent murmur.

Characteristic physical, ECG, and x-ray findings are summarized in Table 2–8.

Systolic murmurs that are audible at the various locations are presented in Figure 2–8 (see also Tables 2–5 through 2–8).

C. Diastolic Murmurs

Diastolic murmurs occur between the S2 and S1. Based on their timing and relation to the heart sounds, they are classified into three types: early diastolic, middiastolic, and presystolic (Fig 2–9).

a. Early diastolic (protodiastolic) decrescendo murmurs occur early in diastole, immediately following the S2, and are caused by incompetence of the aortic or pulmonary valve (see Fig 2–9).

The aorta being a high-pressure vessel, aortic regurgitation murmurs are high pitched, are best heard with the diaphragm of the stethoscope at the 3LICS, and radiate well to the apex. This coincides with the direction of the regurgitation. Bounding peripheral pulses may be present

TABLE 2–8.

Differential Diagnosis of Systolic Murmurs at the Apex

Condition	Important Physical Findings	Chest X-rays	ECG Findings
Mitral regurgitation	*Regurgitant systolic, may not be holosystolic, grade 2–3/6 Transmits to left axilla (less obvious in children) May be loudest in the midprecordium	LAE & LVE	LAH or LVH
Mitral valve prolapse syndrome (MVPS)	*Midsystolic click and late systolic murmur *High incidence of thoracic skeletal anomalies (pectus excavatum, straight back) (85%)	Normal	Inverted T in aVF
Aortic valve stenosis	The murmur and ejection click may be best heard at the apex rather than at 2RICS	(See Table 2–6)	
Hypertrophic obstructive cardiomyopathy (HOCM or IHSS)	The murmur of IHSS may be maximal at the apex (may represent MR) (See Table 2–7)		
Vibratory innocent murmur	This innocent murmur may be loudest at the apex (See Table 2–7)		

LAE = left atrial enlargement; LAH = left atrial hypertrophy; LVE = left ventricular enlargement; LVH = left ventricular hypertrophy; MR = mitral regurgitation; 2RICS = second right intercostal space.
Asterisks (*) indicate findings that are more characteristic of the condition.

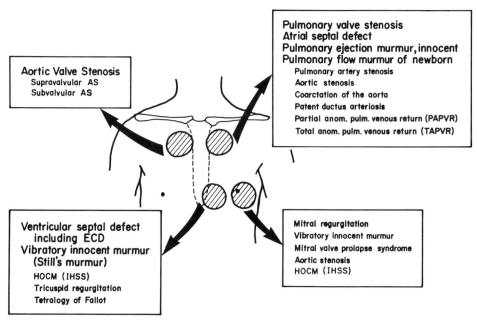

Aortic Valve Stenosis
Supravalvular AS
Subvalvular AS

Pulmonary valve stenosis
Atrial septal defect
Pulmonary ejection murmur, innocent
Pulmonary flow murmur of newborn
Pulmonary artery stenosis
Aortic stenosis
Coarctation of the aorta
Patent ductus arteriosis
Partial anom. pulm. venous return (PAPVR)
Total anom. pulm. venous return (TAPVR)

Ventricular septal defect
including ECD
Vibratory innocent murmur
(Still's murmur)
HOCM (IHSS)
Tricuspid regurgitation
Tetralogy of Fallot

Mitral regurgitation
Vibratory innocent murmur
Mitral valve prolapse syndrome
Aortic stenosis
HOCM (IHSS)

FIG 2–8.
Diagram showing systolic murmurs audible at various locations. Less common conditions are shown in smaller type (see Tables 2–5 through 2–8). AS = aortic stenosis; ECD = endocardial cushion defect; HOCM = hypertrophic obstructive cardiomyopathy; IHSS = idiopathic hypertrophic subaortic stenosis.

if the aortic regurgitation is significant. Aortic regurgitation murmurs are associated with congenital bicuspid aortic valve, subaortic stenosis, post-operative AS (postvalvotomy), and rheumatic heart disease with aortic regurgitation and occasionally subarterial infundibular (supracristal) VSD with prolapsing aortic cusps.

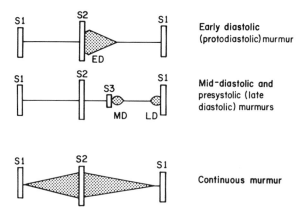

Early diastolic
(protodiastolic) murmur

Mid-diastolic and
presystolic (late
diastolic) murmurs

Continuous murmur

FIG 2–9.
Diagrammatic drawing of diastolic murmurs and the continuous murmur. ED = early diastolic or protodiastolic murmur; LD = late diastolic or presystolic murmur; MD = middiastolic murmur.

Pulmonary regurgitation murmurs also occur early in diastole. They are usually medium pitched but may be high pitched if pulmonary hypertension is present. They are best heard at the 2LICS and radiate along the left sternal border. These murmurs are associated with postoperative tetralogy of Fallot (due to surgically induced pulmonary regurgitation), pulmonary hypertension, postoperative pulmonary valvotomy for PS, and mild, isolated deformity of the pulmonary valve.

b. Middiastolic (or ventricular filling or inflow) murmurs start with a loud S3 and are heard in early or middiastole, but are not temporally midway through diastole (see Fig 2–9). These murmurs are always low pitched and are best heard with the bell of the stethoscope applied lightly to the chest. These murmurs are caused by turbulence in the mitral or tricuspid valve secondary to anatomical stenosis or relative stenosis of these valves (see below).

Mitral middiastolic murmurs are best heard at the apex and are often referred to as "apical rumble," although frequently they are more of a hum than a rumble. These murmurs are associated with mitral stenosis or large left-to-right shunt VSD or PDA, which produce relative mitral stenosis secondary to a large flow across the normal-sized mitral valve.

Tricuspid middiastolic murmurs are best heard along the LLSB. These murmurs are associated with ASD, partial or total anomalous pulmonary venous return, endocardial cushion defect (ECD) (all due to relative tricuspid stenosis), or, rarely, anatomical stenosis of the tricuspid valve.

c. Presystolic (or late diastolic) murmurs are also caused by flow through AV valves during ventricular diastole and are the direct result of active atrial contraction ejecting blood into the ventricle (rather than a passive pressure difference between the atrium and ventricle). These low-frequency murmurs occur late in diastole or just before the onset of systole (see Fig 2–9) and are found with true stenosis of the mitral or tricuspid valve.

D. Continuous Murmur

Continuous murmurs begin in systole and continue without interruption through the S2 into all or part of diastole (see Fig 2–9). Continuous murmurs can be caused by:

1) Aortopulmonary or arteriovenous connection (PDA, AV fistula, or after systemic-pulmonary shunt surgery, or, rarely, persistent truncus arteriosus).

2) Disturbances of flow patterns in veins (venous hum).

3) Disturbance of flow pattern in arteries (COA, pulmonary artery stenosis).

The murmur of PDA has a machinery-like quality, becoming louder during systole (crescendo), peaking at the S2, and diminishing in diastole (decrescendo). This murmur is maximally heard in the left infraclavicular area or along the ULSB. With pulmonary hypertension, only the systolic portion will be audible, but it will be crescendic during systole.

Venous hum is a common innocent murmur audible in the upright position, in the infraclavicular region, unilaterally or bilaterally. The intensity of the murmur changes with the position of the neck, and the murmur usually disappears when the child lies supine. It is usually heard better on the right side.

Less common continuous murmurs of severe COA may be heard over the intercostal collaterals and those of pulmonary artery stenosis over both lung fields and in the back.

The combination of a systolic murmur, such as VSD or PS, and a diastolic murmur, such as from aortic or pulmonary regurgitation, is referred to as a to-and-fro murmur to distinguish it from a machinery-like continuous murmur.

E. Innocent Heart Murmurs

Innocent heart murmurs, also called functional murmurs, are those that arise from cardiovascular structures in the absence of anatomical abnormalities. Innocent heart murmurs are common in children. Over 80% of children will have innocent murmurs of one type or the other sometime during childhood, most commonly beginning about 3–4 years of age. All innocent heart murmurs are accentuated or brought out in high-output states, most importantly with fever.

How do we know which are innocent murmurs? Probably the only way to deal with this problem is to become familiar with more typical forms of innocent heart murmurs by auscultating many innocent murmurs under the supervision of pediatric cardiologists. All innocent heart murmurs are associated with normal ECG and x-ray findings. When one or more of the following are present, the murmur is more likely pathologic and will require cardiac consultation:

1) Symptomatic.

2) Abnormal cardiac size and/or silhouette or abnormal pulmonary vascularity on chest roentgenograms.

3) Abnormal ECG.

4) Diastolic murmur.

5) A systolic murmur that is loud (grade 3/6 or with thrill) and long in duration, which transmits well to other parts of the body.

6) Cyanosis.

7) Abnormally strong or weak pulses.

8) Abnormal heart sounds.

a. Classic Vibratory Murmur (Still's murmur)

Although occasionally detected in infancy, it is not common before the age of 2 years. Most vibratory murmurs are detected between 3 and 6 years of age. It is maximally audible at the mid-left sternal border or between the LLSB and the apex. The murmur is midsystolic in timing and of grade 2–3/6 in intensity. It has a distinctive quality, having been described as "twanging string," groaning, squeaking, buzzing, musical, or vibratory. It is generally of low frequency and best heard with the bell in the supine position. The vibratory quality disappears when the bell is pressed hard, proving its low frequency. It is not accompanied by thrill or ejection click. The intensity of the murmur increases during febrile illness or excitement, after exercise, or in anemic states. The murmur may disappear briefly at maximum Valsalva maneuver. The ECG and chest x-rays are normal (Table 2–9 and Fig 2–10).

An inexperienced examiner may confuse it with the murmur of VSD. The murmur of VSD is usually harsh, grade 2–4/6 in intensity, regurgi-

TABLE 2–9.

Common Innocent Heart Murmurs

Type (Timing)	Description of Murmur	Age Group
Classic vibratory murmur (Still's murmur) (systolic)	Maximal at MLSB or between LLSB and apex Grade 2–3/6 Low-frequency vibratory, "twanging string," groaning, squeaking, or musical	3–6 yr Occasionally in infancy
Pulmonary ejection murmur (systolic)	Maximal at ULSB Early to midsystolic Grade 1–3/6 in intensity Blowing in quality	8–14 yr
Pulmonary flow murmur of newborn (systolic)	Maximal at ULSB Transmits well to the left and right chest, axillae, and back Grade 1–2/6 in intensity	Prematures and fullterm newborns Usually disappears by 3–6 mo. of age
Venous hum (continuous)	Maximal at right (or left) supra- and infra-clavicular areas Grade 1–3/6 in intensity Inaudible in the supine position Intensity changes with rotation of the head and compression of the jugular vein	3–6 yr
Carotid bruit (systolic)	Right supraclavicular area and over the carotids Grade 2–3/6 in intensity Occasional thrill over a carotid	Any age

tant in timing (starting with S1), and often accompanied by a palpable thrill. The ECG and x-rays are often abnormal.

b. **Pulmonary Ejection Murmur (pulmonary flow murmur of children)**
It is common in children 8–14 years of age but most frequent in adolescents. The murmur is maximally audible at the ULSB. The ejection type

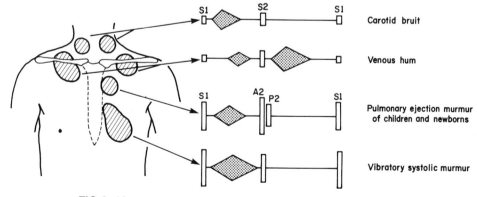

FIG 2–10.
Diagrammatic illustration of innocent heart murmurs in children.

murmur is early to midsystolic in timing, slightly grating (rather than vibratory) in quality, with relatively little radiation. The intensity of the murmur is usually grade 1–3/6. The second heart sound is normal, and there is no associated thrill or ejection click (see Table 2–9 and Fig 2–10).

This murmur may be confused with the murmur of pulmonary valve stenosis or ASD. In pulmonary valve stenosis, there may be an ejection click, systolic thrill, widely split S2, RVH on ECG, and poststenotic dilatation of the main pulmonary artery (MPA) segment on chest x-rays. Important differential points of ASD include widely split and fixed S2, diastolic flow rumble (of relative tricuspid stenosis) at LLSB if the shunt is large, RBBB or mild RVH on ECG (manifested by rsR′ in V1), and chest x-rays revealing increased pulmonary vascular markings and enlargement of the RA, RV, and MPA.

c. **Pulmonary Flow Murmur of Newborn**

This murmur is commonly present in newborn infants, especially those with low birth weight. The murmur usually disappears by 3–6 months of age. If it persists beyond this age, a structural narrowing of the pulmonary arterial tree (pulmonary artery stenosis) must be suspected. It is best audible at the ULSB. Although the murmur is only grade 1–2/6 in intensity, it has an impressive transmission to the right and left chest, both axillae, and the back. There is no ejection click. The ECG and chest x-rays are normal (see Table 2–9 and Fig 2–10).

This murmur originates from the relatively hypoplastic right and left pulmonary arteries at birth. This relative hypoplasia is the result of the small amount of blood flow through these vessels during fetal life (only 15% of combined ventricular output goes to these vessels). The turbulence created in these small vessels near the bifurcation is transmitted along the smaller branches of the pulmonary arteries. Therefore, this murmur is heard well around the chest wall.

The murmur resembles the murmur of organic pulmonary artery stenosis, which may be seen as a component of rubella syndrome or Williams' syndrome. Characteristic noncardiac findings in children with the above syndromes will help one to suspect an organic nature of the pulmonary artery stenosis murmur. Organic pulmonary artery stenosis is frequently associated with other cardiac defects, such as VSD and pulmonary valve stenosis, or seen occasionally as an isolated anomaly. The heart murmur of organic pulmonary artery stenosis will persist beyond infancy, and the ECG may show RVH if the stenosis is severe.

d. **Venous Hum**

This murmur is commonly audible in children between the ages of 3 and 6 years. It originates from turbulence in the jugular venous system. This is a continuous murmur, with the diastolic component louder than the systolic component. The murmur is maximally audible at the right and/or left infra- and supra-clavicular areas (see Table 2–9 and Fig 2–10). The venous hum is heard only in the upright position and disappears in the supine position. It can be obliterated by rotation of the head or by gentle occlusion of the neck veins with the fingers.

The continuous murmur of PDA is loudest at the ULSB or left infra-clavicular area, with bounding peripheral pulses and wide pulse pressure. The systolic component is louder than the diastolic component.

The x-ray films show increased pulmonary vascular markings and cardiac enlargement. The ECG may be normal or show LVH or CVH.

e. **Carotid Bruit**

This is an early systolic ejection murmur, best audible in the supraclavicular fossa or over the carotid arteries (see Table 2–9 and Fig 2–10). It is produced by turbulence in the brachiocephalic or carotid arteries. The murmur is grade 2–3/6 in intensity. Rarely, a faint thrill is palpable over a carotid artery. This bruit may be found in children of any age.

The murmur of aortic stenosis often transmits well to the carotid arteries with a palpable thrill, requiring differentiation from the carotid bruits. In aortic stenosis, the murmur is louder at the URSB, and a systolic thrill is often present in the URSB and suprasternal notch, in addition to the thrill over the carotid artery. An ejection click is often present in aortic valve stenosis. The ECG and chest x-ray may be abnormal.

3 / Electrocardiography I

In clinical diagnosis of congenital or acquired heart disease, detection of hypertrophy of ventricles and atria and ventricular conduction disturbances are often very helpful. These ECG abnormalities may be incorporated into a flow diagram presented in chapter 5 for diagnosis of congenital heart defects. Therefore, this chapter will emphasize hypertrophy of ventricles and atria and ventricular conduction disturbances. A brief discussion of a normal pediatric ECG and the basic measurements that are necessary for routine interpretation of an ECG will also be presented. Other ECG abnormalities such as AV conduction disturbances, arrhythmias, and ST segment and T wave changes will be presented in part 6, Electrocardiography II.

I. NORMAL PEDIATRIC ELECTROCARDIOGRAMS

Electrocardiograms of normal infants and children are quite different from those of normal adults. The most remarkable difference is the right ventricular dominance in infants. The RV dominance is most marked in the newborn, and it gradually changes to LV dominance in the adult. The ECG reflects anatomical differences; the RV is thicker than the LV in the newborn and infant, and the LV is much thicker than the RV in the adult.

Right ventricular dominance of infants is expressed in the ECG by:

a. Right-axis deviation, and

b. Large right ventricular forces (tall R waves in aVR and the right precordial leads [RPLs, such as V4R, V1, and V2] and deep S waves in lead I and the left precordial leads [LPLs, such as V5 and V6]).

An ECG from a 2-week-old infant (Fig 3–1) is compared with that from a young adult (Fig 3–2). The ECG from a normal 2-week-old infant shown in Figure 3–1 demonstrates right-axis deviation (+160°) and dominant R waves in the RPLs (V4R, V1, and V2). The T wave in V1 is almost always negative. Upright T waves in V1 in this age group are suggestive of RVH. Adult-type R/S progression in the precordial leads (deep S waves in V1 and V2 and tall R waves in V5 and V6; see Fig 3–2) is rarely seen in the first month of life.

The normal adult ECG shown in Figure 3–2 demonstrates the QRS axis near +50° and LV dominance manifested by dominant R in the LPLs and dominant S in the RPLs, the adult R/S progression. The T waves are usually anteriorly oriented, resulting in upright T waves in V2 through V6, and sometimes in V1.

II. ROUTINE INTERPRETATION

The following sequence is one of many approaches that can be used in routine interpretation of an ECG.

a. Rhythm (sinus or nonsinus) by considering the P axis.

b. Heart rate (atrial and ventricular rates, if different).

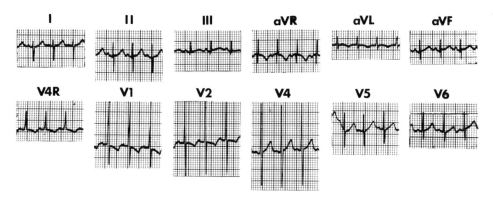

FIG 3–1.
ECG from normal 2-week-old infant.

c. The QRS axis, the T axis, and the QRS-T angle.

d. Intervals: PR, QRS, and QT.

e. The P wave amplitude and duration.

f. The QRS amplitude and R/S ratio; also note abnormal Q waves.

g. ST segment and T wave abnormalities.

Basic measurements that are necessary for routine interpretation will be briefly discussed.

A. Rhythm

Sinus rhythm is the normal rhythm at any age and is characterized by:

a. P waves preceding each QRS complex with a regular (but not necessarily normal) PR interval, and

b. Normal P axis (0 to +90°).

Since the sinoatrial (SA) node is located in the right upper part of the atrial mass, the direction of atrial depolarization is from the right upper part toward the left lower part, producing the P axis in the left lower quadrant (0 to +90°)

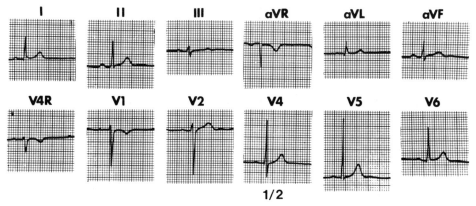

1/2

FIG 3–2.
ECG from normal young adult.

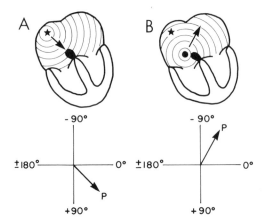

FIG 3–3.
Comparison of P axis in sinus rhythm **(A)** and low atrial rhythm **(B).** In sinus rhythm, the P waves are upright in leads I and aVF. In low atrial rhythm, the P wave is inverted in aVF.

(Fig 3–3,A). This second requirement of normal P axis is important in discriminating sinus from nonsinus rhythm. Some atrial rhythm (nonsinus) may have P waves preceding each QRS complex, but with an abnormal P axis (Fig 3–3,B). For the P axis to be between 0 and +90°, P waves must be upright in leads I and aVF; simple inspection of these two leads will suffice. Normal P axis also results in upright P waves in lead II and inverted P waves in aVR. A method of plotting axes is presented later for the QRS axis.

B. Heart Rate
There are many different ways of calculating the heart rate, but they are all based on the known time scale of ECG papers. At the usual paper speed of 25 mm per second, 1 mm = 0.04 second, and 5 mm = 0.20 second (Fig 3–4). The following methods are often used in calculating the heart rate.

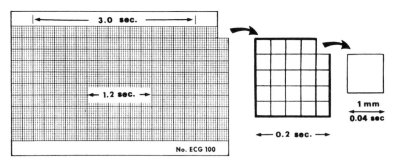

FIG 3–4.
ECG paper. Time is measured on the horizontal axis. Each 1 mm = 0.04 second, and each 5 mm (a large division) = 0.20 second; 30 mm (or 6 large divisions) = 1.2 second or 1/50 minute. Every 7.5 cm marked on the top margin of the paper = 3.0 second or 1/20 minute. (From Park MK, Guntheroth WG: *How to Read Pediatric ECGs,* ed 2. Chicago, Year Book Medical Publishers, 1987. Used by permission.)

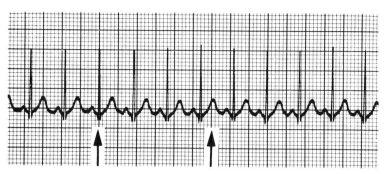

FIG 3–5.
Heart rate of 165/min. There are about 3.3 cardiac cycles (RR intervals) in 6 large divisions. Therefore, the heart rate is 3.3 × 50 = 165. (From Park MK, Guntheroth WG: *How to Read Pediatric ECGs,* ed 2. Chicago, Year Book Medical Publishers, 1987. Used by permission.)

    a. Count the RR cycle in 6 large divisions (1/50 minute) and multiply it by 50 (Fig 3–5).

    b. When the heart rate is slow, count the number of large divisions between two R waves and divide into 300 (1 minute = 300 large divisions) (Fig 3–6).

    c. Count the RR cycles between two markers (3 seconds) on the upper edge of an unmounted tracing and multiply them by 20.

    d. Measure the RR interval (in seconds) and divide 60 by the RR interval. The RR interval is 0.36 second in Figure 3–5: 60 ÷ 0.36 = 166.

    e. Use a convenient ECG ruler.

When the ventricular and atrial rates are different, as in complete heart block or atrial flutter, the atrial rate can be calculated using the same methods as described for the ventricular rate; for atrial rate, use the PP interval rather than the RR interval.

Because of age-related differences in the heart rate, the definition used for adults of bradycardia (less than 60/min) or tachycardia (in excess of 100/min) are not helpful in discriminating normal from abnormal in pediatric patients. Operationally, tachycardia is present when the heart rate is faster than the upper

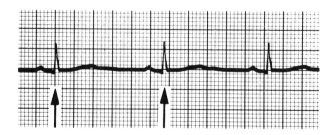

FIG 3–6.
Heart rate of 52/min. There are 5.8 large divisions between the two *arrows.* Therefore, the heart rate is 300 ÷ 5.8 = 52. (From Park MK, Guntheroth WG: *How to Read Pediatric ECGs,* ed 2. Chicago, Year Book Medical Publishers, 1987. Used by permission.)

range of normal, and bradycardia is present when the heart rate is slower than the lower range of normal for that age. Normal resting heart rates per minute according to age are as follows:

Newborn—110–150

2 years—85–125

4 years—75–115

Older than 6 years—60–100

C. The QRS Axis, the T Axis, and the QRS-T Angle

1. The QRS Axis.—The most convenient way of determining the QRS axis is by the use of the hexaxial reference system (Fig 3–7,A). The hexaxial reference system gives information about the left-right and superior-inferior relationship, as in the *frontal* plane of vectorcardiography. The R wave in lead I represents the leftward force and the S wave in lead I the rightward force. The R in aVF is a downward force and the S wave the upward force (see Fig 3–7,A).

An easy way to memorize the system is shown in Figure 3–8 by a superimposition of a body with outstretched arms and legs on the X and Y axes. The right and left hands are the positive poles of the aVR and aVL, respectively. The left and right feet are the positive poles of lead II and lead III, respectively. The bipolar limb leads I, II, and III are clockwise in sequence for the positive electrode.

Successive Approximation Method:
Step 1: Locate a quadrant, using leads I and aVF (Fig 3–9).

From the top panel of Figure 3–9, the net QRS deflection of lead I is positive. This means that the QRS axis is in the left hemicircle (from −90° through 0 to +90°) from the lead I point of view. The net positive QRS deflection in aVF means that the QRS axis is in the lower half of the circle (from 0 through +90 to +180°) from the aVF point of view. Therefore, in order to satisfy the polarity of both leads I and aVF, the QRS axis must be in the left lower quadrant (0 to +90°). Four quadrants can be easily identified based on the net deflections of the QRS complexes in leads I and aVF (see Fig 3–9).

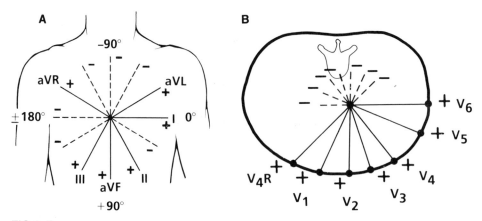

FIG 3–7.
Hexaxial **(A)** and horizontal **(B)** reference systems. (From Park MK, Guntheroth WG: *How to Read Pediatric ECGs,* ed 2. Chicago, Year Book Medical Publishers, 1987. Used by permission.)

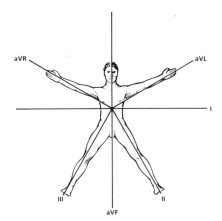

FIG 3–8.
An easy way to memorize the hexaxial reference system. (From Park MK, Guntheroth
WG: *How to Read Pediatric ECGs,* ed 2. Chicago, Year Book Medical Publishers, 1987.
Used by permission.)

> *Step 2: Find a lead with equiphasic QRS complex (in which the height of R
>   wave and the depth of S wave are equal).*

The QRS axis is perpendicular to the lead with equiphasic QRS complex
in the predetermined quadrant.

Example (Fig 3–10): Determine the QRS axis in Figure 3–10.

Step 1: The axis is in the left lower quadrant (0 to +90°), since the R waves
          are upright in both leads I and aVF.

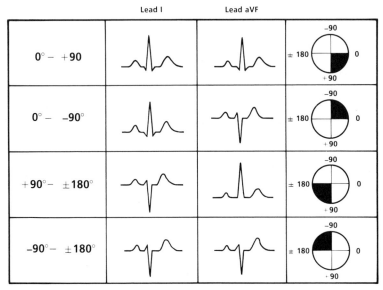

FIG 3–9.
Locating quadrants of mean QRS axis from leads I and aVF. (From Park MK, Guntheroth
WG: *How to Read Pediatric ECGs,* ed 2. Chicago, Year Book Medical Publishers, 1987.
Used by permission.)

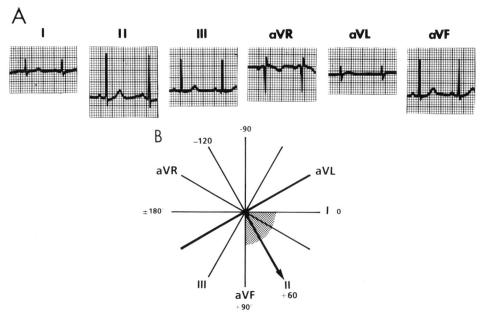

FIG 3–10.
Examples of the ECG strip **(A)** and the hexaxial reference system **(B).**

Step 2: The QRS complex is equiphasic in aVL. Therefore, the QRS axis is
        +60°, which is perpendicular to aVL.

Normal QRS Axis:
    Normal ranges of QRS axis vary with age. The newborn infant normally
has right axis deviation compared with the adult standard. By 3 years of age,
the QRS axis approaches the adult mean value of +50°. The mean and ranges
of normal QRS axis according to age are shown in Table 3–1.
    The QRS axis outside the normal ranges signifies abnormalities in the ven-
tricular depolarization process.

a. Left-axis deviation (LAD) is present when the QRS axis is less than the
   lower limit of normal (LLN) for the patient's age. LAD occurs with LVH,
   LBBB, and left anterior hemiblock.

b. Right-axis deviation (RAD) is present when the QRS axis is greater than
   the upper limit of normal (ULN) for the patient's age. RAD occurs with
   RVH and RBBB.

TABLE 3–1.

Mean and Ranges of Normal QRS Axes

1 wk–1 mo	+110° (+30 to +180)
1–3 mo	+70° (+10 to +125)
3 mo–3 yr	+60° (+10 to +110)
Older than 3 yr	+60° (+20 to +120)
Adults	+50° (−30 to +105)

    c. "Superior QRS" axis is present when the S wave is greater than the R wave in aVF (note the overlap with LAD). It may occur with left anterior hemiblock (in the range of −30° to −90°, seen in endocardial cushion defect or tricuspid atresia) or with RBBB.

Horizontal Reference System:

    While the hexaxial reference system gives information about the left-right and superior-inferior relationships, the horizontal reference system gives information about the anteroposterior and left-right relationship, as in the *horizontal* plane of a vectorcardiogram. The horizontal reference system utilizes precordial leads. Although this system is not used routinely in calculating QRS axis, understanding the system is important in the diagnosis of ventricular hypertrophy based on vectorial approaches.

    The horizontal reference system is not as precise as the hexaxial reference system in which the angle between the two adjacent leads is 30°. The approximate relationship of the system is shown in Figure 3–7,B. The leads V2 and V6 cross at a right angle. The R wave in V2 represents the anterior force, and the S wave in V2 represents the posterior force. The R wave in V6 represents the leftward force, and the S wave represents the rightward force. The R wave in V1 represents the anterior and rightward forces, and the S wave represents the posterior and leftward forces.

2. **The T Axis.**—The T axis can be determined by the same methods used to determine the QRS axis. In normal children, with the exception of the newborn period, the mean T axis is +45°, with a range of 0° to +90°, the same as in normal adults. The T axis outside of the normal quadrant suggests conditions with myocardial dysfunction similar to those listed for abnormal QRS-T angle (see below).

3. **The QRS-T Angle.**—The QRS-T angle is simply the angle formed by the QRS axis and the T axis. A QRS-T angle of more than 60° is unusual, and that of more than 90° is certainly abnormal. An abnormally wide QRS-T angle with the T axis outside the normal quadrant (0° to +90°) is seen in severe ventricular hypertrophy with "strain," ventricular conduction disturbances, and myocardial dysfunction of metabolic or ischemic nature.

D. Intervals

    There are three important intervals that are routinely measured in the interpretation of an ECG: PR interval, QRS duration, and QT interval. The duration of the P wave is also inspected. Figure 3–11 shows these intervals and durations.

1. **PR Interval**

    Normal PR interval varies with *age* and *heart rate* (Table 3–2). Prolongation of the PR interval (first-degree AV block) is seen in myocarditis (rheumatic or viral), digitalis toxicity, CHD (ECD, ASD, Ebstein's anomaly), and other myocardial dysfunctions. A short PR interval is present in preexcitation (Wolff-Parkinson-White syndrome and Lown-Ganong-Levine syndrome).

2. **QRS Duration**

    The QRS duration varies with age (Table 3–3). It is short in the young infant and increases with age. Conditions grouped as ventricular conduction disturbances have in common increased QRS duration; they include (a) bundle branch blocks, right and left; (b) preexcitation (WPW syndrome); (c) intraventricular block (hyperkalemia, toxicity from quinidine or procainamide, myocardial fibrosis, myocardial dysfunction of metabolic or ischemic nature); and

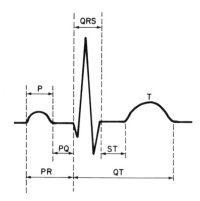

FIG 3–11.
Diagram illustrating important intervals (or durations) and segments of an ECG cycle.

(d) ventricular rhythm (PVCs, ventricular tachycardia, implanted ventricular pacemaker, etc.). Since the QRS duration varies with age, the definition of bundle branch block or other ventricular conduction disturbances should vary with age (see Ventricular Conduction Disturbances below).

3. QT Interval

The QT interval varies primarily with heart rate. The heart rate corrected QT interval (QTc) can be calculated by the use of Bazett's formula:

$$QTc = \frac{QT \text{ measured}}{\sqrt{RR \text{ interval}}}$$

TABLE 3–2.

PR Interval, With Rate and Age (and Upper Limits of Normal)*

Rate	0–1 mo	1–6 mo	6 mo–1 yr	1–3 yr	3–8 yr	8–12 yr	12–16 yr	Adult
<60						0.16 (0.18)	0.16 (0.19)	0.17 (0.21)
60–80					0.15 (0.17)	0.15 (0.17)	0.15 (0.18)	0.16 (0.21)
80–100	0.10 (0.12)				0.14 (0.16)	0.15 (0.16)	0.15 (0.17)	0.15 (0.20)
100–120	0.10 (0.12)			(0.15)	0.13 (0.16)	0.14 (0.15)	0.15 (0.16)	0.15 (0.19)
120–140	0.10 (0.11)	0.11 (0.14)	0.11 (0.14)	0.12 (0.14)	0.13 (0.15)	0.14 (0.15)		0.15 (0.18)
140–160	0.09 (0.11)	0.10 (0.13)	0.11 (0.13)	0.11 (0.14)	0.12 (0.14)			(0.17)
160–180	0.10 (0.11	0.10 (0.12)	0.10 (0.12)	0.10 (0.12)				
>180	0.09	0.09 (0.11)	0.10 (0.11)					

*From Park MK, Guntheroth WG: *How to Read Pediatric ECGs*, ed 2. Chicago, Year Book Medical Publishers, 1987. Used by permission.

TABLE 3–3.

QRS Duration: Average (and Upper Limits) for Age*

	0–1 mo	1–6 mo	6 mo–1 yr	1–3 yr	3–8 yr	8–12 yr	12–16 yr	Adult
Seconds	0.05 (0.07)	0.05 (0.07)	0.05 (0.07)	0.06 (0.07)	0.07 (0.08)	0.07 (0.09)	0.07 (0.10)	0.08 (0.10)

*Modified from Guntheroth WG: *Pediatric Electrocardiography*. Philadelphia, WB Saunders Co, 1965. Used by permission.

According to Bazett's formula, the QTc should not exceed 0.425 second, except in infants. A QTc up to 0.49 second may be normal for the first 6 months of age. Table 3–4 gives averages and upper normal limits of the QT interval.

Long QT intervals may be seen in hypocalcemia, myocarditis, diffuse myocardial diseases, long QT syndrome (Jervell and Lange-Nielsen syndrome and Romano-Ward syndrome), head injury, etc. A short QT interval is a sign of digitalis effect or of hypercalcemia.

E. P Wave Duration and Amplitude

The P wave duration and amplitude are important in the diagnosis of atrial hypertrophy. Normally, the P amplitude is less than 3 mm. The duration of P waves is shorter than 0.09 second in children and shorter than 0.07 second in infants (see Criteria for Atrial Hypertrophy below).

F. The QRS Amplitude, R/S Ratio, and Abnormal Q Waves

The QRS amplitude and R/S ratio are important in diagnosis of ventricular hypertrophy. These values also vary with age (Tables 3–5 and 3–6). Because of normal dominance of RV forces in infants, R waves are taller over the RPLs (V4R, V1, and V2) and S waves are deeper in the LPLs (V5 and V6) in infants and young children. Therefore, the R/S ratio is large in the RPLs and is small in the LPLs in infants and small children.

Abnormal Q waves may manifest themselves as deep and/or wide Q waves or abnormal leads in which they appear. Deep Q waves may be present in ventricular hypertrophy of "volume overload" type, and deep and wide Q waves are seen in myocardial infarction. The presence of Q waves in the RPLs (severe RVH or ventricular inversion) and/or absence of Q waves in the LPLs (LBBB or ventricular inversion) are abnormal. Normal mean Q voltages and upper limits are presented in Table 3–7. The average Q wave duration is 0.02 second and does not exceed 0.03 second.

G. ST Segment and T Waves

The normal ST segment is isoelectric. However, in the limb leads, elevation or depression of the ST segment up to 1 mm is not necessarily abnormal in infants and children. A shift of up to 2 mm is considered normal in the precordial leads.

TABLE 3–4.
Cycle Length, Heart Rate, and QT Interval Average (and Upper Limits)*

Cycle Length (sec)	Heart Rate (per min)	QT Interval (sec)	Cycle Length (sec)	Heart Rate (per min)	QT Interval (sec)
1.50	40	0.45 (0.49)	0.85	70	0.36 (0.38)
1.40	43	0.44 (0.48)	0.80	75	0.35 (0.38)
1.30	46	0.43 (0.47)	0.75	80	0.34 (0.37)
1.25	48	0.42 (0.46)	0.70	86	0.33 (0.36)
1.20	50	0.41 (0.45)	0.65	92	0.32 (0.35)
1.15	52	0.41 (0.45)	0.60	100	0.31 (0.34)
1.10	55	0.40 (0.44)	0.55	109	0.30 (0.33)
1.05	57	0.39 (0.43)	0.50	120	0.28 (0.31)
1.00	60	0.39 (0.42)	0.45	133	0.27 (0.29)
0.95	63	0.38 (0.41)	0.40	150	0.25 (0.28)
0.90	67	0.37 (0.40)	0.35	172	0.23 (0.26)

*From Guntheroth WG: *Pediatric Electrocardiography*. Philadelphia, WB Saunders Co, 1965. Used by permission.

TABLE 3–5.

R and S Voltages According to Lead and Age: Mean (and Upper Limits)*

	Lead	0–1 mo	1–6 mo	6 mo–1 yr	1–3 yr	3–8 yr	8–12 yr	12–16 yr	Young Adults
R voltage†	I	4 (8)	7 (13)	8 (16)	8 (16)	7 (15)	7 (15)	6 (13)	6 (13)
	II	6 (14)	13 (24)	13 (27)	13 (23)	13 (22)	14 (24)	14 (24)	9 (25)
	III	8 (16)	9 (20)	9 (20)	9 (20)	9 (20)	9 (24)	9 (24)	6 (22)
	aVR	3 (7)	3 (6)	3 (6)	2 (6)	2 (5)	2 (4)	2 (4)	1 (4)
	aVL	2 (7)	4 (8)	5 (10)	5 (10)	3 (10)	3 (10)	3 (12)	3 (9)
	aVF	7 (14)	10 (20)	10 (16)	8 (20)	10 (19)	10 (20)	11 (21)	5 (23)
	V4R	6 (12)	5 (10)	4 (8)	4 (8)	3 (8)	3 (7)	3 (7)	
	V1	15 (25)	11 (20)	10 (20)	9 (18)	7 (18)	6 (16)	5 (16)	3 (14)
	V2	21 (30)	21 (30)	19 (28)	16 (25)	13 (28)	10 (22)	9 (19)	6 (21)
	V5	12 (30)	17 (30)	18 (30)	19 (36)	21 (36)	22 (36)	18 (33)	12 (33)
	V6	6 (21)	10 (20)	13 (20)	12 (24)	14 (24)	14 (24)	14 (22)	10 (21)
S voltage†	I	5 (10)	4 (9)	4 (9)	3 (8)	2 (8)	2 (8)	2 (8)	1 (6)
	V4R	4 (9)	4 (12)	5 (12)	5 (12)	5 (14)	6 (20)	6 (20)	
	V1	10 (20)	7 (18)	8 (16)	13 (27)	14 (30)	16 (26)	15 (24)	10 (23)
	V2	20 (35)	16 (30)	17 (30)	21 (34)	23 (38)	23 (38)	23 (48)	14 (36)
	V5	9 (30)	9 (26)	8 (20)	6 (16)	5 (14)	5 (17)	5 (16)	
	V6	4 (12)	2 (6)	2 (4)	2 (4)	1 (4)	1 (4)	1 (5)	1 (13)

*From Park MK, Guntheroth WG: *How to Read Pediatric ECGs*, ed 2, Chicago, Year Book Medical Publishers, 1987. Used by permission.
†Voltages are measured in millimeters, when 1 mV = 10 mm paper.

TABLE 3–6.

R/S Ratio According to Age: Mean, Lower, and Upper Limits of Normal*

	Lead	0–1 mo	1–6 mo	6 mo–1 yr	1–3 yr	3–8 yr	8–12 yr	12–16 yr	Adult
V1	LLN†	0.5	0.3	0.3	0.5	0.1	0.15	0.1	0.0
	Mean	1.5	1.5	1.2	0.8	0.65	0.5	0.3	0.3
	ULN‡	19	S = 0	6	2	2	1	1	1
V2	LLN	0.3	0.3	0.3	0.3	0.05	0.1	0.1	0.1
	Mean	1	1.2	1	0.8	0.5	0.5	0.5	0.2
	ULN	3	4	4	1.5	1.5	1.2	1.2	2.5
V6	LLN	0.1	1.5	2	3	2.5	4	2.5	2.5
	Mean	2	4	6	20	20	20	10	9
	ULN	S = 0	S = 0	S = 0	S = 0	S = 0	S = 0	S = 0	S = 0

*From Guntheroth WB: *Pediatric Electrocardiography*. Philadelphia, WB Saunders Co, 1965. Used by permission.
†Lower limits of normal.
‡Upper limits of normal.

Abnormal shift of ST segment occurs in pericarditis, myocardial ischemia or infarction, digitalis effect, etc. (see also chap. 24). Associated T wave changes are commonly present.

Tall peaked T waves may be seen in hyperkalemia and LVH ("volume overload"). Flat or low T waves may occur in normal newborns or with hypothyroidism, hypokalemia, pericarditis, myocarditis, myocardial ischemia, etc.

TABLE 3–7.

Q Voltages According to Lead and Age: Mean (and Upper Limits)*

Lead†	0–1 mo	1–6 mo	6 mo–1 yr	1–3 yr	3–8 yr	8–12 yr	12–16 yr	Adult
III	2 (5)	3 (8)	3 (8)	3 (8)	1.5 (6)	1 (5)	1 (4)	0.5 (4)
aVF	2 (4)	2 (5)	2 (6)	1.5 (5)	1 (5)	1 (3)	1 (3)	0.5 (2)
V5	1.5 (5)	1.5 (4)	2 (5)	2 (6)	2 (6)	2 (4.5)	1 (4)	0.5 (3.5)
V6	1.5 (4)	1.5 (4)	2 (5)	2 (4.5)	1.5 (4.5)	1.5 (4)	1 (2.5)	0.5 (3)

*From Guntheroth WG: *Pediatric Electrocardiography.* Philadelphia, WB Saunders Co, 1965. Used by permission.
†Voltages measured in millimeters, when 1 mV = 10 mm paper.

III. ATRIAL HYPERTROPHY

A. Right atrial hypertrophy (RAH)
Tall P waves (greater than 3 mm) are an indication of right atrial hypertrophy ("p-pulmonale") (Fig 3–12).

B. Left atrial hypertrophy (LAH)
Wide P wave duration (greater than 0.10 second in children and 0.08 second in infants) is seen in left atrial hypertrophy ("p-mitrale") (see Fig 3–12).

C. Combined atrial hypertrophy (CAH)
In combined atrial hypertrophy, a combination of an increase in amplitude and duration of the P waves is present. (see Fig 3–12).

IV. VENTRICULAR HYPERTROPHY

Ventricular hypertrophy produces abnormalities in one or more of the following areas: the QRS axis, the QRS voltages, the R/S ratio, the T axis, and miscellaneous areas.

a. Changes in the QRS Axis
The QRS axis is usually directed toward the ventricle that is hypertrophied. Although RAD is present with RVH, marked LAD is rare with LVH and is

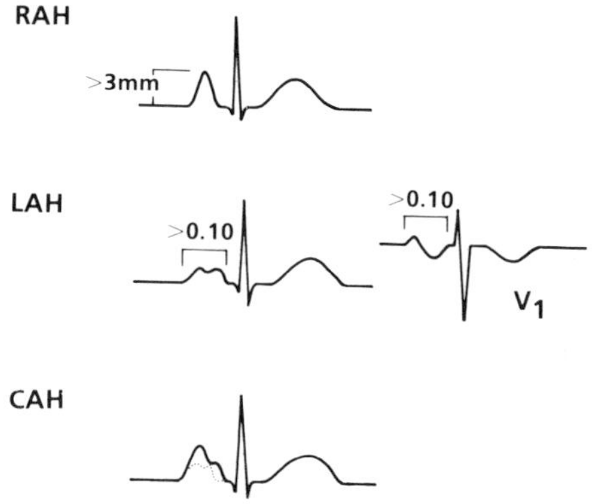

FIG 3–12.
Criteria for atrial hypertrophy. (From Park MK, Guntheroth WG: *How to Read Pediatric ECGs,* ed 2. Chicago, Year Book Medical Publishers, 1987. Used by permission.)

usually indicative of ventricular conduction disturbances (left anterior hemiblock or "superior" QRS axis).

b. Changes in QRS Voltages

Anatomically, the RV occupies the right and anterior aspect, and the LV the left and posterior aspect of the ventricular mass. With ventricular hypertrophy, there is an increase in the voltage of the QRS complex toward the direction of the respective ventricle.

In the frontal plane (Fig 3–13,A), LVH will show increased R voltages in leads I, II, aVL, aVF, and sometimes III, especially in small infants. RVH will show increased R voltages in aVR and III and increased S voltages in lead I (see Table 3–5 for normal QRS voltages).

In the horizontal plane (Fig 3–13,B), tall R waves in V4R, V1, and V2 or deep S waves in V5 and V6 are seen in RVH. With LVH, tall R waves in V5 and V6 and/or deep S waves in V4R, V1, and V2 are present (see Table 3–5).

c. Changes in R/S Ratio

An increase in the R/S ratio in the RPLs suggests RVH and a decrease in the R/S ratio in these leads suggests LVH. By the same token, an increase in the R/S ratio in the LPLs suggests LVH and a decrease in the ratio suggests RVH (see Table 3–6).

d. Changes in the T Axis

Changes in the T axis are seen in severe ventricular hypertrophy with relative ischemia of the hypertrophied myocardium. In the presence of other criteria of ventricular hypertrophy, a wide QRS-T angle (90° or greater) with the T axis outside the normal range indicates "strain" pattern. When the T axis remains in the normal quadrant (0° to +90°), a wide QRS-T angle alone indicates a *possible* "strain" pattern.

e. Miscellaneous Nonspecific Changes

RVH: (a) A true q wave in V1 (either qR or qRs) is suggestive of RVH. (Make sure it is not an rsR' with a very small or isoelectric r wave, giving an erroneous appearance of qR pattern.)

(b) An upright T wave in V1 after 3 days of age is a sign of probable RVH.

LVH: Deep Q waves (5 mm or greater) and/or tall T waves in V5 and V6 are said to be signs of LVH of "volume overload" type.

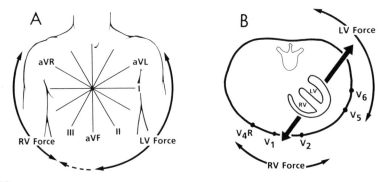

FIG 3–13.
Diagrammatic representation of left and right ventricular forces on the frontal projection or hexaxial reference system **(A)** and the horizontal plane **(B)**. (From Park MK, Guntheroth WG: *How to Read Pediatric ECGs,* ed 2. Chicago, Year Book Medical Publishers, 1987. Used by permission.)

A. Criteria for Right Ventricular Hypertrophy (RVH)

1. RAD for the patient's age (see Table 3–1).

2. Increased rightward and anterior QRS voltages.

   a. R in V1, V2, or aVR greater than the ULN for the patient's age (see Table 3–5).

   b. S in I and V6 greater than the ULN for the patient's age (see Table 3–5).

3. Abnormal R/S ratio in favor of the RV (in the absence of BBB) (see Table 3–6).

   a. R/S ratio in V1 and V2 greater than the ULN for age.

   b. R/S ratio in V6 less than 1 after one month of age.

4. Upright T in V1 in patients more than 3 days of age, provided that the T is upright in the LPLs (V5, V6). Upright T in V1 is not abnormal in patients 6 years or older.

5. A q wave in V1 (qR or qRs patterns) is suggestive of RVH (make sure that there is not a small r in an rsR' configuration).

6. In the presence of RVH, a wide QRS-T angle with T axis outside the normal range, usually in the 0° to −90° quadrant, indicates "strain" pattern.

In general, the greater the number of positive, independent criteria, the greater the probability of an abnormal degree of RVH.

Figure 3–14 is an example of RVH. There is RAD for the patient's age (+150°). The T axis is −10°, and the QRS-T angle is abnormally wide (160°) with the T axis in an abnormal quadrant. The R waves in III and aVR and the S waves in I and V6 are beyond the ULN, indicating abnormal rightward force. The R/S ratio in V1 and V2 is larger than the ULN, and the ratio in V6 is smaller than the LLN, again indicating RVH. This tracing, therefore, shows RVH with "strain."

Right Ventricular Hypertrophy in the Newborn:

The diagnosis of RVH in newborn infants is particularly difficult because of the normal dominance of the RV during that period of life. The following clues, however, are helpful in the diagnosis of RVH in newborn infants.

a. Pure R wave (with no S wave) in V1 greater than 10 mm.

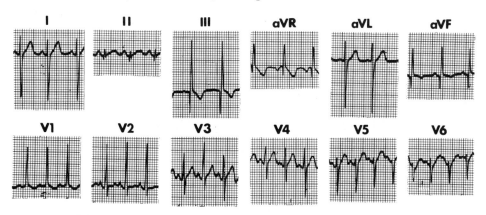

FIG 3–14.
Tracing from a 10-month-old infant with severe tetralogy of Fallot.

    b. R in V1 greater than 25 mm, or R in aVR greater than 8 mm.

    c. A qR pattern in V1 (also seen in 10% of healthy newborn infants).

    d. Upright T in V1 in neonates more than 3 days of age (with upright T in V6) is strongly suggestive of RVH.

    e. RAD greater than +180°.

B. Criteria for Left Ventricular Hypertrophy (LVH)

    1. LAD for the patient's age (see Table 3–1).

    2. QRS voltages in favor of the LV:

        a. R in I, II, III, aVL, aVF, V5, or V6 greater than the ULN for age (see Table 3–5).

        b. S in V1 or V2 greater than the ULN for age (see Table 3–5).

    3. Abnormal R/S ratio in favor of the LV: R/S ratio in V1 and V2 less than the LLN for the patient's age (see Table 3–6).

    4. Q in V5 and V6, 5 mm or more, coupled with tall symmetric T waves in the same leads ("LV diastolic overload").

    5. In the presence of LVH, a wide QRS-T angle with the T axis outside the normal range indicates "strain" pattern. This is manifested by flat or inverted T waves in lead I or aVF.

    The greater the number of positive, independent criteria, the greater the probability of an abnormal degree of LVH.

    Figure 3–15 is an example of LVH. There is LAD for the patient's age (0 degrees). The R waves in I, aVL, V5, and V6 are beyond the ULN, indicating abnormal LV force. The T vector (+55°) remains in the normal quadrant. This tracing shows LVH (without "strain").

C. Criteria for Combined Ventricular Hypertrophy (CVH)

    1. Positive voltage criteria for right *and* left ventricular hypertrophy (in the absence of BBB or preexcitation).

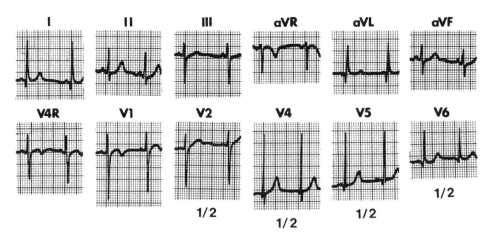

FIG 3–15.
Tracing from a 4-year-old child with moderate VSD. Note that some precordial leads are in ½ normal standardization.

2. Positive voltage criteria for RVH or LVH and relatively large voltages for the other ventricle.

3. Large equiphasic QRS complexes in two or more of the limb leads and in the midprecordial leads (V2 through V5), called Katz-Wachtel phenomenon.

Figure 3–16 is an example of CVH. It is difficult to plot the QRS axis because of large diphasic QRS complexes in limb leads and in the LPLs (Katz-Wachtel phenomenon). The S waves in I and V6 are abnormally deep (abnormal rightward force) and the R in V1 (rightward and anterior force) is also abnormally large, suggesting RVH. The R waves in leads I and aVL (leftward force) are also abnormally large. Therefore, this tracing shows CVH.

V. VENTRICULAR CONDUCTION DISTURBANCES

Conditions that are grouped together as ventricular conduction disturbances have in common abnormal prolongation of QRS duration. Ventricular conduction disturbances include:

a. Bundle branch blocks, right and left.

b. Preexcitation (WPW syndrome).

c. Intraventricular block.

d. Ventricular rhythms, including artificial ventricular pacemaker, ventricular tachycardia, and ventricular premature beats.

In bundle branch blocks and ventricular rhythms, the prolongation is in the terminal portion of the QRS complex ("terminal slurring"). In the preexcitation, the prolongation is in the initial portion of the QRS complex ("initial slurring"), producing "delta" waves. In intraventricular block, the prolongation is throughout the duration of the QRS complex (Fig 3–17). Note that the QRS duration varies with age; it is shorter in infants than in older children or adults (see Table 3–3). In adults, a QRS duration greater than 0.10 second is required for diagnosis of a bundle branch block (or ventricular conduction disturbances), but in infants, a QRS duration of 0.08 second meets the requirement for a BBB.

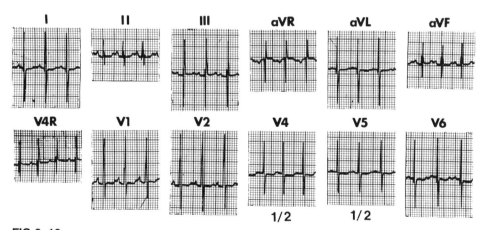

FIG 3–16.
Tracing from a 2-month-old infant with large-shunt VSD, PDA, and severe pulmonary hypertension.

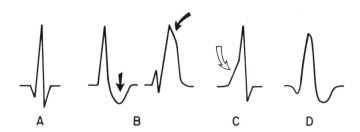

FIG 3–17.
Schematic diagram of three types of ventricular conduction disturbances. **A,** normal QRS complexes. **B,** QRS complex in RBBB or premature ventricular contractions with prolongation of the QRS duration in the terminal portion (terminal slurring; *black arrows*). **C,** a preexcitation with delta wave (initial slurring, *open arrow*). **D,** intraventricular block in which the prolongation of the QRS complex is throughout the duration of the QRS complex.

By far the most commonly encountered form of ventricular conduction disturbance is RBBB (see below for detailed discussion). Although uncommon, the WPW syndrome is a well-defined entity deserving a brief description. LBBB is extremely rare in children, although common in adults with ischemic and hypertensive heart disease. Intraventricular block is associated with metabolic disorders and diffuse myocardial diseases.

A. Right Bundle Branch Block (RBBB)

In RBBB, delayed conduction through the right bundle branch prolongs the time required for a depolarization of the RV. When the LV is completely depolarized, RV depolarization is still in progress. This produces prolongation of the QRS duration, more specifically the terminal portion of the QRS complex ("terminal slurring") (Fig 3–17,B). The terminal slurring of the QRS complex is directed to the *right* and *anteriorly*, because the RV is located rightward and anteriorly in relation to the LV.

Criteria for Right Bundle Branch Block:

a. RAD, at least for terminal portion of QRS complex.

b. QRS duration longer than the ULN for the patient's age (see Table 3–3).

c. Terminal slurring of the QRS complex directed to the right and usually, but not always, anteriorly:

  1) Wide and slurred S in I, V5, and V6

  2) Terminal, slurred R′ in aVR and the RPLs (V4R, V1, and V2)

d. ST segment shift and T wave inversion are common in adults but not in children.

Because there is asynchrony of the opposing electromotive forces of each ventricle in RBBB, a greater manifest potential for both ventricles results, making it unsafe to make a diagnosis of ventricular hypertrophy in the presence of RBBB. This also applies to LBBB and the WPW syndrome.

Figure 3–18 is an example of RBBB. The terminal QRS axis is in the right upper quadrant (about −160°). The QRS duration is increased (0.11 second), indicating a ventricular conduction disturbance. There is slurring of the terminal portion of the QRS complex (indicating a BBB), and the slurring is directed to

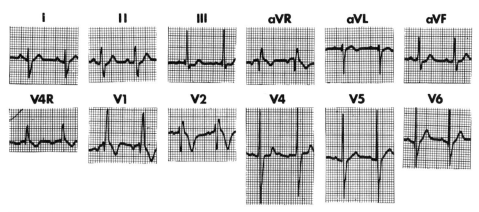

FIG 3–18.
Tracing from a 6-year-old boy who had corrective surgery for tetralogy of Fallot that involved right ventriculotomy for repair of VSD and resection of infundibular narrowing.

the right (slurred S in I and V6, and slurred R in aVR) and anteriorly (slurred R in V4R and V1), satisfying criteria for RBBB. Although the S waves in I, V5 and V6 are abnormally deep and the R/S ratio in V1 is abnormally large, one cannot interpret it as RVH in the presence of RBBB.

Two most common pediatric conditions that present with RBBB are atrial septal defect and conduction disturbances following open heart surgery involving ventriculotomy. Other conditions that are often associated with RBBB include Ebstein's anomaly, coarctation of the aorta in infants less than 6 months of age, endocardial cushion defect, partial anomalous pulmonary venous return, and occasional normal children. The significance of RBBB in children is different from that in adults. In several pediatric examples of RBBB, the right bundle is intact. In ASD, the longer QRS duration is due to a longer pathway through a dilated RV. Right ventriculotomy for repair of VSD or tetralogy of Fallot disrupts the right ventricular subendocardial Purkinje network and causes prolongation of the QRS duration, without necessarily injuring the main right bundle, although the latter may occasionally also be disrupted.

Some pediatricians are concerned with the rsR′ pattern in V1. Although it is unusual to see this in adults, the rsR′ pattern in V1 is *normal* in infants and small children provided that:

a. The QRS duration is not prolonged, and

b. The voltage of the primary or secondary R waves is not abnormally large.

The reason why the rsR′ pattern may be seen in healthy children is that the terminal QRS vector is more rightward and anterior in infants and children than it is in adults.

B. Intraventricular Block
In this condition, the prolongation is throughout the duration of the QRS complex (see Fig 3–17,D). It is associated with metabolic disorders (hyperkalemia), myocardial ischemia as seen during cardiopulmonary resuscitation, quinidine or procainamide toxicity, and diffuse myocardial diseases (myocardial fibrosis, systemic diseases with myocardial involvement).

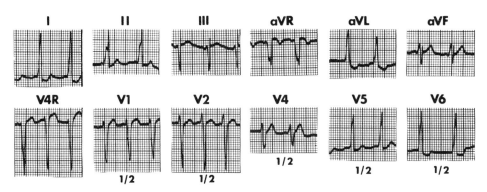

FIG 3–19.
Tracing from a 6-month-old infant with possible glycogen storage disease.

C. Wolff-Parkinson-White syndrome

The WPW syndrome is a form of preexcitation. It results from an anomalous conduction pathway (bundle of Kent) between the atrium and the ventricle, bypassing the normal delay of conduction in the AV node. The premature depolarization of a ventricle produces a delta wave and results in prolongation of the QRS duration (Fig 3–17,C).

Criteria for Wolff-Parkinson-White syndrome:

a. Short PR interval, less than the LLN for the patient's age.
Lower limit of normal PR interval:

Less than 3 years	0.08 second
3–16 years	0.10 second
More than 16 years	0.12 second

b. Delta wave (initial slurring of the QRS complex).

c. Wide QRS duration (beyond the ULN).

Patients with WPW syndrome are prone to attacks of paroxysmal supraventricular tachycardia (see chap. 23). The WPW syndrome may mimic other ECG abnormalities such as ventricular hypertrophy, RBBB, or myocardial disorders. In the presence of this syndrome, diagnosis of ventricular hypertrophy cannot be made safely. There are two other forms of preexcitation:

1. Lown-Ganong-Levine (LGL) syndrome is characterized by short PR and normal QRS duration. In this condition, James fibers bypass the upper AV node, producing a short PR interval, but the ventricles are depolarized normally through the His-Purkinje system.

2. Mahaim-type preexcitation syndrome is characterized by normal PR interval and long QRS duration with delta wave. There is an abnormal Mahaim fiber between the His bundle and one of the ventricles producing delta waves.

Figure 3–19 is an example of WPW syndrome. The QRS duration is increased to 0.10 second (ULN = 0.07). The PR interval is short (0.07 second). There are delta waves in the initial portion of the QRS complexes, best seen in I, aVL, and V5. The leftward and posterior QRS voltages are abnormally large, but the diagnosis of LVH cannot be made in the presence of the WPW syndrome.

4 / Chest Roentgenography

The chest roentgenogram is an essential part of cardiac evaluation. Information to be gained from x-ray films is: (1) heart size and silhouette, (2) enlargement of specific cardiac chambers, (3) pulmonary blood flow (PBF) or pulmonary vascular markings (PVM), and (4) other information regarding lung parenchyma, spine, bony thorax, abdominal situs, etc. Posteroanterior (PA) and lateral views are routinely obtained in most institutions. Special cardiac views (PA, lateral, right anterior oblique, and left anterior oblique views) with barium swallow (barium esophagogram) are seldom indicated in initial evaluation of infants and children.

I. HEART SIZE AND SILHOUETTE

A. Heart Size

Measurement of the cardiothoracic ratio (CT ratio) is, by far, the simplest way to estimate the heart size (Fig 4–1) in older children. The CT ratio is obtained by relating the largest transverse diameter of the heart to the widest internal diameter of the chest:

$$CT\ ratio = (A + B)/C$$

where A and B are maximal cardiac dimensions to the right and to the left of the midline, respectively, and C is the widest internal diameter of the chest. A CT ratio of more than 0.5 is considered to indicate cardiomegaly. However, the CT ratio cannot be used with any accuracy in newborns and small infants, in whom a good inspiratory chest film is rarely obtained. Therefore, estimation of the cardiac volume from the PA and lateral views is as valid as the CT ratio in this situation.

In determining the presence or absence of cardiomegaly, the lateral view of the heart should also be taken into consideration. For example, an isolated RV enlargement may not be obvious on a PA film, but will be on a lateral film. In a patient with a flat chest (or narrow anteroposterior diameter of the chest), a PA film may erroneously show cardiomegaly.

Remember that an enlarged heart on chest x-rays more reliably reflects a volume overload than a pressure overload; the pressure overload is better represented in the ECG.

B. Normal Cardiac Silhouette

The structures that form the cardiac borders in the PA projection of a chest roentgenogram are as follows. The right cardiac silhouette is formed by the superior vena cava (SVC) superiorly and by the right atrium (RA) inferiorly. The left cardiac border is formed from the top to the bottom by the aortic knob, the main pulmonary artery (MPA), and the left ventricle (LV). The left atrial appendage (LAA) is located between the MPA and the LV and is *not* prominent in a normal heart. The right ventricle (RV) does not form the cardiac border in the PA view. The lateral projection of the cardiac silhouette is formed anteriorly

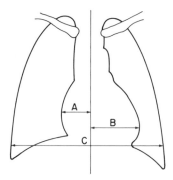

FIG 4–1.
Diagram showing how to measure the cardiothoracic ratio (CT ratio) from the PA view of a chest x-ray film. The CT ratio is obtained by dividing the largest horizontal diameter of the heart *A + B)* by the longest internal diameter of the chest *(C).*

by the RV and posteriorly by the left atrium (LA) above and the LV below. Note that, in a normal heart, the lower posterior cardiac border (LV) crosses the inferior vena cava (IVC) line above the diaphragm (Fig 4–2).

In the newborn, however, a typical normal cardiac silhouette as shown in Figure 4–2 is rarely seen because of the presence of a large thymus and because the films are often exposed during expiration. The thymus is situated in the superior-anterior mediastinum. Therefore, the base of the heart may be widened, with resulting alteration in the normal silhouette in the PA view. In the lateral view, the retrosternal space, which is normally clear in older children, may be obliterated by the large thymus.

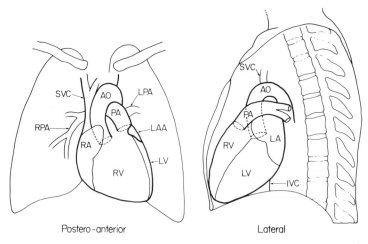

Postero-anterior   Lateral

FIG 4–2.
Posteroanterior and lateral projections of normal cardiac silhouette. Note that in the lateral projection, the RV is contiguous with the lower third of the sternum and that the LV normally crosses the posterior margin of the inferior vena cava above the diaphragm. AO = aorta; IVC = inferior vena cava; LA = left atrium; LAA = left atrial appendage; LV = left ventricle; PA = pulmonary artery; LPA and RPA = left and right pulmonary arteries; RA = right atrium; RV = right ventricle; SVC = superior vena cava.

C. Abnormal Cardiac Silhouette

Although discerning individual chamber enlargement is often helpful in determining acyanotic heart defect, the overall shape of the heart sometimes provides important clues to the type of defect, particularly in dealing with cyanotic infants and children. A few examples are presented below with the status of pulmonary blood flow (PBF).

a. "Boot-shaped" heart with decreased PBF is a typical shape of the heart in infants with cyanotic tetralogy of Fallot (TOF). This is also seen in some infants with tricuspid atresia. Typical of both conditions is the presence of hypoplastic MPA segment (Fig 4–3,A). The ECGs are helpful in differentiating these two conditions: the ECG shows RAD, RVH, and occasional RAH in TOF, while it shows "superior" QRS axis (left anterior hemiblock), RAH, and LVH in tricuspid atresia.

b. Narrow waist and "egg-shaped" heart with increased PBF in a cyanotic infant is strongly suggestive of transposition of the great arteries (TGA). The narrow waist is due to the absence of a large thymus and to the abnormal relationship of the great arteries (Fig 4–3,B).

c. "Snowman" sign with increased PBF is seen in infants with the supracardiac type of total anomalous pulmonary venous return (TAPVR). The head of the "snowman" is made up of the vertical vein (left superior vena cava), the left innominate vein, and the dilated SVC (Fig 4–3,C).

II. EVALUATION OF CARDIAC CHAMBERS AND GREAT ARTERIES

A. Individual Chamber Enlargement

Identification of individual chamber enlargement is important in deriving a diagnosis of a specific lesion, particularly in dealing with acynotic heart defects. Although enlargment of a single chamber is discussed here, in a real situation, more than one chamber is usually involved.

a. Left Atrial Enlargement.—An enlarged LA causes alterations not only of the cardiac silhouette, but also of the various adjacent structures (Fig 4–4). (1) Mild LA enlargement can be best appreciated in the lateral projection by the posterior protrusion of the LA border. (2) An enlargement of the LA may

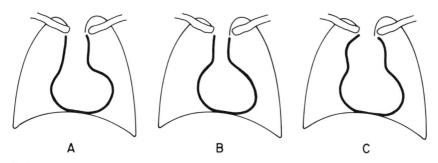

A   B   C

FIG 4–3.
Abnormal cardiac silhouette. **(A),** "Boot-shaped" heart seen in cyanotic tetralogy of Fallot or tricuspid atresia. **(B),** "egg-shaped" heart seen in transposition of the great arteries, and **(C),** "snowman" sign seen in total anomalous pulmonary venous return (supracardiac type).

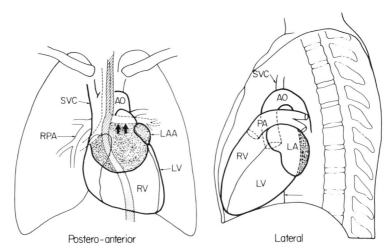

FIG 4–4.
Schematic diagram showing roentgenographic findings of LA enlargement in the PA and lateral projections. *Arrows* show left main-stem bronchus elevation. The isolated enlargement of the LA shown here is only hypothetical, since it usually accompanies other changes. Abbreviations are the same as in Figure 4–2.

produce "double density" on the PA view. (3) With further enlargement, the left atrial appendage (LAA) becomes prominent on the left cardiac border. (4) The left main-stem bronchus is elevated. (5) The barium-filled esophagus is indented to the right.

    b. Left Ventricular Enlargement.—(1) In the PA view, the apex of the heart is not only farther to the left but it is also downward. (2) In the lateral view, the lower posterior cardiac border is displaced further posteriorly, and it meets the IVC line below the diaphragm level (Fig 4–5).

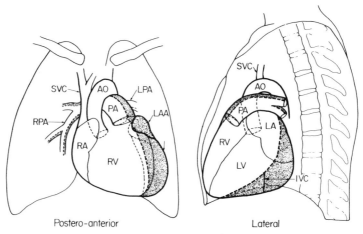

FIG 4–5.
Diagrammatic representation of VSD, which demonstrates LV enlargement in addition to the enlargement of the LA and a prominent MPA segment. Abbreviations are the same as those in Figure 4–2.

   c. **Right Atrial Enlargement.**—The RA enlargement is most obvious in the PA projection as an increased prominence of the right lower cardiac silhouette (Fig 4–6). This is, however, not an absolute finding, as both false positive and false negative results are possible.

   d. **Right Ventricular Enlargement.**—An isolated RV enlargement may not be obvious in the PA projection, and the normal CT ratio may be maintained, since the RV does not make up the cardiac silhouette in the PA projection. The RV enlargement is best appreciated in the lateral view, by the filling of the retrosternal space (Fig 4–6).

B. **The Size of the Great Arteries**
   As in the enlargement of specific cardiac chambers, the size of the great arteries is often helpful in making a specific diagnosis.

   a. **Prominent MPA Segment:** Prominence of a normally placed pulmonary artery in the PA view (Fig 4–7,A) is due to one of the following:

   1) Poststenotic dilatation (pulmonary valve stenosis).

   2) Increased blood flow through the PA (ASD, VSD).

   3) Increased pressure in the PA (pulmonary hypertension).

   4) Occasional normal adolescence, especially in girls.

   b. **Hypoplasia of the PA:** A concave MPA segment with resulting "boot-shaped" heart is seen in (1) tetralogy of Fallot and (2) tricuspid atresia (Fig 4–7,B). Obviously, malposition of the PA must be ruled out.

   c. **Dilatation of the aorta.** An enlarged ascending aorta may be observed in the frontal projection as a rightward bulge of the right upper mediastinum, but a mild degree of enlargement may easily escape detection. Aortic enlargement is seen in tetralogy of Fallot and aortic stenosis (poststenotic dilatation) and less often in PDA, COA, or systemic hypertension. When the ascending aorta and aortic arch are enlarged, the aortic knob may become prominent on the PA view (Fig 4–7,C).

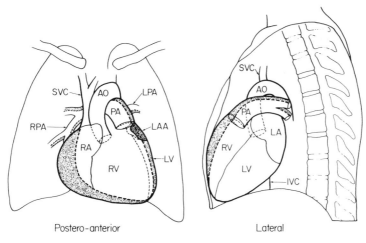

Postero-anterior   Lateral

FIG 4–6.
Schematic diagrams of PA and lateral chest roentgenograms of ASD. Enlargement of the RA and RV and an increased pulmonary vascularity. Abbreviations are the same as those in Figure 4–2.

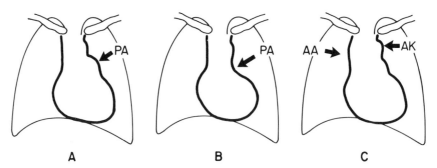

FIG 4–7.
Abnormalities of the great arteries. **A,** prominent main pulmonary artery *(PA)* segment. **B,** concave pulmonary artery segment *(PA)* due to hypoplasia. **C,** dilatation of the aorta may be seen as a bulge on the right upper mediastinum by a dilated ascending aorta *(AA)* or as a prominence of the aortic knob *(AK)* on the left upper cardiac border.

III. PULMONARY VASCULAR MARKINGS (PVM)

One of the major goals of radiologic examination is the assessment of the pulmonary vasculature. Although many textbooks explain how to detect the increased PBF, this is one of the more difficult aspects of interpretation of chest x-rays of cardiac patients. Nothing can substitute for the experience gained by looking at many chest x-rays with normal and abnormal PBF.

A. Increased Pulmonary Blood Flow

Increased pulmonary vascularity is present when (a) the pulmonary arteries appear enlarged and extend into the lateral third of the lung field, where they are not usually present, (b) there is an increased vascularity to the lung apices where the vessels are normally collapsed, (c) the external diameter of the right pulmonary artery visible in the right hilus is wider than the internal diameter of the trachea.

An increased PBF in an acyanotic child represents either ASD, VSD, PDA, endocardial cushion defect (ECD), partial anomalous pulmonary venous return (PAPVR), or any combination of these. In a cyanotic infant, increased pulmonary vascular markings may indicate transposition of the great arteries (TGA), total anomalous pulmonary venous return (TAPVR), hypoplastic left heart syndrome, persistent truncus arteriosus, or single ventricle.

B. Decreased Pulmonary Blood Flow

A decreased PBF is suspected when the hilum appears small, the remaining lung fields appear black, and the vessels appear small and thin. Ischemic lung fields are seen in cyanotic heart diseases with decreased PBF such as critical stenosis or atresia of the pulmonary or tricuspid valves, including tetralogy of Fallot (TOF).

C. Pulmonary Venous Congestion

Pulmonary venous congestion is characterized by hazy and indistinct margin of the pulmonary vasculature. This is caused by pulmonary venous hypertension owing to left ventricular failure or obstruction to pulmonary venous drainage, such as hypoplastic left heart syndrome (HLHS), mitral stenosis, total anomalous pulmonary venous return (TAPVR), cor triatriatum, etc. Kerley's B lines are short, transverse strips of increased density best seen in the costophrenic

sulci. This is caused by engorged lymphatics and interstitial edema of the inter-
lobular septa secondary to pulmonary venous congestion.

D. Normal Pulmonary Vasculature
Pulmonary vascularity is normal in patients with obstructive lesions, such as PS
or AS. Unless the stenosis is extremely severe, pulmonary vascularity remains
normal in PS. Patients with small left-to-right shunt lesions also show normal
pulmonary vascular markings.

IV. SYSTEMATIC APPROACH

The interpretation of chest x-ray films should include a systematic routine to avoid
overlooking important anatomical changes relevant to cardiac diagnosis.

A. Location of the Liver and Stomach Gas Bubble
The cardiac apex should be on the same side as the stomach or opposite the
hepatic shadow. When there is heterotaxia, with the apex on the right and the
stomach on the left, or vice versa, the likelihood of serious heart defect is great.
An even more ominous situation exists with a "midline" liver, associated with
asplenia (Ivemark's) syndrome, or polysplenia syndrome (see Fig 25–1). These
infants usually have uncorrectable heart defects.

B. Skeletal Aspect of Chest X-ray Film
Pectus excavatum may flatten the heart in the anteroposterior dimension and
cause a compensatory increase in its transverse diameter, creating the false
impression of cardiomegaly. Thoracic scoliosis and vertebral abnormalities are
frequent findings in cardiac patients. Rib notching is a specific finding of coarctation of the aorta in the older child (usually older than 5 years) and is usually
found between the 4th and 8th ribs.

C. Identification of the Aorta
Identification of the descending aorta along the left margin of the spine usually
indicates a left aortic arch, and that along the right margin of the spine a right
aortic arch. When the descending aorta is not directly visible, the position of
the trachea (and esophagus) may help locate the descending aorta. If the trachea
(and esophagus) is located slightly to the right of the midline, the aorta usually
descends normally on the left (left aortic arch). In the right aortic arch, the
trachea and esophagus are shifted to the left. Right aortic arch is frequently
associated with tetralogy of Fallot or persistent truncus arteriosus. In a heavily
exposed film, the precoarctation and postcoarctation dilatation of the aorta may
be seen as a "figure of 3." This may be confirmed by barium esophagogram with
E-shaped indentation (Fig 4–8).

D. Upper Mediastinum
The thymus is prominent in healthy infants and may give a false impression of
cardiomegaly. It may give the classic "sail sign" (Fig 4–9). The thymus often
has a wavy border because this structure becomes indented by the ribs. On the
lateral view, the thymus occupies the superior anterior mediastinum, obscuring
the upper retrosternal space. In cyanotic infants or infants under severe stress
from CHF, the thymus shrinks. In transposition of the great arteries, the mediastinal shadow is narrow ("narrow waist"), partly due to the shrinkage of the
thymus gland. Infants with DiGeorge syndrome have absent thymic shadow and
a high incidence of aortic arch anomalies. "Snowman figure" (figure-of-eight
configuration) is seen in infants (usually older than 4 months) with anomalous

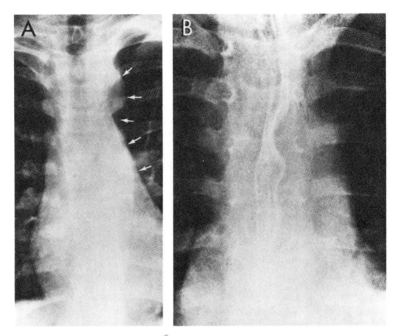

FIG 4–8.
A, the figure-of-3 configuration indicates the site of coarctation with the large proximal segment of aorta and/or prominent left subclavian artery above and the poststenotic dilatation of the descending aorta below it. **B,** barium esophagogram reveals the E-shaped indentation or reversed figure-of-3 configuration. (From Caffey J: *Pediatric X-Ray Diagnosis,* ed 7. Chicago, Year Book Medical Publishers, 1978. Used by permission.)

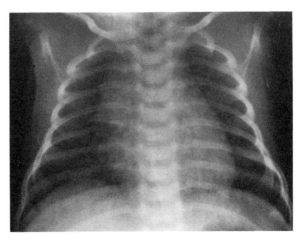

FIG 4–9.
A roentgenogram showing the typical "sail sign" on the right mediastinal border.

pulmonary venous return draining into the SVC via the left superior vena cava (vertical vein) and the left innominate vein (see Fig 4–3,C).

E. Pulmonary Parenchyma

Pneumonia is a common complication in patients with high pulmonary venous pressure, such as a large PDA or VSD. A long-standing density, particularly in the right lower lung field, suggests bronchopulmonary sequestration in which a segment of the lung is supplied directly by an artery from the descending aorta. A vertical vascular shadow along the right lower cardiac border may suggest partial anomalous pulmonary venous return from the lower lobe and sometimes from the middle lobe of the right lung (the scimitar syndrome). Bronchopulmonary sequestration is often associated with the scimitar syndrome.

5 / Flow Diagram

A flow diagram that often helps in arriving at a diagnosis of congenital heart disease is shown in Table 5–1. It is based on the presence or absence of cyanosis and the status of pulmonary blood flow (PBF), whether normal, increased, or decreased. Presence of either right or left ventricular hypertrophy or of both further narrows down the possibilities. Only common entities are listed in the flow diagram.

TABLE 5–1.

Flow Diagram of Congenital Heart Disease

Acyanotic defects	
Increased PBF	
LVH or CVH	Ventricular septal defect (VSD)
	Patent ductus arteriosus (PDA)
	Complete endocardial cushion defect (ECD)
RVH	Atrial septal defect (ASD) (often RBBB)
	Partial anomalous pulmonary venous return (PAPVR)
	Eisenmenger's physiology secondary to VSD, PDA, etc.
Normal PBF	
LVH	Aortic stenosis (AS) or aortic regurgitation (AR)
	Coarctation of the aorta (COA)
	Primary myocardial disease (endocardial fibroelastosis)
	Mitral regurgitation (MR)
RVH	Pulmonary stenosis (PS)
	COA in infants
	Mitral stenosis (MS)
Cyanotic defects	
Increased PBF	
LVH or CVH	Persistent truncus arteriosus
	Single ventricle (common ventricle)
	Transposition of the great arteries (TGA) plus VSD
RVH	TGA
	Total anomalous pulmonary venous return (TAPVR)
	Hypoplastic left heart syndrome (HLHS)
Decreased PBF	
CVH	TGA plus PS
	Persistent truncus arteriosus with hypoplastic PA
	Single ventricle with PS
LVH	Tricuspid atresia
	Pulmonary atresia with hypoplastic RV
RVH	Tetralogy of Fallot (TOF)
	Eisenmenger's physiology (secondary to ASD, VSD, PDA)
	Ebstein's anomaly (RBBB)

CVH = combined ventricular hypertrophy; LVH = left ventricular hypertrophy; PBF = pulmonary blood flow; RBBB = right bundle branch block; RVH = right ventricular hypertrophy.

In using this flow diagram, certain adjustments are often necessary. For example, in some instances in which pulmonary vascularity on chest x-rays may be interpreted as normal or at the upper limit of normal, one may need to check the list under both normal and increased PBF. Likewise, an ECG may show RV dominance but not meet strict criteria for RVH. Such a case may need to be treated as RVH. It should also be remembered that normal ECG and normal pulmonary vas-

TABLE 5–2.

Common ECG Manifestations of Some Congenital Heart Defects

Congenital Defects	ECG Findings
Anomalous origin of the left coronary artery from the pulmonary artery	Myocardial infarction, anterolateral
Anomalous pulmonary venous return	
Total	RAD, RVH, and RAH
Partial	Mild RVH or RBBB
Aortic stenosis	
Mild to moderate	Normal or LVH
Severe	LVH with or without "strain"
Atrial septal defect	
Primum type	Left anterior hemiblock (superior QRS axis) rsR′ pattern in V1 and aVR (RBBB or RVH) First-degree AV block (>50%) Counterclockwise QRS loop in the frontal plane of vectorcardiogram
Secundum type	RAD, RVH, or RBBB (rsR′ in V1 and aVR) First-degree AV block (10%)
Coarctation of the aorta	
Infants younger than 6 mo.	RBBB or RVH
Older children	LVH, normal, or RBBB

Common ventricle or single ventricle	Abnormal Q waves
	  Q in V1 and no Q in V6
	  No Q in any precordial leads
	  Q in all precordial leads
	Stereotype RS complex in most or all precordial leads
	WPW syndrome or PAT
	First- or second-degree AV block

Cor triatriatum	Same as for mitral stenosis
Ebstein's anomaly	RAH, RBBB First-degree AV block WPW syndrome No RVH
Endocardial cushion defect	
Complete	Left anterior hemiblock (superior QRS axis) RVH or CVH, RAH First-degree AV block, RBBB
Partial	See ASD, primum type

(Continued.)

TABLE 5–2. *(cont.)*.

Congenital Defects	ECG Findings
Endocardial fibroelastosis	LVH Abnormal T waves Myocardial infarction patterns
Hypoplastic left heart syndrome (aortic and/or mitral atresia)	RVH
Mitral stenosis, congenital or acquired	RAD, RVH, RAH, LAH (±)
Patent ductus arteriosus	
Small shunt	Normal
Moderate shunt	LVH, LAH (±)
Large shunt	CVH, LAH
Eisenmenger's syndrome (pulmonary vascular obstructive disease)	RVH or CVH
Persistent truncus arteriosus	LVH or CVH
Pulmonary atresia (with hypoplastic RV)	LVH
Pulmonary stenosis	
Mild	Normal or mild RVH
Moderate	RVH
Severe	RVH with "strain," RAH
Pulmonary vascular obstructive disease (Eisenmenger's syndrome)	RVH or CVH
Tetralogy of Fallot	RAD RVH, moderate or severe RAH (±)
D-Transposition of the great arteries (complete transposition)	
Intact ventricular septum	RVH, RAH
VSD and/or PS	CVH, RAH, or CAH
L-Transposition of the great arteries (congenitally "corrected" transposition)	AV block, first- to third-degree Atrial arrhythmias (PAT, atrial fibrillation) WPW syndrome Absent Q in V5 and V6 and qR pattern in V1 LAH or CAH
Tricuspid atresia	Left anterior hemiblock (superior QRS axis) LVH, RAH
Ventricular septal defect	
Small shunt	Normal
Moderate shunt	LVH, LAH (±)
Large shunt	CVH, LAH
Pulmonary vascular obstructive disease (Eisenmenger's syndrome)	RVH

cular markings on chest x-rays do not rule out CHD. In fact, many mild, acyanotic heart defects do not show abnormalities on the ECG or chest x-rays. Diagnosis of these defects rests primarily on findings from the physical examination, particularly on auscultation.

In addition to ventricular hypertrophy seen on ECGs, other ECG findings are occasionally helpful in making the diagnosis. For example, a superiorly oriented QRS axis (left anterior hemiblock) in an acyanotic infant suggests endocardial cushion defect, while in a cyanotic infant it suggests tricuspid atresia. Common ECG manifestations of some congenital heart diseases are summarized in Table 5–2.

Chest x-ray findings other than pulmonary vascular markings are also helpful in suspecting a certain type of CHD. A few examples are listed below (refer to chap. 4 for further discussion).

a. Heart size.

   1) A large heart indicates large shunt lesions or myocardial failure.

   2) A large heart almost always rules out tetralogy of Fallot (TOF).

b. Cardiac silhouette.

   1) "Boot-shaped" heart suggests TOF or tricuspid atresia.

   2) "Egg-shaped" heart with increased pulmonary vascularity suggests transposition of the great arteries.

   3) "Snowman" sign suggests anomalous pulmonary venous return.

c. Right aortic arch is commonly seen in TOF or persistent truncus arteriosus.

d. Midline liver strongly suggests complex cardiac defects associated with the asplenia or polysplenia syndrome.

PART II

Special Tools in Evaluation of Cardiac Patients

Some readers may want to skip this section at this time and come back later as the need arises. Special tools to be discussed in this section may be considered too specialized. Omission of this section will not affect the understanding of pathophysiology and most clinical aspects of pediatric cardiac problems.

A number of special tools are available to the cardiologist in the evaluation of cardiac patients. Some tools are readily available and frequently used in tertiary centers, while others are more specialized and infrequently used. Only those tests that noncardiologists have the opportunity to be exposed to will be briefly discussed. Echocardiography (M-mode, two-dimensional, and Doppler), exercise tolerance test (stress test), and ambulatory electrocardiography (Holter monitor) are noninvasive tests, while cardiac catheterization and angiocardiography are invasive. Although catheter intervention procedures are not diagnostic, they will be discussed in this section, as they are usually performed in conjunction with cardiac catheterization.

Several other tests are rarely performed or are too specialized and therefore will not be discussed. They are phonocardiography, vectorcardiography, electrophysiologic study, nuclear cardiology (radionuclide cineangiography, myocardial scintigraphy), and magnetic resonance imaging (MRI).

6 / Noninvasive Techniques of Cardiac Evaluation

I. ECHOCARDIOGRAPHY

Echocardiography (ECHO) is an extremely useful, safe, and noninvasive method for the diagnosis and management of heart disease. ECHO, which utilizes ultrasound, provides not only anatomical diagnosis but also functional information, especially with the incorporation of Doppler echocardiography.

The M-mode ECHO which provides an "ice-pick" view of the heart has limited capability in demonstrating the spatial relationship of structures, but remains an important tool in the evaluation of certain cardiac conditions and function, particularly for dimensions and timing. The two-dimensional (2D) ECHO (or cross-sectional ECHO) provides enhanced ability to demonstrate the spatial relationship of structures and, therefore, a more accurate anatomical diagnosis of abnormalities of the heart and great vessels. The Doppler study has added to the ECHO examination the ability to detect valve regurgitation and cardiac shunts and to provide some quantitative information such as pressure gradient across a valve, cardiac output, and shunt calculation. A discussion of instruments and techniques is beyond the scope of this book. Only a brief discussion of normal ECHO images and their role in diagnosis of common cardiac problems in pediatric patients will be presented.

I. M-Mode Echocardiography

An M-mode ECHO is obtained with the ultrasonic transducer placed along the left sternal border and directed toward the part of the heart to be examined. In Figure 6–1, the ultrasound is depicted as passing through three important structures of the left side of the heart. The line (1) passes through the aorta (AO) and left atrium (LA), where the dimension of these structures is measured. The line (2) transverses through the mitral valve. The line (3) goes through the main body of the right and left ventricles. Along the line (3) is where the dimensions of the right ventricle (RV) and left ventricle (LV) and thickness of the interventricular septum and posterior LV wall are measured. Pericardial effusion is also best detected at this level.

Although 2D ECHO has replaced many roles of the M-mode ECHO in the diagnosis of cardiac diseases, the M-mode ECHO still maintains many important applications, including:

a) Measurement of the dimensions of cardiac chambers and vessels, thickness of the ventricular septum and free walls,

b) Left ventricular systolic function,

c) Study of the motion of valves (mitral valve prolapse, mitral stenosis, pulmonary hypertension, etc.) and the interventricular septum, and

d) Detection of pericardial fluid.

69

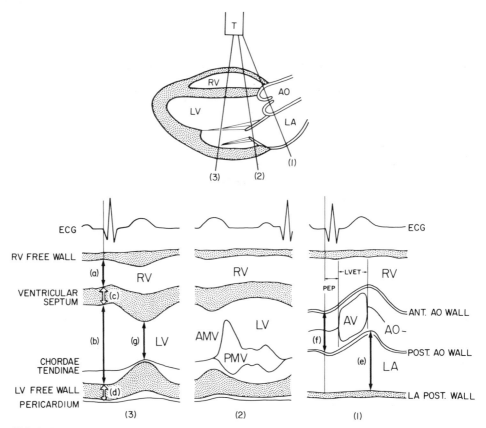

FIG 6–1.
A cross-sectional view of the left side of the heart along the long axis *(top)* through which "ice-pick" views of the M-mode ECHO recordings are made *(bottom).* Many other M-mode views are possible, but only three are shown in this figure. The dimension of the aorta *(AO)* and left atrium *(LA)* is measured along the line *(1).* Systolic time intervals for the left side are also measured at the level of the aortic valve *(AV).* The line *(2)* passes through the mitral valve. Measurements made at this level are not useful in pediatric patients. Measurement of chamber dimensions and wall thickness of right and left ventricles is made along the line *(3).* Normal values of these measurements are shown in Table 6–1. *(a)* = RV dimension; *(b)* = LV diastolic dimension; *(c)* = interventricular septal thickness; *(d)* = LV posterior wall thickness; *(e)* = LA dimension; *(f)* = aortic dimension; *(g)* = LV systolic dimension. Abbreviations: AMV = anterior mitral valve; LV = left ventricle; LVET = left ventricular ejection time; PEP = preejection period; PMV = posterior mitral valve; RV = right ventricle.

A. Normal Electrocardiographic Values

Dimensions of cardiac chambers and the aorta increase with increasing age. Table 6–1 shows mean values and ranges of common M-mode ECHO measurements according to the weight of the patient. Methods of measurement are shown in Figure 6–1. Most dimensions are measured during diastole, coincident with the onset of the QRS complex; LA dimension and LV systolic dimension are exceptions.

TABLE 6–1.
Normal M-Mode Echocardiographic Values (mm) by Weight (lb): Mean (Ranges)*

	0–25 lb	26–50 lb	51–75 lb	76–100 lb	101–125 lb	126–200 lb
RV dimension	9 (3–15)	10 (4–15)	11 (7–18)	12 (7–16)	13 (8–17)	13 (12–17)
LV dimension	24 (13–32)	34 (24–38)	38 (33–45)	41 (35–47)	43 (37–49)	49 (44–52)
LV free wall (or septum)	5 (4–6)	6 (5–7)	7 (6–7)	7 (7–8)	7 (7–8)	8 (7–8)
LA dimension	17 (7–23)	22 (17–27)	23 (19–28)	24 (20–30)	27 (21–30)	28 (21–37)
Aortic root	13 (7–17)	17 (13–22)	20 (17–23)	22 (19–27)	23 (17–27)	24 (22–28)

*Adapted from Feigenbaum H: *Echocardiography*, ed. 4. Philadelphia, Lea & Febiger, 1986.

B. Left Ventricular Function

Left ventricular systolic function is evaluated by fractional shortening (FS) and systolic time intervals. Ejection fraction is a derivative of fractional shortening and offers no advantage over the fractional shortening. Serial determinations of these measurements are important in conditions in which LV function may change, such as in patients with chemotherapy-induced LV dysfunction and those with chronic or acute myocardial disease.

1) Fractional shortening of the left ventricle:
Fractional shortening (FS) is derived by:

$$FS\ (\%) = \frac{Dd - Ds}{Dd} \times 100$$

where Dd = end-diastolic dimension, and Ds = end-systolic dimension. Mean normal value is 36% with 95% prediction limits of 28%–44%. Ejection fraction (EF) is also a function of ventricular dimensions and is obtained by the formula:

$$EF\ (\%) = \frac{(Dd)^3 - (Ds)^3}{(Dd)^3} \times 100$$

Normal mean ejection fraction is 74%, with 95% prediction limits of 64%–83%. Fractional shortening (or ejection fraction) is decreased in a poorly compensated LV regardless of etiology (pressure overload, volume overload, primary myocardial disorders, doxorubicin (Adriamycin) cardiotoxicity, etc). It is increased in compensated LV function, such as volume overload (VSD, PDA, aortic regurgitation, mitral regurgitation) and pressure overload lesions (moderately severe aortic valve stenosis or hypertrophic obstructive cardiomyopathy [or IHSS], etc).

2) Systolic time intervals:
The systolic time interval of a ventricle includes the preejection period (PEP) and the ventricular ejection time (VET). The PEP (from the onset of the Q wave of the ECG to the opening of the semilunar valve [see Fig 6–1]) usually reflects the rate of pressure rise in the ventricle during isovolumic systole (dp/dt). The VET is measured from the valve cusp opening to cusp closing. Although the PEP and VET are affected by the heart rate, the ratio of PEP/VET for both right (RPEP/RVET) and left (LPEP/LVET) sides is little affected by changes in the heart rate (RPEP

= right preejection period; RVET = right ventricular ejection time; LPEP = left preejection period; LVET = left ventricular ejection time). The method of measuring LPEP and LVET is shown in Figure 6–1. Measurement of RPEP and RVET is sometimes difficult as only the posterior part of the pulmonary valve is normally recorded on the M-mode ECHO. Normal values (and ranges) are:

$$RPEP/RVET = 0.24 (0.16 - 0.30)$$
$$LPEP/LVET = 0.35 (0.30 - 0.39)$$

RPEP/RVET is elevated in children with large-shunt VSD and pulmonary hypertension and in persistent pulmonary hypertension of the newborn (PPHN, or PFC syndrome) and in RBBB. In persistent pulmonary hypertension of the newborn, the ratio is almost always greater than 0.50. LPEP/LVET is elevated in congestive heart failure and in LBBB.

II. Two-dimensional echocardiography

Two-dimensional (2D) ECHO examinations are performed by directing the plane of the transducer beam along several cross-sectional planes through the heart. Routine 2D ECHO is obtained from four transducer locations: parasternal, apical, subcostal, and suprasternal notch positions. Figures 6–2 through 6–5 illustrate some standard images of the heart and great vessels. Many other views are possible with different transducer positions and angulations.

A. Parasternal views

Parasternal long-axis view: This most basic view shows the left ventricular inflow and outflow tracts (Fig 6–2,A) and is most important in evaluating the following structures and abnormalities in or near these structures: the mitral valve, left atrium, left ventricle, LV outflow tract, aortic valve, ascending aorta, and ventricular septum. Pericardial effusion, VSD (of TOF and persistent truncus arteriosus), and overriding of the aorta are best evaluated in this view.

Parasternal short-axis view: This projection provides cross-sectional images of the heart and the great arteries at different levels. Important views are those taken at the levels of the semilunar valves, mitral valve, and papillary muscles (Fig 6–2,B–E). Parasternal short-axis views are important in the evaluation of the aortic valve (bicuspid or tricuspid), pulmonary valve, pulmonary artery and its branches, RV outflow tract, coronary arteries (absence, aneurysm), left atrium, left ventricle, ventricular septum, LV outflow tract, the AV valves, and the right side of the heart. Patent ductus arteriosus is usually visualized in a plane similar to Figure 6–2,B (see Fig 26–4). Doppler interrogation of the ductal shunt is performed in that plane.

B. Apical Views

The apical four-chamber view (Fig 6–3,A) is used in the evaluation of atrial and ventricular septa, atrial and ventricular chambers, AV valves, pulmonary venous return, identification of anatomical RV and LV, and detection of pericardial effusion. Endocardial cushion defect (ECD) is well imaged in this view. The apical four-chamber view which shows LV outflow tract (Fig 6–3,B) is useful in the visualization of the perimembranous ventricular septum (where the VSD is most frequently found), LV outflow tract, and ascending aorta, in addition to those structures seen in the regular apical four-chamber view. The apical long-axis view (Fig 6–3,C) shows structures similar to those shown in the parasternal long-axis view.

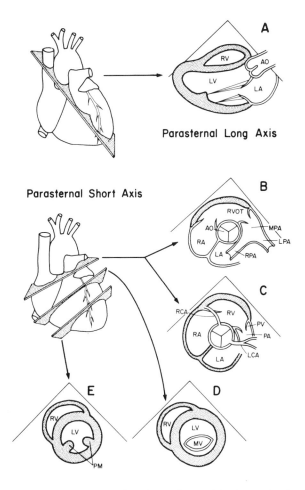

FIG 6–2.
Diagrammatic illustration of important 2D echocardiographic views obtained from the parasternal transducer position. Parasternal long-axis view **(A)** is shown at the top. Parasternal
short-axis views obtained at various levels: the semilunar valve and great artery level
(B,C); the mitral valve level **(D)**; and the papillary muscle level **(E)**. AO = aorta; MPA =
main pulmonary artery; MV = mitral valve; LA = left atrium; LCA = left coronary artery;
LPA = left pulmonary artery; LV = left ventricle; PA = pulmonary artery; PM = papillary
muscle; PV = pulmonary valve; RA = right atrium; RCA = right coronary artery; RPA =
right pulmonary artery; RV = right ventricle.

C. Subcostal Views

The subcostal four-chamber view (Fig 6–4,A) demonstrates atrial and ventricular septa, AV valves, atrial and ventricular chambers, and the drainage
of systemic and pulmonary veins. This is the best view for the evaluation of
an ASD. With further anterior angulation (Fig 6–4,B and C), or turning the
transducer 90° (Fig 6–4,D), the ventricular outflow tract of both ventricles
and the great arteries can be imaged.

D. Suprasternal Notch Views

The suprasternal long-axis (Fig 6–5,A) and short-axis (Fig 6–5,B) views are
important in the evaluation of anomalies in the ascending and descending

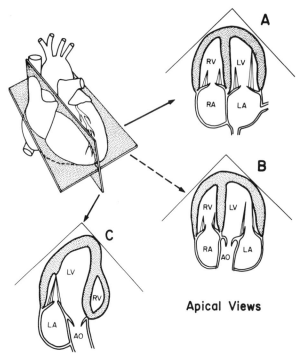

FIG 6–3.
Diagrammatic illustration of 2D ECHO views obtained with the transducer at the apical position. **A,** apical four-chamber view; **B,** apical four-chamber view with LV outflow tract; **C,** apical long-axis view. Abbreviations are same as in Figure 6–2.

aortas (COA), aortic arch (interruption), and the size of the pulmonary arteries, and anomalies of systemic veins.

E. **Indications**

Indications for 2D ECHO studies are expanding with its increasing accuracy of diagnostic imaging. The following are some selected indications for 2D ECHO examination.

1. Routine screening of infants who appear to have cyanotic CHD.

2. To rule out cyanotic CHD in newborn infants with clinical findings of persistent pulmonary hypertension of the newborn (PPHN, or PFC syndrome).

3. To confirm diagnosis in infants and children with findings atypical of certain defects.

4. To rule in or rule out certain important conditions which are raised by routine evaluation (physical examination, chest x-rays, and ECG).

5. Follow-up of certain conditions which may change with time and/or treatment (PDA in premature infants before and after indomethacin treatment, CHF, LV function studies, etc.).

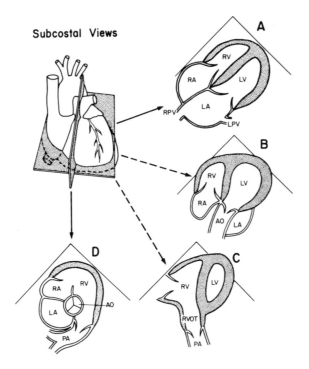

FIG 6–4.
Diagrammatic illustration of 2D ECHO views obtained with the transducer at the subcostal position. **A,** subcostal four-chamber view; **B,** the view showing the LV outflow tract and the proximal aorta; **C,** the view that shows the RV outflow tract and the proximal MPA; **D,** subcostal short-axis view. Abbreviations are same as in Figure 6–2. LPV = left pulmonary vein; RPV = right pulmonary vein.

   6. Before cardiac catheterization and angiocardiography.

      (a) Having prior knowledge of certain information can reduce the amount of time spent in the cardiac catheterization laboratory and the amount of the radiopaque dye injected.

      (b) It can supply some information which angiocardiography cannot. 2D ECHO is superior to angiocardiography in demonstrating small, thin structures (such as subaortic membrane, cor triatriatum, eustachian valve, straddling AV valves, Ebstein's anomaly) which may be easily missed by angiocardiography.

   7. It can replace cardiac catheterization and angiocardiography in certain situations.

   8. Postoperative evaluation.

III. Contrast Echocardiography
   Injection of indocyanine green, dextrose in water, saline, or the patient's own blood into a peripheral or central vein produces microcavitations and creates a cloud of echoes on the echocardiogram. Structures of interest are visualized and/or recorded by either M-mode or 2D ECHO at the time of the injection.

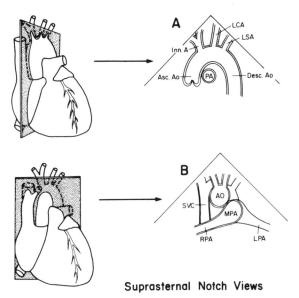

Suprasternal Notch Views

FIG 6-5.
Diagrammatic drawing of suprasternal notch 2D ECHO views. **A,** long-axis view; **B,** short-axis view. AO = aorta; Asc. Ao = ascending aorta; Desc. Ao = descending aorta; Inn. A = innominate artery; LCA = left carotid artery; LPA = left pulmonary artery; LSA = left subclavian artery; MPA = main pulmonary artery; PA = pulmonary artery; RPA = right pulmonary artery; SVC = superior vena cava.

This technique has been used successfully to detect intracardiac shunt, validate structures, and identify flow patterns within the heart. For example, an injection of any liquid into an IV line may confirm the presence of a right-to-left shunt at the atrial or ventricular level. This technique is frequently used in diagnosis of cyanosis due to a right-to-left shunt at the atrial level (such as seen with persistent pulmonary hypertension of the newborn; see Fig 26-1) or in postoperative patients with persistent arterial desaturation. Numerous other applications have been described. It has been replaced to a large extent by Doppler echocardiography.

IV. Doppler Echocardiography

Doppler ECHO combines the study of cardiac structures and blood flow profiles. The Doppler effect is a change in the observed frequency of sound due to motion of the source or of the target. When the moving object or column of blood is moving toward the ultrasonic transducer, there is an apparent increase in the frequency of the reflected sound wave (a positive Doppler shift). Conversely, when blood moves away from the transducer, there is a decreasing frequency (a negative Doppler shift). Doppler ultrasound equipment detects frequency shifts and thus determines the direction and velocity of red blood cell flow with respect to the ultrasound beam.

Two Doppler techniques are in common use: continuous wave (CW) and pulsed wave (PW). In pulsed-wave Doppler technique, a short burst of ultrasound is emitted, and the echo-Doppler receiver "listens" for returning information. Continuous-wave Doppler emits a constant ultrasound beam with one crystal and continuously receives returning information with another crystal.

Both techniques have advantages and disadvantages. The major advantage of PW Doppler is the ability to control the site at which Doppler signals are sampled, but the maximum detectable velocity is limited, so that it cannot be used for quantification of severe obstruction. On the other hand, the advantage of the CW Doppler is the capability of measuring very high velocities (for the estimation of severe stenosis), but it cannot localize the site of sampling; it picks up the signal anywhere along the Doppler beam. When these two techniques are used in combinations, much wider clinical applications can be obtained. Doppler ECHO determines the direction of flow and flow disturbances. Flow disturbances are seen with stenosis or regurgitation of cardiac valves or narrowing of blood vessels. By multiplying the mean velocity of flow and the cross-sectional area, blood flow (cardiac output) can be estimated. Abnormal connections produce turbulence and alteration of the direction of normal flows, allowing detection of cardiac shunts (PDA, VSD, ASD).

Color-coded Doppler is now being used in some centers, providing images of the distribution of flow disturbances superimposed on the ECHO structural image. The same information can be obtained by systematic mapping with the conventional pulsed Doppler equipment.

II. EXERCISE TEST

Exercise testing has come to play an important, although infrequent, role in evaluating cardiac symptoms, quantifying the severity of the cardiac abnormality and assessing the effectiveness of management. There are basically two types of equipment used in exercise testing: bicycle ergometers and treadmills. Bicycle ergometer protocols have been developed by various laboratories but are not widely performed. Treadmill protocols are more widely used and well standardized, and normal values for children are now available for the Bruce protocol (Table 6–2).

TABLE 6–2.
Bruce Treadmill Test Endurance Times (min)*

Age Group (yr)	Percentile					Mean	SD
	10	25	50	75	90		
Boys							
4–5	8.1	9.0	10.0	12.0	13.3	10.4	1.9
6–7	9.7	10.0	12.0	12.3	13.5	11.8	1.6
8–9	9.6	10.5	12.4	13.7	16.2	12.6	2.3
10–12	9.9	12.0	12.5	14.0	15.4	12.7	1.9
13–15	11.2	13.0	14.3	16.0	16.1	14.1	1.7
16–18	11.3	12.1	13.6	14.5	15.8	13.5	1.4
Girls							
4–5	7.0	8.0	9.0	11.2	12.3	9.5	1.8
6–7	9.5	9.6	11.4	13.0	13.0	11.2	1.5
8–9	9.9	10.5	11.0	13.0	14.2	11.8	1.6
10–12	10.5	11.3	12.0	13.0	14.6	12.3	1.4
13–15	9.4	10.0	11.5	12.0	13.0	11.1	1.3
16–18	8.1	10.0	10.5	12.0	12.4	10.7	1.4

*Adapted from Cumming GR, Everatt D, Hastman L: Bruce treadmill test in children: Normal values in a clinic population. *Am J Cardiol* 1978; 41:69–75.

During stress testing, the patient is continuously monitored for ischemic changes or arrhythmias by ECG and for symptoms such as chest pain or faintness. In the Bruce protocol, the level of exercise is increased by increasing the speed and grade of the treadmill for each 3-minute stage. The following three functions are measured every minute or two throughout the test and for 10 minutes following the test.

1) Heart rate response: Mean maximum exercise heart rate is 190–200/min. Inadequate increments may be seen with sinus node dysfunction. A very high rate at low levels of work may indicate physical deconditioning or marginal circulatory compensation.

2) Blood pressure response: Systolic pressure in the arm may rise to 180 mm Hg with little change in diastolic pressure. Failure of arterial blood pressure to rise reflects an inadequate increase in cardiac output and is commonly seen with cardiomyopathy, LV outflow tract obstructive lesions, or coronary artery disease.

3) ECG monitoring: Arrhythmias and ischemic changes are monitored. ST-segment depression of 2 mm or greater lasting at least 1 minute postexercise in leads with dominant R waves is evidence of subendocardial ischemia. False positive (hypokalemia, mitral valve prolapse, WPW syndrome, digitalis, psychoactive drugs) and false negative (β-blockers or coronary vasodilators) results are possible.

Endurance time has been shown to be the best predictor of exercise capacity in children by the Bruce protocol. Normal endurance times for children are shown in Table 6–2. A time of 13 minutes indicates that the subject completed Stage IV and 1 minute of Stage V.

Stress testing has been particularly useful in children for the following conditions:

1) Aortic stenosis: Ischemic changes are considered an indication for surgical intervention.

2) Evaluation of arrhythmias and AV conduction: PVCs increasing in frequency with exercise may require initiation of antiarrhythmic therapy. AV blocks which worsen with exercise warrant therapy.

3) Postoperative evaluation of TOF and other cyanotic CHD.

4) Adolescent chest pain (to rule out cardiac cause).

5) Postcoarctectomy patients who may have an abnormal blood pressure response to exercise.

6) Appropriate exercise prescription for participation in vocational, recreational, and competitive activities.

III. AMBULATORY ELECTROCARDIOGRAPHY

Electrocardiographic electrodes are attached to the chest wall, and ECG rhythm is continually recorded for 8–24 hours or longer using a transistorized tape recorder (Holter monitor). The patient is given a diary into which symptoms and activities are recorded during the period of monitoring. The tape is scanned manually or by computer, and the number, types, and duration of arrhythmias are reported. Arrhythmias are correlated with the patient's activities and symptoms. Important portions of the rhythm are printed out on an ECG paper for permanent record.

Ambulatory ECG monitoring is obtained (1) to document the presence of arrhythmias, (2) to determine the frequency, duration, and types of arrhythmias, (3) to relate symptoms to an arrhythmia, (4) to determine precipitating or terminating events of arrhythmias, (5) to evaluate efficacy of antiarrhythmic agents, and (6) to screen high-risk cardiac patients (postoperative TGA and TOF). Ambulatory ECG monitoring is not very helpful in detecting an episode that occurs infrequently (i.e., once a week or once a month) and is unnecessary for asymptomatic extrasystoles.

Ambulatory ECGs on normal adolescent boys reveal the maximum awake heart rate to be as high as 200 beats/min and the minimum rate 45/min. During sleep, the maximum rate is 110 and the minimum rate as low as 30/min. Sinus rhythm is seen consistently. Sinus pause, first-degree AV block, and premature atrial and ventricular contractions are frequently recorded. In the newborn, short runs of supraventricular tachycardia are often seen.

7 / Invasive Procedures

I. CARDIAC CATHETERIZATION AND ANGIOCARDIOGRAPHY

Cardiac catheterization and angiocardiography usually constitute the final definitive diagnostic tests for most cardiac patients. They are carried out under general sedation using various sedatives. A mixture of meperidine (Demerol), chlorpromazine (Thorazine), and promethazine (Phenergan) is widely used. Smaller doses of sedatives are used in cyanotic infants. Using local anesthesia and strict aseptic preparation of skin, catheters are placed in peripheral (most commonly the femoral) vessels, usually through the percutaneous technique.

The catheter is manipulated into different cardiac chambers and great vessels under fluoroscopy, with image intensification to reduce radiation exposure. At each location, values of pressure and oxygen saturation of blood are obtained. The oxygen saturation data provide information on the site and magnitude of the left-to-right or right-to-left shunt, if any. The pressure data provide information on the site and severity of obstruction. Cardiac output may be obtained from oxygen saturation data (the Fick principle; see below), or by indicator dilution (indocyanine green dye) or thermodilution (cold saline injection) technique. Selective angiocardiography is usually performed as a part of the catheterization procedure (see below).

A. Normal Hemodynamic Values

Normal oxygen saturation in the right side of the heart varies between 65% and 80%, depending on cardiac output. Left-sided saturations are usually 95%–98% in room air. In newborns and heavily sedated children, the oxygen saturation may be lower. Pressures are lower in the right side than in the left side of the heart, with systolic pressures in the right ventricle and pulmonary artery about 20%–30% of those in the left side of the heart (Fig 7–1). The following calculations are routinely obtained: flow and resistance for systemic and pulmonary circuits and left-to-right or right-to-left shunt.

1. Flows (cardiac output) and shunts

Flow is calculated by the use of the Fick formula:

$$\text{Pulmonary flow } (\dot{Q}p) = \frac{V_{O_2}}{C_{PV} - C_{PA}}$$

$$\text{Systemic flow } (\dot{Q}s) = \frac{V_{O_2}}{C_{AO} - C_{MV}}$$

where flows are in L/min, V_{O_2} = oxygen consumption (ml/min), C = oxygen content (ml/L) at various positions, PV = pulmonary vein, PA = pulmonary artery, AO = aorta, and MV = mixed systemic venous blood (SVC or RA).

80

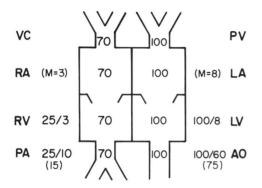

FIG 7–1.
Pressure and oxygen saturation values in normal children.

Oxygen consumption is either directly measured during the procedure or estimated from a table. Oxygen content (ml/100 ml) is derived by multiplying oxygen capacity by percent saturation. Oxygen capacity (ml/100 ml) refers to the total content of oxygen that hemoglobin contains when it is 100% saturated (1.36 × hemoglobin gm/100 ml).

When there is a pure left-to-right or right-to-left shunt, the magnitude of the shunt is calculated as follows:

$$\text{Left-to-right shunt} = \dot{Q}p - \dot{Q}s$$

$$\text{Right-to-left shunt} = \dot{Q}s - \dot{Q}p$$

The flow data are subject to much error because of difficulties involved in measuring accurate oxygen consumption or because of the frequent use of assumed oxygen consumption (140–160 ml/m^2/min) in pediatric patients. Therefore, the ratio of pulmonary-to-systemic flow ($\dot{Q}p/\dot{Q}s$) is frequently used, which does not require an oxygen consumption value. The ratio provides information on the magnitude of the shunt. Left-to-right shunts greater than 2:1 are usually surgical candidates. Normal systemic flow (or pulmonary flow in the absence of shunt) is 3.1 ± 0.4 L/min/m^2 (cardiac index).

2. Resistance
Hydraulic resistance (R) is defined by analogy to Ohm's law as the ratio of the mean pressure drop (ΔP) to flow (Q) between two points in a liquid flowing in a tube (R = ΔP/Q). Therefore, pulmonary vascular resistance (PVR) and systemic vascular resistance (SVR) are calculated using the following formulas:

$$\text{PVR} = \frac{\text{mean PA pressure} - \text{mean LA pressure}}{Qp}$$

$$\text{SVR} = \frac{\text{mean aortic pressure} - \text{mean RA pressure}}{Qs}$$

The normal SVR varies between 15 and 30 units/m^2. The normal PVR is high at birth but reaches values near adult values after 2–4 months. Normal values in children and adults are 1–3 units/m^2. Obviously, the ratios of PVR/SVR will range from 1/10 to 1/20. High values of PVR increase the risk of corrective surgery for many congenital cardiac defects.

B. Selective Angiocardiography

Information derived from echocardiography and the oxygen saturation and pressure data from catheterization help to determine the number and sites of selective angiocardiograms required to delineate anatomy of cardiovascular structures. A radiopaque dye is rapidly injected into a certain site, and angiograms are recorded on motion picture film at 60 or 90 frames per second, often on biplane views. Depending on the cardiovascular anomaly under study, special views are obtained either by moving the fluoroscopic camera or by positioning the patient at desired angles. Multiple injection sites are often necessary to obtain a complete anatomical diagnosis (see Fig 7–2,A).

C. Risks

Cardiac catheterization and angiocardiography can lead to serious complications, including death, rarely. Complications related to catheter insertion and manipulation include serious arrhythmias, heart block, cardiac perforation, hypoxic spells, arterial obstruction, hemorrhage, and infection. Complications related to contrast injection include reactions to the contrast material, intramyocardial injection, and renal complications (hematuria, proteinuria, oliguria, anuria). Complications related to exposure, sedation, and medications include hypothermia, acidemia, hypoglycemia, convulsions, hypotension, and respiratory depression and are more likely to occur in the newborn infant.

In general, the risk of cardiac catheterization and angiocardiography varies with the age and illness of the patient, the type of lesion, and the experience of those doing the procedure. The reported rate of fatal complications varies between lower than 1% and as high as 5% in the newborn period. About 3%–5% of patients may have significant but nonfatal complications, such as arrhythmias and arterial complications. However, with more careful preparation and monitoring (see below) and the use of prostaglandin infusion in selected newborns, the mortality and morbidity can be kept to a minimum.

D. Indications

Indications for these invasive studies vary from institution to institution as well as cardiologist to cardiologist. With improved capability of noninvasive techniques (2D ECHO and Doppler studies), many cardiac problems are adequately diagnosed and managed without the invasive studies. The following are considered indications by most but not all cardiologists.

1. Newborns with cyanotic CHD who may require palliative surgery or those who may require balloon atrial septostomy during the procedure.

2. Newborns with CHF from CHD.

3. Children with CHD when the lesion is severe enough to require surgical intervention.

4. Children who appear to have had unsatisfactory results from cardiac surgery.

5. Infants and children with lesions amenable to balloon angio/valvuloplasty.

E. Preparation and Monitoring

Adequate preparation of the patient before the procedure and careful monitoring during the procedure can minimize possible complications and fatality from the invasive studies. Following areas are particularly important.

1. Increasing temperature in the cardiac catheterization laboratory when an infant is being studied.

2. Using a warming blanket and a rectal thermistor to monitor rectal temperature and to avoid hypothermia.

3. Checking arterial blood gases and pH and correcting acidemia and hypoxemia.

4. Correcting hypoglycemia or hypocalcemia before the start of the procedure. Administering glucose during the procedure if hypoglycemia is found.

5. Administering oxygen, if indicated, during the procedure.

6. Intubating or readiness for intubating in infants with respiratory difficulties.

7. Having emergency medications (atropine, epinephrine, bicarbonate, etc.) drawn up and ready.

8. Initiating prostaglandin infusion in cyanotic infants who appear to be ductus dependent.

9. Whenever possible, having another physician available to monitor noncardiac aspects of the patient, so that the operator can concentrate on the procedure.

II. CATHETER INTERVENTION PROCEDURES

Recent technical advances have allowed for the development of a variety of therapeutic procedures, utilizing specially modified catheters, which can be performed in the cardiac catheterization laboratory. These procedures may be lifesaving in critically ill neonates or may eliminate or delay elective surgical procedures in children with certain CHD.

A. Balloon Atrial Septostomy (Rashkind's Procedure)

This procedure remains the standard initial palliation of TGA. It has also been used in selected patients with TAPVR, critical PS, pulmonary atresia with intact ventricular septum, and mitral atresia and stenosis, conditions in which a large atrial communication is desirable. A special balloon-tipped catheter is introduced into the LA from the RA through a patent foramen ovale or an existing ASD. The balloon is inflated with diluted contrast material, and the catheter is rapidly pulled back to the RA through the interatrial communication, creating a large opening in the atrial septum.

B. Blade Atrial Septostomy

In older infants and children, the atrial septum is too thick for the Rashkind procedure to be successful, but the septum can be opened in some cases with a blade catheter. The blade catheter uses a small blade that unfolds from the tip of the catheter to actually incise the atrial septum as the catheter tip is withdrawn from the LA to the RA. This procedure may eliminate the need for surgical atrial septectomy (the Blalock-Hanlon operation).

C. Balloon Valvuloplasty and Angioplasty

These balloon intervention procedures use balloons which are constructed of special plastic polymers and have the unique feature of retaining their pre-

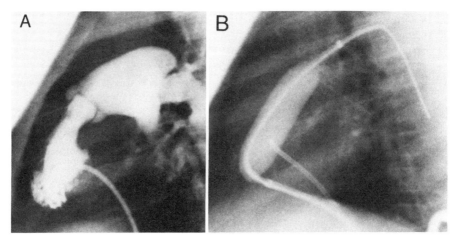

FIG 7–2.
Angiocardiography and balloon valvuloplasty. **A,** lateral view of right ventriculogram showing a thick, dome-shaped pulmonary valve and a marked poststenotic dilatation of the
pulmonary artery. **B,** a maximally inflated sausage-shaped valvuloplasty balloon is seen,
which suggests the stenotic pulmonary valve has been widened. The balloon catheter was
introduced over a guide wire, which was positioned in the left pulmonary artery.

determined diameters. The elongated, sausage-shaped balloon is placed precisely in the position desired with the use of a guide wire. The balloon is
then inflated with a diluted contrast material to relieve obstruction at a valve
or a vessel.

This technique is the treatment of choice for valvular PS, and has replaced, to a large extent, surgical pulmonary valvotomy (Fig 7–2,B). The
procedure is usually successful in recurrent COA, but the long-term effects
of the procedure for native coarctation are not clear. Selected cases of valvular aortic stenosis, peripheral pulmonary artery stenosis, and vena caval
baffle obstruction have received favorable results. Indications for the procedure will undoubtedly increase as our experience grows.

D. More complicated catheter procedures for closing PDA, ASD, and VSD are
in the experimental stage.

PART III
Pathophysiology

In this section discussion of fetal and perinatal circulation and the circulatory changes that take place after birth is followed by discussion of pathophysiology of some representative congenital and acquired heart diseases.

The knowledge of fetal and perinatal circulation is very helpful in understanding clinical manifestations and natural history of congenital heart diseases. A few examples of clinical importance in relation to fetal and perinatal circulation will be pointed out. In discussing pathophysiology of congenital and acquired heart disease, attempts were made to explain why particular ECG, chest x-ray, and physical findings are associated with each defect based on hemodynamic abnormalities. In doing so, it was necessary to use a simplistic approach and avoid controversies. Careful study of the pathophysiology section will enable readers not only to explain, but also to recall and predict physical findings and abnormalities of ECG and chest x-rays of many cardiac anomalies.

8 / Fetal and Perinatal Circulation

The knowledge of fetal and perinatal circulation is an integral part of understanding the pathophysiology and natural history of congenital heart disease. Only a brief discussion of clinically important aspects of fetal and perinatal circulation will be presented.

I. FETAL CIRCULATION

Fetal circulation differs from the adult circulation in several ways, almost all attributable to the fundamental difference in the site of gas exchange. In the adult, the lung is the site of gas exchange, whereas in the fetus, the placenta provides the exchange of gases and nutrients.

A. Course of Fetal Circulation

The general course of fetal circulation is shown in Figure 8–1. There are four shunts in the fetal circulation: placenta, ductus venosus, foramen ovale, and ductus arteriosus. Some important aspects of fetal circulation are summarized below:

   a. The placenta receives the largest amount of combined (right and left) ventricular output (55%) and has the lowest vascular resistance in the fetus.

   b. The superior vena cava (SVC) drains the upper part of the body, including the brain (15% of combined ventricular output), while the inferior vena cava (IVC) drains the lower part of the body and the placenta (70% of combined ventricular output). Since the blood is oxygenated in the placenta, the O_2 saturation in the IVC (70%) is higher than that in the SVC (40%). The highest PO_2 is found in the umbilical vein (32 mm Hg) (see Fig 8–1).

   c. Most of the SVC blood goes to the RV. About one-third of the IVC blood with higher oxygen saturation is directed by the crista dividens to the LA through the foramen ovale, while the remaining two-thirds enters the RV and MPA. The end result is that the brain and coronary circulation receive blood with higher oxygen saturation (PO_2 of 28 mm Hg) than the lower half of the body (PO_2 of 24 mm Hg) (see Fig 8–1).

   d. Less oxygenated blood in the PA flows through the widely open ductus arteriosus to the descending aorta and then to the placenta for oxygenation.

B. Dimensions of Cardiac Chambers

The proportions of the combined cardiac output traversing the heart chambers and the major blood vessels are reflected in the relative dimensions of these chambers and vessels (see Fig 8–1). For example:

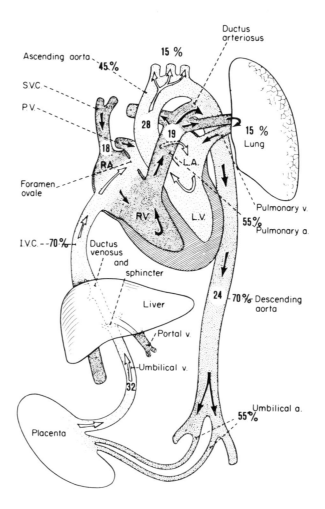

FIG 8–1.
Diagram of the fetal circulation showing the four sites of shunt: placenta, ductus venosus, foramen ovale, and ductus arteriosus. Intravascular *shading* is in proportion to oxygen saturation, with the lightest shading representing the highest Po_2. The numerical value inside the chamber or vessel is the Po_2 for that site in mm Hg. The percentages outside the vascular structures represent the relative flows in major tributaries and outlets for the two ventricles. The combined output of the two ventricles represents 100%. a = artery; v = vein; IVC = inferior vena cava; PV = pulmonary vein; SVC = superior vena cava. (From Guntheroth WG, et al: Physiology of the circulation: Fetus, neonate and child, in Kelley VC (ed): *Practice of Pediatrics,* Philadelphia, Harper and Row, 1982–83, vol 8, chap 23. Used by permission.)

    a. Because the lungs receive only 15% of combined ventricular output, the branches of the PA are small. This is important in the genesis of the pulmonary flow murmur of the newborn (see Innocent Heart Murmurs in chap. 2 and 26).

    b. The RV is the dominant ventricle, as it handles 55% of combined ventricular output, while the LV handles 45% of combined ventricular output. In addition, the pressure in the RV is identical to that in the LV, unlike in the adult.

This fact is reflected in the ECG of the newborn, which shows more RV force than that of the adult.

C. Fetal Cardiac Output

Unlike the adult heart, which increases its stroke volume when the heart rate decreases, the fetal heart is unable to increase stroke volume when the heart rate falls. Therefore, the fetal cardiac output is dependent on the heart rate; when the heart rate drops, as in fetal distress, a serious fall in cardiac output results.

II. CHANGES IN CIRCULATION AFTER BIRTH

The primary change in the circulation after birth is a shift of the blood flow for gas exchange from the placenta to the lungs. The placental circulation disappears, and the pulmonary circulation is established.

A. Interruption of the umbilical cord results in:

    a. an increase in systemic vascular resistance (SVR) as a result of removal of the very-low-resistance placenta, and

    b. closure of the ductus venosus as a result of lack of blood return from the placenta.

B. Expansion of the lungs results in:

    a. a reduction of pulmonary vascular resistance (PVR), an increase in pulmonary blood flow (PBF), and a fall in pulmonary artery pressure.

    b. functional closure of the foramen ovale as a result of increased pressure in the LA in excess of RA pressure. LA pressure increases secondary to increased pulmonary venous return. RA pressure falls with closure of the ductus venosus.

    c. closure of patent ductus arteriosus (PDA) as a result of increased arterial O_2 saturation (see below for further discussion).

III. CHANGES IN PVR AND CLOSURE OF PDA

Changes in PVR and closure of the PDA are so important in understanding many congenital heart diseases that further discussion is necessary.

A. Pulmonary Vascular Resistance

The pulmonary vascular resistance (PVR) is as high as systemic vascular resistance (SVR) near or at term. This high resistance is maintained by an increased amount of smooth muscle in the walls of the pulmonary arterioles, the collapsed lungs, and the alveolar hypoxia.

With expansion of the lungs and resulting increase in the alveolar oxygen tension, there is an initial rapid fall in PVR. This rapid fall in PVR is secondary to the vasodilating effect of oxygen on the pulmonary vasculature (Fig 8–2). In 6–8 weeks after birth, there is a slower fall in PVR and in the pulmonary artery pressure, associated with thinning of the medial layer of the pulmonary arterioles. There is further decline in PVR after the first 2 years. This may be related to the increase in the number of alveolar units and their associated vessels.

Many conditions that involve inadequate oxygenation may interfere with the normal maturation (thinning) of the pulmonary arterioles, resulting in persistent

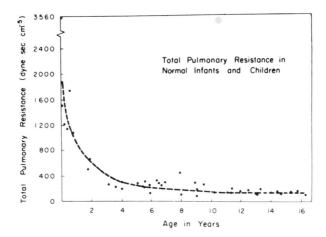

FIG 8–2.
Postnatal changes in pulmonary vascular resistance. (From Moller JH, et al: *Congenital Heart Disease.* Kalamazoo, Mich, The Upjohn Company, 1974. Used by permission.)

pulmonary hypertension or delay in the fall of PVR (Table 8–1). A few examples of clinical importance are presented below.

a. Infants with a large VSD may not develop congestive heart failure (CHF) while living at a high altitude but may develop CHF if they move to sea level. This is because of the delayed fall in PVR associated with altitude.

b. Premature infants with severe hyaline membrane disease usually do not develop CHF because their PVR is high, which restricts the left-to-right shunt. Acidosis, which is often present in these infants, may contribute to maintaining a high PVR. CHF may develop as their hyaline membrane disease improves because the resulting increase in arterial Po_2 dilates pulmonary vasculature.

c. Direct transmission of high pulmonary artery pressure resulting from large VSD delays the fall in PVR. Therefore, CHF does not develop until 6–8 weeks of age or later. In contrast, PVR falls normally in infants with small VSD, since direct transmission of systemic pressure to the PA does not occur through a restrictive VSD.

B. Closure of Ductus Arteriosus
Functional closure of the ductus arteriosus occurs 10–15 hours after birth, and anatomical closure is accomplished by 2–3 weeks of age. What closes the ductus? Increased oxygen saturation in the systemic circulation is the strongest

TABLE 8–1.

Conditions That May Interfere With the Normal Maturation of Pulmonary Arterioles

Hypoxia and/or altitude
Lung disease such as hyaline membrane disease
Acidemia
Increased pulmonary artery pressure due to large VSD or PDA
Increased pressure in the LA or pulmonary vein

stimulus for the constriction of the ductal smooth muscle, leading to the closure of the ductus. Less importantly, acetylcholine and bradykinin also constrict the ductus. Gestational age also plays an important role in closure of the ductus. The responsiveness of the ductal smooth muscle to oxygen is lower in the premature infant than in the full-term infant. This lack of response to oxygen of the immature ductus is not due to lack of smooth muscle development, since acetylcholine contracts the immature ductus.

It has been established that prostaglandins E_1 and E_2 are important in the maintenance of patency of the ductus arteriosus in the fetus. There are a few important clinical situations worth mentioning.

a. A decrease in prostaglandin E level results in closure of the PDA. Prostaglandin synthetase inhibitors (indomethacin, aspirin) will constrict the ductus by reducing the prostaglandin level. Indomethacin has been used successfully to close the PDA in premature infants with a significant ductal shunt (see heart failure in premature infants with PDA in chap. 26).

b. Prolonged patency of the ductus can be maintained by intravenous (IV) infusion of prostaglandin E in infants whose survival depends on the patency of the ductus, such as those with pulmonary atresia.

c. Maternal ingestion of a large amount of aspirin, an inhibitor of prostaglandin synthetase, may be harmful to the fetus, as it may constrict the ductus during fetal life, with resulting pulmonary hypertension in the newborn infant. It has been suggested that some cases of persistent pulmonary hypertension of the newborn (PFC syndrome) may be caused by a premature constriction of the ductus arteriosus.

IV. RESPONSE OF PULMONARY ARTERY AND DUCTUS ARTERIOSUS TO VARIOUS STIMULI

It is important to remember that the responses of the pulmonary artery and the ductus arteriosus to oxygen and acidosis are opposite. Hypoxia and acidosis relax the ductus arteriosus but constrict the pulmonary arterioles. Oxygen relaxes pulmonary arterioles but constricts the ductus.

Pulmonary arteries are also constricted by sympathetic stimulation and α-adrenergic stimulation (epinephrine, norepinephrine). Vagal stimulation, β-adrenergic stimulation (isoproterenol), and bradykinin dilate pulmonary arteries.

V. PREMATURE NEWBORN INFANTS

Two important problems that premature infants may face need to be addressed briefly. They are related to the rate at which PVR falls and the responsiveness of the ductus arteriosus to oxygen.

A. In premature infants, the pulmonary vascular smooth muscle is less well developed than in full-term infants. Therefore, the fall in PVR occurs more rapidly than in the mature infant, thus allowing early onset of large left-to-right shunt and CHF (see chaps. 25 and 26).

B. The ductus arteriosus may not close immediately after birth because of its decreased responsiveness to oxygen.

9 / Pathophysiology of Left-to-Right Shunt Lesions

Before we discuss hemodynamic abnormalities of common left-to-right shunt lesions, let us familiarize ourselves with the model that will be used throughout this section. Figure 9–1 is a block diagram of a normal heart in which one arrow represents a "unit" of normal cardiac output. Let us assume that cardiac chambers and great arteries and veins with one arrow are normal in size. If a cardiac chamber or great artery has more than one arrow in it, that chamber or blood vessel will be dilated. A diagram of a normal cardiac roentgenogram was presented in a previous chapter (see Fig 4–2). Modification in the appearance of chest roentgenograms owing to enlargement (or reduction) of cardiac chambers or great vessels will be presented in diagrammatic drawings to aid in interpreting chest x-ray films.

A. Atrial Septal Defect (ASD)

In ASD, the magnitude of the left-to-right shunt is determined by the *size* of the defect and the relative *compliance* of the RV and LV. Because the compliance of the RV is greater than that of the LV, a left-to-right shunt is present. The magnitude of the shunt is reflected in the degree of cardiac enlargement.

Let us assume that there is a left-to-right shunt of one arrow at the atrial level. As can be seen in the block diagram (Fig 9–2), the chambers that are enlarged are the RA, RV, and MPA and its branches. These findings are translated into the chest x-rays (Fig 9–3), which reveal enlargement of the RA, RV, and MPA and an increase in pulmonary vascular markings. Note that the LA is not enlarged (see Figs 9–2 and 9–3). This is because the increased pulmonary venous return to the LA does not stay in that chamber, but is shunted immediately to the RA. The absence of LA enlargement is one of the helpful x-ray signs of differentiating ASD from VSD (see below).

The dilated RV cavity prolongs the time required for depolarization of the RV because of its longer pathway, producing RBBB pattern (rsR′ in V1) in the ECG. The RBBB pattern in children with an ASD is not due to actual block in the right bundle. If the duration of the QRS complex is not abnormally prolonged, the ECG may be read as mild RVH. Therefore, one sees either RBBB or mild RVH on the ECG of children with ASD (see RBBB in chap. 3).

The heart murmur in ASD is not due to the shunt at the atrial level. Since the pressure gradient between the atria is so small and the shunt occurs throughout the cardiac cycle, both in systole and diastole, the left-to-right shunt is silent. The heart murmur in ASD originates from the pulmonary valve because of the increased blood flow through this normal-sized valve (relative pulmonary stenosis) (see Fig 9–2), and, therefore, the murmur is systolic in timing. An increased blood flow through the tricuspid valve (2 arrows) results in a relative stenosis of this valve and a diastolic rumble at the tricuspid valve area (LLSB). The widely split and fixed S2 that is typical of an ASD results in part from the RBBB (electric delay in RV depolarization). In addition, the large atrial

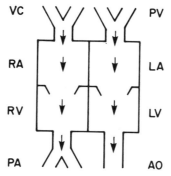

FIG 9–1.
Diagram of a normal heart. *One arrow* represents a unit of normal cardiac output. AO = aorta; LA = left atrium; LV = left ventricle; PA = pulmonary artery; PV = pulmonary vein; RA = right atrium; RV = right ventricle; VC = venae cavae.

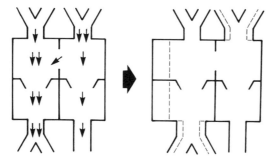

FIG 9–2.
Block diagram of an atrial septal defect. The number of arrows in each chamber represents the amount of blood to be handled by that particular chamber. When one redraws the chambers with two arrows larger than normal, one can predict which chambers will be enlarged.

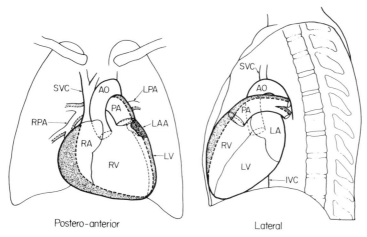

Postero-anterior   Lateral

FIG 9–3.
Posteroanterior (PA) and lateral view diagrams of chest roentgenograms. Enlargement of the RA and MPA segment and increased pulmonary vascular markings are present in the PA view. The RV enlargement is best seen in the lateral view.

shunt tends to abolish respiration-related fluctuation in systemic venous return to the right side of the heart, resulting in a large venous return to the RA throughout the respiratory cycle, and, therefore, the fixed S2.

Congestive heart failure (CHF) is extremely rare in children. Even in the presence of a large left-to-right shunt, pulmonary artery pressure remains normal for many years. Pulmonary arteries handle increased amount of PBF (without direct transmission of systemic pressure) very well for a long time. However, CHF and pulmonary hypertension eventually develop in the 3rd and 4th decade of life.

B. Ventricular Septal Defect (VSD)

The direction of the shunt in acyanotic VSD is left-to-right. The magnitude of the shunt is determined by the *size* (not the location) of the defect and the level of *pulmonary vascular resistance*. With a small defect, a large resistance to the left-to-right shunt is offered at the defect, and the shunt does not depend on the level of pulmonary vascular resistance (PVR). With a large VSD, the resistance offered by the defect is minimal, and the left-to-right shunt is dependent on the level of PVR: the lower the PVR, the greater the magnitude of left-to-right shunt. This type of left-to-right shunt is called "dependent" shunt. Even in the presence of a large VSD, the decrease in PVR to a critical level does not occur until the age of 6–8 weeks, so that the onset of CHF is delayed until that age.

Let us first consider which cardiac chambers become enlarged in a VSD of moderate size, using the block diagram shown in Figure 9–4. The chambers or vessels that will become enlarged are those with two arrows. Therefore, there will be enlargement of the MPA, LA, and LV and increased pulmonary vascular markings. In VSD, it is the LV that does volume overwork, not the RV, resulting in LV enlargement. Note the absence of RV enlargement. Since the shunt of VSD occurs mainly during systole when the RV also contracts, the shunted blood goes out directly to the PA rather than remaining in the RV cavity. Therefore, there is no significant volume overload to the RV and the RV remains relatively normal in size (Figs 9–4 and 9–5). Note the difference between VSD and ASD with respect to the presence of LA enlargement. Also note the similarities between VSD and PDA as to the presence of enlarged LA and LV (see Fig 9–8).

Figure 9–6 summarizes the hemodynamics of VSDs of different sizes and helps in understanding the clinical manifestations. The size of the chamber is

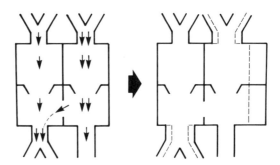

FIG 9–4.
Block diagram of VSD that shows the chambers and vessels that will be enlarged. There is an enlargement of the LA and LV. The MPA is prominent and the pulmonary vascularity increased. Note the absence of RV enlargement (see text for explanation).

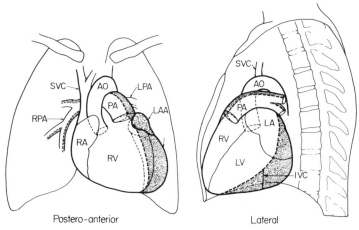

FIG 9–5.
PA and lateral view diagrams of chest roentgenograms of a moderate VSD. Enlargement of the LA, LV, and MPA and increased pulmonary vascular markings are present. Note the presence of LA enlargement, which is absent in ASD.

directly related to the amount of blood handled by the chamber or the number of arrows, and the overall heart size is also determined by the number of arrows.

With a *small* VSD, there is only one-half of an arrow coming from the LV to the MPA, and the degree of pulmonary vascular congestion and the chamber enlargement is either minimal or too small to result in a significant change on

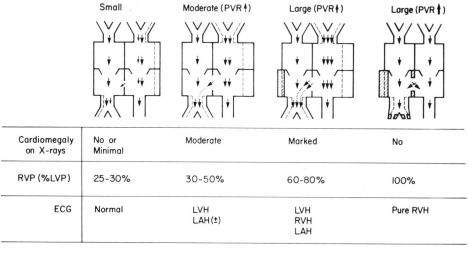

	Small	Moderate (PVR ↑)	Large (PVR ↑)	Large (PVR ↑)
Cardiomegaly on X-rays	No or Minimal	Moderate	Marked	No
RVP (%LVP)	25–30%	30–50%	60–80%	100%
ECG	Normal	LVH LAH(±)	LVH RVH LAH	Pure RVH

FIG 9–6.
Diagrammatic summary of pathophysiology of VSD. Most of the x-ray and ECG findings can be deduced from this diagram (see text for full description). LAH = left atrial hypertrophy; LVH = left ventricular hypertrophy; LVP = left ventricular pressure; RVH = right ventricular hypertrophy; RVP = right ventricular pressure; PVR = pulmonary vascular resistance.

chest x-rays. The degree of volume work imposed on the LV is also too small to produce LVH on the ECG (see Fig 9–6). The shunt itself will produce a heart murmur (regurgitant systolic), and the intensity of P2 will be normal, as the PA pressure is normal.

With a VSD of moderate size *(moderate VSD)*, one arrow shunts from the LV, and all the chambers that are enlarged handle two arrows. Therefore, the cardiomegaly on the x-ray will be of significant degree. The volume overwork done by the LV is significant so that the ECG will produce LVH (of "volume overload" type). Although the shunt is large, the RV is not significantly dilated (as discussed above), and the pressure in this chamber is only slightly elevated (see Fig 9–6). In other words, in moderate VSD the RV is under no significant volume or pressure overload, and, therefore, ECG signs of RVH are absent. As in a small VSD, a heart murmur (regurgitant systolic type) is produced by the left-to-right shunt itself. The normal-sized mitral valve handles two arrows. This relative mitral stenosis will produce a middiastolic rumble at the apex. The PA pressure is mildly elevated; therefore, the intensity of P2 may be slightly increased.

With a *large VSD*, the overall heart size is greater than that seen with moderate VSD, as there is a much greater shunt. Since there is direct transmission of the LV pressure through the large defect to the RV along with a much greater shunt, the RV becomes enlarged and hypertrophied. Therefore, the x-ray will show biventricular enlargement, LA enlargement, and greatly increased pulmonary vascularity. The ECG will show combined ventricular hypertrophy (CVH) and sometimes LAH (see Fig 9–6). Large VSD usually results in CHF.

When large VSD is left untreated, irreversible changes take place in the pulmonary arterioles. With gradual development of the *pulmonary vascular obstructive disease* (PVOD) or *Eisenmenger's syndrome*, which may take years, striking changes occur in the heart size, ECG, and clinical findings. Since the PVR is notably elevated at this stage, approaching systemic level, the magnitude of the left-to-right shunt decreases. This results in the removal of a volume overload placed on the LV. Therefore, the size of the LV and the overall heart size decreases and the ECG evidence of LVH disappears, leaving RVH because of the persistence of pulmonary hypertension. Although the heart size becomes small, the MPA segment remains enlarged because of persistent pulmonary hypertension. In other words, with development of PVOD, the heart size returns toward normal except for a prominent MPA segment and pure RVH on ECG results. A bidirectional shunt will cause cyanosis. Since the shunt is small, the loudness of the murmur decreases or the murmur may even disappear. The S2 is loud and single because of the pulmonary hypertension.

C. Patent Ductus Arteriosus (PDA)

The hemodynamics of PDA are similar to those of VSD. The magnitude of the left-to-right shunt is determined by the *resistance* offered by the ductus (diameter and length, as well as tortuosity) when the ductus is small, and by the level of *pulmonary vascular resistance* when the ductus is large (dependent shunt). Therefore, the onset of CHF with a PDA is similar to that with VSD.

As can be seen in Figure 9–7, the chambers and vessels that are enlarged are the same as in VSD, with the exception of an enlarged aorta up to the level of PDA (enlarged ascending aorta). Therefore, in PDA chest x-rays will show enlargement of LA and LV, and large ascending aorta and MPA in addition to an increase in pulmonary vascular markings (Fig 9–8). Although the aorta is enlarged, since the aorta does not form the cardiac silhouette, it usually does not

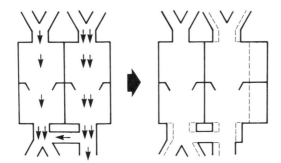

FIG 9–7.
Block diagram of the heart in PDA. Note the similarities between PDA and VSD as to the chamber enlargement. There is an enlargement of the aorta to the level of the ductus arteriosus.

produce an abnormal cardiac silhouette. Therefore, chest x-rays of PDA are indistinguishable from those of VSD.

Hemodynamic consequences of PDA are similar to those of VSD, which have already been discussed. In PDA with a small shunt, the LV enlargement is minimal, and therefore the ECG and chest x-ray findings are near normal. As there is a significant pressure gradient between the aorta and the PA both in systole and diastole, the left-to-right shunt occurs throughout the cardiac cycle, producing the characteristic continuous murmur of this condition. The intensity of the P2 is normal, as the PA pressure is normal.

In PDA with a moderately large shunt, the heart size is moderately enlarged with increased PBF. The chambers enlarged are the LA, LV, and the MPA segment. The ECG shows LVH as in moderate VSD. In addition to the characteristic continuous murmur, there may be an apical diastolic flow rumble owing to relative mitral stenosis. The P2 is slightly increased in intensity, if it can be separated from the loud heart murmur.

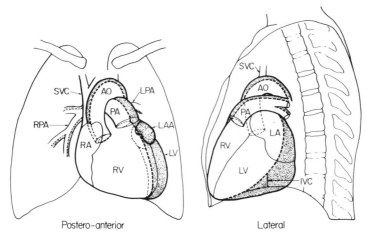

Postero-anterior   Lateral

FIG 9–8.
Diagrammatic drawing of the PA and lateral chest x-rays of PDA. Note the similarities in chest x-rays between PDA and VSD.

In large PDA, marked cardiomegaly and increased pulmonary vascular markings will be present. The volume overload is on the LV and LA, producing LVH and occasional LAH on the ECG. The free transmission of aortic pressure to the PA produces pulmonary hypertension and RV hypertension, with resulting RVH on the ECG. Therefore, the ECG shows CVH and LAH as in a large VSD. The continuous murmur is present with a loud apical diastolic rumble owing to a relative mitral stenosis. The P2 is accentuated in intensity because of pulmonary hypertension.

An untreated large PDA can also produce PVOD, with resulting bidirectional (right-to-left and left-to-right) shunt at the ductus level. The bidirectional shunt will produce cyanosis only in the lower half of the body (differential cyanosis). As in VSD with Eisenmenger's syndrome, the heart size returns to normal because of the reduced magnitude of the shunt. The peripheral pulmonary vascularity decreases, but the central hilar vessels and the MPA segment are greatly dilated because of severe pulmonary hypertension. The ECG shows pure RVH because the LV is no longer under volume overload. Auscultation no longer reveals the continuous murmur or the apical rumble as a result of the reduced shunt. The S2 is single and loud because of pulmonary hypertension.

D. Endocardial Cushion Defect (ECD)

During fetal life, the endocardial cushion tissue contributes to the closure of the lower part of the atrial septum (ostium primum) and of the upper part of the ventricular septum, and to the formation of the mitral and tricuspid valves. The failure of this tissue to develop may be complete or partial. A simplistic way of understanding the complete form of ECD is that the tissue in the center of the heart is missing, with resulting VSD, primum-type ASD, and clefts in the mitral and tricuspid valves. In the partial form of the defect, only an ASD is present at the site of ostium primum (primum-type ASD), often associated with a cleft in the mitral valve.

Hemodynamic abnormalities of primum-type ASD are similar to those of secundum-type ASD, in which the RA and RV are dilated with increased PBF (Fig 9–9), and this will be expressed in the chest x-rays (see Fig 9–3). The cleft mitral valve is usually not significant from a hemodynamic point of view because blood regurgitated into the LA is immediately shunted to the RA, decompressing the LA. The physical findings are also similar to those of secundum ASD: a widely split and fixed S2, a systolic ejection murmur at the ULSB, and a mid-diastolic rumble (of relative tricuspid stenosis) at the LLSB. In addition, a systolic murmur of mitral regurgitation may also be present. The ECG findings are also similar—RBBB (rsR′ in V1) or mild RVH. One exception, important in differentiating between the two types of ASD, is the presence of "superior" QRS axis or left anterior hemiblock (in the range of $-20°$ to $-150°$) in the primum-type ASD. The abnormal QRS axis seen in ECD (both partial and complete forms) is not due to any of the hemodynamic abnormalities mentioned, but to a primary abnormality in the development of the His bundle and the bundle branches.

Hemodynamic changes seen with complete ECD are the sum of those of ASD and VSD. The magnitude of the left-to-right shunt in both ASD and VSD is determined by the level of PVR (dependent shunt). It has volume overload on the LA and LV as in VSD and in part owing to mitral regurgitation. In addition, it has volume overload of the RA and RV as in ASD (see Fig 9–9). This is translated to chest x-rays as biatrial and biventricular enlargement (Fig 9–10). The ECG also reflects these changes as combined ventricular hypertrophy

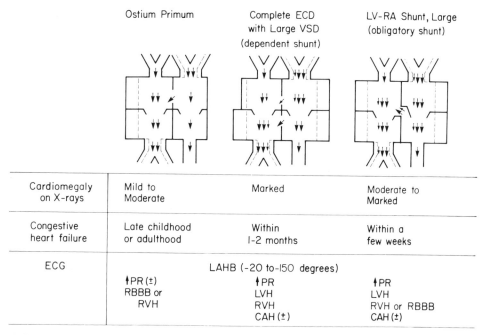

	Ostium Primum	Complete ECD with Large VSD (dependent shunt)	LV-RA Shunt, Large (obligatory shunt)
Cardiomegaly on X-rays	Mild to Moderate	Marked	Moderate to Marked
Congestive heart failure	Late childhood or adulthood	Within 1-2 months	Within a few weeks
ECG	LAHB (-20 to-150 degrees)		
	↕PR (±) RBBB or RVH	↕PR LVH RVH CAH (±)	↕PR LVH RVH or RBBB CAH (±)

FIG 9–9.
Hemodynamic changes in different types of ECD. Hemodynamics of the ostium primum-type ASD are identical to those of the secundum-type ASD. The cleft mitral valve is usually not significant from a hemodynamic point of view. In complete ECD, the hemodynamic changes are the sum of those of VSD and ASD, resulting in enlargement of all four cardiac chambers and increased PBF. Again, the cleft mitral valve is not significant, and its effect is not shown here. The shunt is dependent on the level of the pulmonary vascular resistance (dependent shunt). In the LV–RA shunt, the shunt is not dependent on the level of PVR, but on the size of the defect (obligatory shunt). Therefore, CHF may occur within the first weeks of life. CAH = combined atrial hypertrophy; LVH = left ventricular hypertrophy; LAHB = left anterior hemiblock; RBBB = right bundle branch block; RVH = right ventricular hypertrophy.

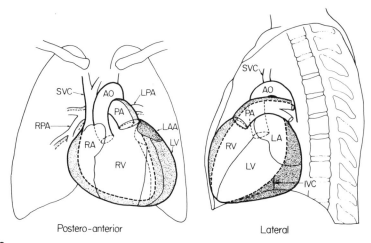

FIG 9–10.
Diagrammatic drawing of chest roentgenograms in the complete form of ECD. All four cardiac chambers are enlarged with increased pulmonary vascular markings.

99

(CVH) and occasional combined atrial hypertrophy (CAH). Left anterior hemiblock is characteristic of ECD. Physical examination is characterized by a hyperactive precordium and systolic murmurs of VSD and mitral regurgitation, loud and narrowly split S2 (because of pulmonary hypertension), apical and/or tricuspid diastolic rumble, and signs of CHF. Those who survive infancy may develop PVOD as has been discussed for large VSD or large PDA.

A direct communication between the LV and RA may occur either as part of ECD or as an isolated defect unrelated to ECD. The direction of the shunt is from the high-pressure LV to the low-pressure RA, and the magnitude of the shunt is determined by the *size* of the defect, regardless of the state of PVR; blood shunted to the RA must go forward through the lungs even if the PVR is high. This type of shunt, which is independent of the status of PVR, is called "obligatory" shunt (see Fig 9–9). Congestive heart failure occurs within a few weeks, much earlier than in the usual VSD. The chambers enlarged are identical to those of the complete form of ECD. Therefore, the chest x-rays and ECG findings are similar to those seen in complete ECD. Physical findings are also similar to those of complete ECD, although the holosystolic murmur may be more prominent at the MRSB.

10 / Pathophysiology of Obstructive and Valvular Regurgitant Lesions

In this chapter hemodynamic abnormalities of obstructive and valvular regurgitant lesions of both congenital and acquired etiologies will be discussed. For convenience, they will be divided into the following three groups based on hemodynamic similarities:

1. Ventricular outflow obstructive lesions (AS, PS, COA).

2. Stenosis of atrioventricular (AV) valves (mitral stenosis, tricuspid stenosis).

3. Valvular regurgitant lesions (mitral regurgitation, aortic regurgitation, pulmonary regurgitation).

I. OBSTRUCTION TO VENTRICULAR OUTPUT

Common congenital obstructive lesions to ventricular output are aortic stenosis (AS), pulmonary stenosis (PS), and coarctation of the aorta (COA). All of these obstructive lesions produce the following three pathophysiologic changes (Fig 10–1):

a. An ejection systolic murmur (auscultation).

b. Hypertrophy of the responsible ventricle (ECG).

c. Poststenotic dilatation (chest x-rays). The poststenotic dilatation is not seen with subvalvular stenosis, isolated infundibular stenosis, or with supravalvular stenosis.

A. Aortic and Pulmonary Valve Stenoses

An ejection type systolic murmur is best audible when the stethoscope is placed over the area distal to the obstruction. Therefore, the murmur of AS is usually loudest over the ascending aorta (URSB or aortic valve area), and the murmur of PS is loudest over the main pulmonary artery (ULSB or pulmonary valve area). However, the actual location of the aortic valve is under the sternum at the level of 3LICS, and the murmur of AS may be quite loud at 3LICS.

In isolated stenosis of the pulmonary or aortic valve, the intensity and duration of the ejection type systolic murmur are directly proportional to the severity of the stenosis. In mild stenosis of a semilunar valve, the murmur is of low intensity (grade 1–2/6) and occurs early in systole, with the apex of the "diamond" in the first half of the systole. With increasing severity of the stenosis, the murmur becomes louder (often with a thrill), and the apex of the murmur moves toward the S2. With mild pulmonary valve stenosis, the S2 either is normal or may split widely because of prolonged "hangout time" (see splitting

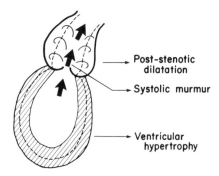

FIG 10–1.
Three secondary changes in ventricular outflow obstructive lesions. A normal-sized ventricle and a great artery are shown in broken lines.

of S2, chap. 2). With severe PS, the murmur may go beyond the A2, the S2 splits widely, and the intensity of the P2 decreases (Fig 10–2,A). With severe AS, the S2 becomes either single or split paradoxically, because of the delayed A2 in relation to the P2 (see Fig 10–2,B). In semilunar valve stenosis an ejection click may be present, which is produced by a sudden checking of the valve motion, or possibly, the sudden distention of the dilated great arteries.

If the obstruction is severe enough, the ventricle that has to pump blood against the obstruction will hypertrophy. The LV will hypertrophy in aortic stenosis and the RV in pulmonary stenosis, resulting in LVH and RVH, respectively, on the ECG. Cardiac output is maintained unless myocardial failure occurs in very severe cases, and, therefore, the heart size remains normal.

Poststenotic dilatation of a significant degree is the hallmark of an obstruction at the valvular level. It is not seen with subvalvular stenosis, and it is seen only mildly or not at all with supravalvular stenosis. The mechanism of poststenotic dilatation is believed to be the result of fatigue of collagen fibers owing to sustained vibration of the vessel distal to the narrowing. In pulmonary valve stenosis, a prominent MPA segment is visible on chest x-rays (see Fig 4–7,A). In aortic valve stenosis, a dilated aorta may be seen as a bulge on the right upper mediastinum or as a prominence of the aortic knob on the left upper medias-

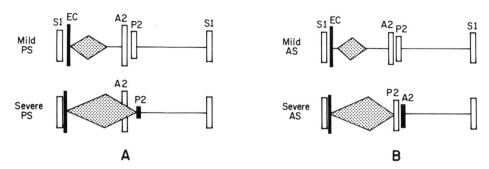

FIG 10–2.
Systolic murmurs of pulmonary **(A)** and aortic **(B)** valve stenoses. The duration and intensity of the murmur increase with increasing severity of the stenosis. Note the changes in the splitting of S2 (see text). An ejection click *(EC)* is present in both conditions. Abnormal heart sounds are shown as *black bars.*

tinum (see Fig 4–7,C). Mild dilatation of the ascending aorta secondary to aortic valve stenosis is usually not visible on the plain chest x-ray films, since the ascending aorta does not form the cardiac border.

B. Coarctation of the Aorta (COA)

The murmur of COA is maximally audible over the descending aorta distal to the site of coarctation (left interscapular area). A large percentage of these patients also have aortic valve abnormalities (bicuspid aortic valve), with aortic stenosis murmurs and occasional aortic regurgitation murmurs. The arterial pulses in the lower extremities are weak or absent on palpation. The weak pulse is primarily due to a slow rise of the upstroke of the pulse.

In coarctation of the aorta, LVH is present on ECG for obvious reasons in older children. However, it is RVH or RBBB (rather than LVH) that is seen in infants, especially those with preductal type of COA. It is not difficult to understand why the preductal COA produces RVH rather than LVH. During fetal life, the RV normally performs 55% and the LV 45% of combined ventricular volume work (RV:LV volume work ratio of 55:45). If the COA is preductal (Fig 10–3,A) during fetal life, the LV sees an increased level of resistance to the forward cardiac output than does the RV during fetal life. More volume work, therefore, is delegated to the RV; for example, RV:LV volume work ratio of 65:35, resulting in a greater dominance of the RV. RVH seen in the preductal type of COA is primarily due to increased volume overload of the RV during fetal life. This RVH is gradually replaced by LVH by 2 years of age.

On chest x-rays, the poststenotic dilatation of the descending aorta distal to the coarctation often produces the figure-of-3 sign on the plain film or E sign on the barium esophagogram (see Fig 4–8).

There are two major differences between the preductal and postductal COA with respect to the degree of development of collateral circulation and the incidence of associated intracardiac defects. These account for the differences in clinical manifestations between the two types of COA. First, the presence of a pressure gradient between the proximal and distal portions of the aorta during fetal life is a strong stimulus for the development of collaterals. Such a pressure gradient is absent in the preductal type, since the descending aorta is perfused by the RV at the systemic pressure through the ductal right-to-left shunt during fetal life (see Fig 10–3,A), resulting in little or no collateral development. When the ductus closes after birth, there is a sudden decrease in perfusion of the descending aorta, with resulting circulatory shock and renal shutdown. However, in the postductal type of COA, a marked pressure difference is present

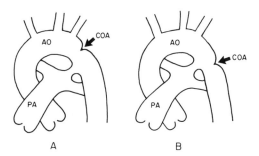

FIG 10–3.
Two types of coarctation of the aorta in relation to the patent ductus arteriosus. **A,** preductal; and **B,** postductal.

between the ascending and descending aortas during fetal life, resulting in well-developed collateral circulation at the time of birth (Fig 10–3,B). In these infants, closure of the ductus after birth will not result in dramatic decrease in the perfusion of the descending aorta and the kidneys. Second, there is a higher incidence of intracardiac anomalies in the preductal COA. The combination of the absence of collaterals at birth and the presence of other intracardiac defects is responsible for the early onset of severe CHF in infants with the preductal type of COA.

Occasionally, a combination of COA and PDA may exist. If the COA is distal to the PDA (postductal COA), there will be a varying degree of left-to-right shunt through the ductus. The magnitude of the shunt will be determined by the size of the ductus and the severity of the coarctation. The majority of the patients develop CHF in early infancy. If there is a combination of preductal COA (usually tubular hypoplasia of the aortic arch) and a permanent distal ductus (in association with PVOD and RV hypertension), the lower half of the body will receive unoxygenated blood from the RV through a right-to-left ductal shunt, producing differential cyanosis (cyanosis only in the lower half of the body). If the ductus is large, peripheral pulses (or blood pressure) in the legs may be normal or only slightly diminished.

II. STENOSIS OF ATRIOVENTRICULAR VALVES

Stenosis of atrioventricular valves produces obstruction to pulmonary or systemic venous return. Clinical manifestations are the result of passive congestion in the pulmonary or systemic venous system.

A. Mitral Stenosis (MS)

Stenosis of the mitral valve is more often rheumatic than congenital in origin. It produces a diastolic rumble and certain changes in the LA, pulmonary vein and artery, and the RV—structures proximal to the point of obstruction.

When significant mitral stenosis is present, the LA becomes dilated and hypertrophied (Fig 10–4). The pressure in the LA is raised with a pressure gradient between the LA and LV during diastole. The elevated LA pressure in turn raises pulmonary venous and capillary pressures. Pulmonary edema may result if the hydrostatic pressure in the capillaries exceeds the osmotic pressure of the blood. Therefore, chest x-rays may reveal pulmonary venous congestion or pulmonary edema in addition to LA enlargement. This produces dyspnea, with or without exertion, and orthopnea. The high pulmonary capillary pressure results in reflex arteriolar constriction. The pulmonary arteriolar constriction may help prevent pulmonary edema, but causes pulmonary arterial hypertension (reflected as RVH on ECG and as a prominent MPA segment on x-rays) and ultimate right heart failure (cardiomegaly on x-rays).

The pressure gradient during diastole produces a middiastolic rumble that is best audible at the apex on auscultation. When the mitral valve is mobile (not severely stenotic), an opening snap precedes the murmur (see Fig 21–1). During the last part of diastole, the pressure gradient persists and the LA contracts, producing a presystolic murmur. At the time of the onset of ventricular contraction, the mitral valve leaflets are relatively wide apart because of prolonged atrial contraction, thereby producing a loud S1. If cardiac output is significantly reduced, thready pulses result. The dilated LA contributes to the frequent occurrence of atrial fibrillation in the adult, which would result in the loss of the presystolic phase of the murmur.

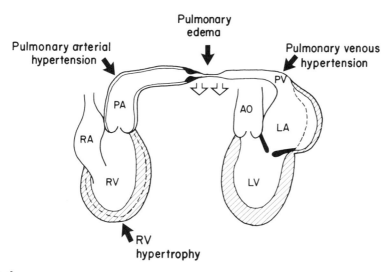

FIG 10–4.
Hemodynamic changes in severe mitral stenosis. Left atrial enlargement and hypertrophy, pulmonary venous hypertension, and possible pulmonary edema result. Reflex vasoconstriction of pulmonary arterioles leads to pulmonary arterial hypertension and right ventricular hypertrophy.

The following conditions, which are characterized by an elevated pulmonary venous pressure, have similar pathophysiology and require differentiation from mitral stenosis:

a. Total anomalous pulmonary venous return with obstruction (see chap. 14).

b. Cor triatriatum (see chap. 17).

c. Stenosis of individual pulmonary vein.

d. Hypoplastic left heart syndrome (see chap. 28).

e. Left atrial myxoma (see chap. 18).

B. Tricuspid Stenosis (TS)
Stenosis of the tricuspid valve is rare and usually congenital. It produces dilatation and hypertrophy of the RA for obvious reasons. Therefore, chest x-rays reveal RA enlargement, and the ECG shows RAH.

Increased pressure in the systemic veins produces hepatomegaly, distended neck veins, and occasional splenomegaly. A middiastolic murmur is produced by a pressure gradient present across this valve during diastole. A prolonged contraction of the RA in order to push blood through the narrow valve may produce a presystolic murmur. It may be associated with hypoplasia of the RV, which exaggerates the obstruction to pulmonary blood flow.

III. VALVULAR REGURGITANT LESIONS

Important valvular regurgitant lesions are aortic and mitral regurgitation. Severe pulmonary valve regurgitation is relatively rare and tricuspid valve regurgitation is rare.

In general, when regurgitation is severe, chambers both proximal *and* distal to a regurgitant valve become dilated with volume overload of these chambers. With mitral regurgitation, both the LV and LA dilate, whereas with aortic regurgitation, the LV enlarges and the aorta either enlarges or increases its pulsation. If the regurgitation is minimal, only auscultatory abnormalities will indicate its presence.

A. Mitral Regurgitation (MR)

The major problem in mitral regurgitation is a volume overload of both the LA and LV with resulting enlargement of these chambers (Fig 10–5). Therefore, chest x-rays reveal enlargement of both the LA and LV, and the ECG may show LVH and LAH.

Regurgitation of blood from the LV to the LA produces a regurgitant systolic murmur that is best audible near the apex. Because of an abnormal increase in the flow across the mitral orifice during the rapid filling phase, the S3 is usually loud. When the regurgitation is significantly large, a middiastolic rumble may be present because of "relative" mitral stenosis in handling an excessive amount of left atrial blood through the normal-sized mitral orifice. The dilated LA chamber tends to dampen the transmission of the pressure from the LV, and the pressure in the LA is usually not notably elevated. Therefore, marked pulmonary hypertension occurs only occasionally.

B. Tricuspid Regurgitation (TR)

Hemodynamic changes similar to those described for mitral stenosis result. The RA and RV enlarge for obvious reasons. The ECG may show RAH and RVH (or RBBB).

A systolic regurgitant murmur, a loud S3, and a diastolic rumble develop as in mitral regurgitation, but they are audible at the tricuspid area (both sides of lower sternal border) rather than at the apex. When the regurgitation is severe, pulsation of the liver and neck veins may occur.

C. Aortic Regurgitation (AR)

There is volume overload of the LV, since this chamber must handle normal cardiac output in addition to that which leaks back to the LV (Fig 10–6). This is represented as LV enlargement on x-rays and LVH on the ECG. Because of the increase in stroke volume that is received by the aorta, although it does not retain all of it, the aorta becomes somewhat dilated.

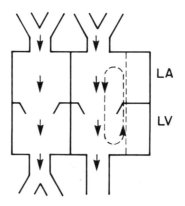

FIG 10–5.
Diagrammatic representation of hemodynamic changes in mitral regurgitation. Note that the chambers with *two arrows* (LA and LV) are enlarged.

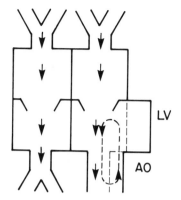

FIG 10–6.
Diagrammatic representation of hemodynamic changes in aortic regurgitation. Note that the LV and aorta, with *two arrows,* are enlarged.

There is an increase in stroke volume with resulting increase in systolic pressure. The diastolic pressure is lower because of continuous leak back to the LV during diastole. This results in a wide pulse pressure and bounding peripheral pulse. The regurgitation during diastole produces a high-pitched decrescendo diastolic murmur immediately following the S2 (see Fig 21–4). The regurgitant flow is directed toward the apex, and the diastolic decrescendo murmur may be audible along the same direction. The aortic regurgitant flow produces flutter motion of the mitral valve coincident with the forward flow of the left atrial blood, producing an Austin-Flint murmur. With severe aortic regurgitation, a high LV end-diastolic pressure approximates the mitral valve leaflets at the onset of the ventricular systole, resulting in a reduced intensity of the S1.

D. Pulmonary Regurgitation (PR)
Pathophysiology of pulmonary regurgitation is similar to that of aortic regurgitation. The RV dilates and the PA may enlarge. This is represented in x-rays as RV enlargement and a prominence of the MPA segment. The ECG may show RVH or RBBB.

Because of the low diastolic pressure of the pulmonary artery, the murmur of pulmonary regurgitation is low-pitched, and the gap between the S2 and the onset of the decrescendo diastolic murmur is wider than that seen in aortic regurgitation. However, in the presence of pulmonary hypertension, the murmur of pulmonary regurgitation resembles that of aortic regurgitation. The direction of the regurgitation is to the body of the RV; therefore, the pulmonary regurgitation murmur is audible along the left sternal border (rather than toward the apex as in aortic regurgitation). This is a helpful auscultatory finding in differentiating pulmonary regurgitation from aortic regurgitation.

11 / Pathophysiology of Cyanotic Congenital Heart Defects

I. RECOGNITION OF CYANOSIS

Cyanosis means a bluish color of the skin and mucous membrane owing to an increased concentration of reduced hemoglobin. About 5 gm/100 ml of reduced hemoglobin in the cutaneous veins is required for clinical recognition of cyanosis. The presence of so much reduced hemoglobin in the cutaneous veins may result from (a) the desaturation of arterial blood or (b) an increased extraction of oxygen by peripheral tissue in the presence of normal arterial oxygen saturation, due to a sluggish flow of blood (such as seen in circulatory shock, hypovolemia, or vasoconstriction from cold). The former is called "central" cyanosis and the latter "peripheral" cyanosis. The manifestation of cyanosis is greatly influenced by the level of hemoglobin. Cyanosis is appreciated with a lesser degree of arterial desaturation (or a higher oxygen saturation) in patients with polycythemia and at a much lower oxygen saturation in patients with anemia. Indeed, adult patients with polycythemia vera and newborn infants with physiologic polycythemia may look cyanotic in the presence of normal oxygen saturation. On the other hand, some patients with anemia who have clear arterial desaturation may have no cyanosis by clinical inspection.

Cyanosis may result from a range of causes. Table 11–1 is a classification of cyanosis based on its mechanism. Early detection of cyanosis of cardiac origin is very important, but detection of mild cyanosis is not easy. In a newborn, acrocyanosis, a normal finding in some newborn infants, may be a source of confusion. In addition, these infants are polycythemic, which adds to the appearance of cyanosis. True cyanosis is more difficult to detect in children with dark pigmentation, and it is perceived better in natural than in artificial light. In older infants and children, chronic cyanosis of mild degree, which may be difficult to detect, will produce clubbing. When in doubt, a hemoglobin or hematocrit should be checked for polycythemia, which occurs with even mild cyanosis. Arterial blood gas values may also be obtained: they will not only detect a mild degree of cyanosis, but also repeated arterial blood gas values in 100% oxygen (hyperoxitest) will help differentiate cyanosis owing to cyanotic heart disease from that owing to lung disease (see also chap. 26). In the presence of lung diseases, inhalation of 100% oxygen for 10 minutes will often increase the arterial Po_2 to 300–400 mm Hg or greater, and almost always raises it above 100 mm Hg. However, in cyanotic heart disease, the arterial Po_2 usually does not rise above 50 mm Hg. Clinically, cyanosis improves on crying in children with lung problems, and it worsens with crying in children with cyanotic heart disease.

TABLE 11–1.

Causes of Cyanosis

Reduced arterial oxygen saturation (central cyanosis)
    Inadequate alveolar ventilation
        CNS depression
        Inadequate ventilatory drive (obesity, pickwickian syndrome)
        Obstruction of the airway, congenital or acquired
        Structural changes in the lungs and/or ventilation-perfusion mismatch (pneumonia,
           cystic fibrosis, hyaline membrane disease, pulmonary edema, congestive heart
           failure, etc.)
        Weakness of the respiratory muscles
    Desaturated blood bypassing effective alveolar units
        Intracardiac right-to-left shunt (cyanotic congenital heart disease)
        Intrapulmonary shunt (pulmonary AV fistula, chronic hepatic disease resulting in
           multiple micro-AV fistulas in the lungs)
        Pulmonary hypertension with the resulting right-to-left shunt at the atrial, ventricular,
           or ductal levels (Eisenmenger's syndrome, persistent pulmonary hypertension of the
           newborn)
Increased deoxygenation in the capillaries (peripheral cyanosis)
    Circulatory shock
    Congestive heart failure
    Acrocyanosis of newborns
Abnormal hemoglobin (unrelated to the degree of oxygenation)
    Methemoglobinemia (well-water ingestion, aniline dye, congenital methemeglobinemia)
    Carbon monoxide poisoning

II. CONSEQUENCES AND COMPLICATIONS OF LONG-STANDING CYANOSIS

A. Polycythemia

Low arterial oxygen content stimulates bone marrow through erythropoietin release from the kidneys, and produces an increased number of red blood cells. Polycythemia, with resulting increase in oxygen-carrying capacity, is beneficial to cyanotic children. However, when the hematocrit reaches 65% or higher, there is a sharp increase in the viscosity of blood, and the polycythemic response becomes disadvantageous, particularly if there is congestive heart failure. Some cyanotic infants have relative anemia with normal or lower than normal hematocrit and hypochromia on blood smear. Although less cyanotic, these infants are usually more symptomatic and improve when the hematocrit is raised by iron therapy.

B. Clubbing

Clubbing is a hypertrophic osteoarthropathy as a consequence of central cyanosis. It usually does not appear until a child is 6 months or older, and is seen first and most pronounced on the thumb. In the early stage, it appears as shininess and redness of the tips of the fingers. When fully developed, the fingers and toes become thick and wide and have convex nail beds (see Fig 2–1). Clubbing is also seen in patients with liver disease, subacute bacterial endocarditis, and on a hereditary basis without cyanosis.

C. Hypoxic Spells and Squatting

Although seen most frequently in infants with tetralogy of Fallot, the hypoxic spell may occur in infants with other forms of cyanotic heart disease. It is characterized by a period of uncontrollable crying, rapid and deep breathing (hyperpnea), deepening of cyanosis, limpness or convulsions, and, occasionally, death. (The mechanism of the hypoxic spell will be discussed in detail under tetralogy of Fallot in this chapter.) A special posture, squatting, is commonly seen in children with right-to-left shunt. This posture has been shown to increase arterial oxygen saturation, probably by a temporary trapping of desaturated blood in the lower extremities.

D. CNS Complications

Cyanotic infants, particularly those with severe hypoxia, are prone to develop CNS disorders: brain abscess or cerebrovascular accident (CVA). Brain abscess tends to occur in infants older than 2 years who have polycythemia and severe cyanosis. CVA occurs more often in infants younger than 2 years who have cyanosis and relative iron-deficiency anemia. A possible explanation for this finding is that hyperviscosity resulting from polycythemia is further aggravated by microcytosis.

E. Bleeding Disorders

Disturbances of hemostasis are frequently present in children with severe cyanosis and polycythemia. Most frequently noted are thrombocytopenia and defective platelet aggregation. Other abnormalities include prolonged PT and PTT and lower levels of fibrinogen and factors V and VIII. Clinical manifestations may include easy bruising, petechiae of skin and mucous membrane, epistaxis, and gingival bleeding. Red cell reduction and replacement with an equal volume of plasma tends to correct the hemorrhagic tendency and lower blood viscosity.

III. COMMON CYANOTIC DEFECTS

A. D-Transposition of the Great Arteries

D-Transposition of the great arteries (D-TGA), commonly called complete transposition of the great arteries, is the most common cyanotic CHD in newborn infants. In this condition, the aorta arises from the RV and the pulmonary artery from the LV. Therefore, the normal anteroposterior relationship of the great arteries is reversed so that the aorta is anterior to the PA (transposition), but the aorta remains to the right of the PA; hence the prefix D is used for dextroposition. In levo-transposition of the great arteries (L-TGA), the aorta is anterior to and to the left of the PA; hence, the prefix L is used (see chap. 14 for further discussion). The atria and ventricles are normally related. The coronary arteries arise from the aorta as in a normal heart. Desaturated blood returning from the body to the RA goes out the aorta, without being oxygenated in the lungs, and returns to the RA. Therefore, tissues including such vital organs as the brain and the heart are perfused by blood with a low oxygen saturation. On the other hand, well-oxygenated blood returning to the LA goes out the pulmonary artery and returns to the LA. The end result is a complete separation of the two circuits. The two circuits are said to be "in parallel" rather than "in series," as in the normal circulation (Fig 11–1). This defect is incompatible with life unless there is a communication between the two circuits to provide the necessary oxygen to the body. This communication can occur at the atrial, ventricular, or ductal level or at any combination of these levels.

The most frequently encountered form of D-TGA is the one in which only a small communication exists between the atria, usually a patent foramen ovale (PFO) (Fig 11–2,A). The newborn infant is notably cyanotic from birth, with

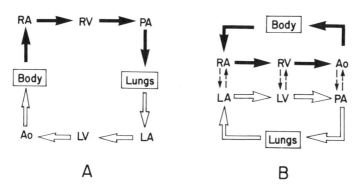

FIG 11–1.
Circulation pathways of normal "in series" circulation **(A)** and the "in parallel" circulation of transposition of the great arteries **(B)**. *Open arrows* indicate oxygenated blood and *closed arrows* desaturated blood.

arterial oxygen saturation of 30%–50%. The low arterial PO_2, which is in the range of 20–30 mm Hg, causes an anaerobic glycolysis, with resulting metabolic acidosis. The hypoxia and acidosis are detrimental to myocardial function. Normal postnatal decrease in pulmonary vascular resistance (PVR) results in increased pulmonary blood flow (PBF) and volume overload to the LA and LV. The severe hypoxia and acidosis (with resulting decrease in myocardial function) and the volume overload to the left side of the heart cause CHF in the first week of life. Therefore, chest x-rays show cardiomegaly and increased pulmonary vascularity. Unless hypoxia and acidosis are eliminated, these infants deteriorate rapidly. Hypoxia and acidosis stimulate the carotid and cerebral chemoreceptors, causing hyperventilation (and a low PCO_2 in the pulmonary circulation). Other metabolic problems encountered are hypoglycemia (probably secondary to pancreatic islet hypertrophy and hyperinsulinism) and a tendency toward hypothermia. The ECG shows RVH, but it may be difficult to diagnose in the first days of life. There is usually no heart murmur, a characteristic finding. The S2 is single, mainly because the pulmonary valve is farther from the

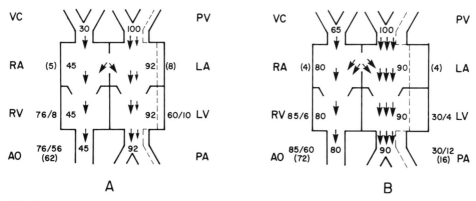

FIG 11–2.
Diagrammatic representation of hemodynamics of TGA with inadequate mixing **(A)** and with a good mixing at the atrial level **(B)**. Numbers within the diagram denote O_2 saturation values and those outside the diagram pressure values.

chest wall, and, therefore, the P2 is not audible. A deeply cyanotic newborn infant with increased pulmonary vascular markings and cardiomegaly without heart murmur can be considered to have TGA until proved otherwise.

The presence of a large ASD is most desirable in infants with TGA. The incidence of these occurring naturally is low, but when they occur together the infants have good arterial O_2 saturation, as high as 80%–90%, because of good mixing (Fig 11–2,B). Therefore hypoxia and metabolic acidosis are not the problems in these children. In fact, the idea of the balloon atrial septostomy (Rashkind procedure) was derived from the natural history of infants with TGA and large ASD. Infants who have had a successful balloon atrial septostomy behave like those with a naturally occurring ASD. As the PVR falls after birth, PBF increases with an increase in the size of the LA and LV. Although these infants are not hypoxic or acidotic, CHF develops because of volume overload to the left side of the heart. Since the RV is the systemic ventricle, RVH becomes evident on the ECG.

When associated with a large VSD, only minimal arterial desaturation is present, and cyanosis may be missed (Fig 11–3,A). Metabolic acidosis, therefore, does not develop, but left heart failure results within the first few weeks of life as the PBF increases with decreasing pulmonary vascular resistance. Chest x-rays will reflect this, showing cardiomegaly with increased pulmonary vascular markings. The ECG may show CVH when the VSD is large: RVH because of the systemic RV, and LVH because of volume overload of the left side of the heart (see Fig 11–3,A). A heart murmur of VSD is present and the S2 is single either because the P2 is inaudible or pulmonary hypertension is present.

The next important group is that associated with VSD and pulmonary stenosis (Fig 11–3,B). Although the VSD helps good mixing, because of pulmonary stenosis, the volume of fully saturated blood returning from the lungs to be shunted to the systemic circulation is inadequate. Likewise, even after a well-performed Rashkind procedure, the arterial oxygen saturation does not increase because of the decreased PBF. These infants have severe hypoxia and acidosis and may succumb early in life. This is a good illustration of how the magnitude of PBF affects the arterial oxygen saturation in a given cyanotic congenital heart defect (see Pathophysiology of Total Anomalous Pulmonary Venous Return for

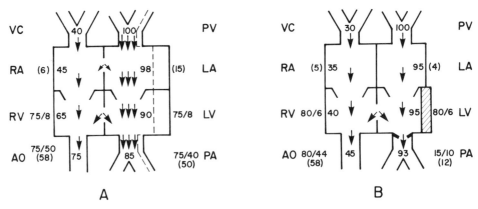

                                A   B

FIG 11–3.
Diagrammatic representation of hemodynamic abnormalities in TGA with a large VSD **(A)** and with VSD and PS **(B)**. Numbers within the diagram denote O_2 saturation values and those outside the diagram pressure values.

further discussion). Since PBF is not increased, the left cardiac chambers are not under increased volume work; therefore, cardiac enlargement and CHF do not develop. This will be reflected in x-rays as a normal heart size and normal or decreased pulmonary vascularity. The ECG will show evidence of CVH: LVH component is present because of pulmonary stenosis and RVH because of the nature of TGA. Physical examination reveals a pulmonary stenosis murmur and a single S2 in addition to cyanosis.

B. Persistent Truncus Arteriosus and Single Ventricle

In persistent truncus arteriosus (Fig 11–4,A), a single arterial blood vessel (truncus arteriosus) arises from the heart. The pulmonary artery or its branches arise from the truncus arteriosus, and the truncus continues as the aorta. A large VSD is always present in this condition. In single (or common) ventricle (Fig 11–4,B), two AV valves empty into a single ventricular chamber from which a great artery (either the aorta or PA) arises. The other great artery arises from a rudimentary ventricular chamber attached to the main ventricle. No ventricular septum of significance is present (see Fig 14–29).

There are similarities between persistent truncus arteriosus and single ventricle from the hemodynamic point of view:

a. There is almost complete mixing of systemic and pulmonary venous blood in the ventricle, and the oxygen saturation of blood in the two great arteries is similar.

b. Pressures in both ventricles are identical.

c. The level of oxygen saturation in the systemic circulation is proportional to the magnitude of PBF.

In addition to the level of PVR, the magnitude of PBF is determined by the caliber of the PA in the case of persistent truncus arteriosus and by the presence or absence of pulmonary stenosis in the case of single ventricle. When the PBF is large, the patient is minimally cyanotic but may develop CHF because of an excessive volume overload placed on the ventricle. In contrast, when the PBF

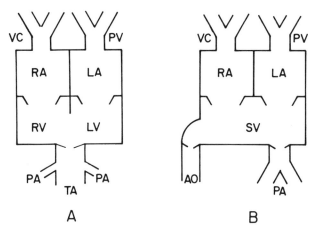

FIG 11–4.
Diagrammatic representation of persistent truncus arteriosus **(A)** and a common form of single ventricle **(B).** SV = single ventricle; TA = truncus arteriosus. Other abbreviations are the same as in Figure 9–1.

is small, the patient is severely cyanotic and does not develop CHF, as there is no volume overload (note the similarity between this latter group and those with tetralogy of Fallot).

Physical examination reveals varying degrees of cyanosis depending on the magnitude of PBF. There is rarely a heart murmur of the VSD because of the huge defect. There may be a stenotic semilunar valve ejection murmur. A diastolic murmur of truncal valve regurgitation may be heard. The ECG usually shows combined ventricular hypertrophy (CVH) in both conditions. In persistent truncus arteriosus, the ECG is similar to that of the large VSD that produces CVH. In single ventricle, the QRS complexes of all precordial leads (V1 through V6) are recorded over *one* ventricle, unopposed by the other ventricle. Therefore, QRS complexes over the entire precordial leads are similar (poor R/S progression), suggesting CVH. Chest x-ray findings are determined by the magnitude of PBF: if large, the heart size is large and the pulmonary vascularity is increased. If small, the heart size is small and the pulmonary vascularity is decreased. With increased PBF and resulting pulmonary hypertension, CHF and later pulmonary vascular obstructive disease (Eisenmenger's syndrome) may develop.

C. Tetralogy of Fallot

The classic description of tetralogy of Fallot (TOF) includes four abnormalities: VSD, pulmonary stenosis, right ventricular hypertrophy, and overriding of the aorta. From a physiologic point of view, TOF requires only two abnormalities— a VSD that is large enough to equalize systolic pressures in both ventricles (as well as in the aorta) and a stenosis of the RV outflow tract (in the form of infundibular stenosis, valvular stenosis, or both). Right ventricular hypertrophy is secondary to pulmonary stenosis, and the overriding of the aorta is not always present. Depending on the severity of the RV outflow tract obstruction, the direction and the magnitude of the shunt through the VSD vary. With mild stenosis, the shunt is left-to-right, and the clinical pictures resemble those of VSD. This is called "acyanotic" or "pink" tetralogy of Fallot (Fig 11–5,A). With

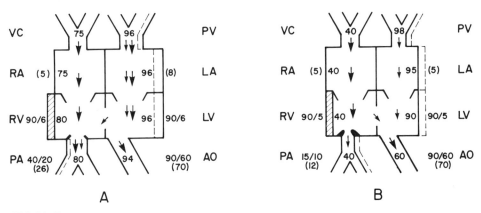

FIG 11–5.
Hemodynamics of acyanotic **(A)** and cyanotic **(B)** tetralogy of Fallot. Numbers within the diagram denote oxygen saturation values and those outside the diagram pressure values. In both conditions, the systolic pressure in the RV is identical to that in the LV and the aorta, and there is a significant pressure gradient between the RV and the PA. In acyanotic form **(A)**, PBF is slightly to moderately increased, whereas in cyanotic form **(B)**, PBF is decreased.

a more severe stenosis, the shunt is right-to-left, resulting in "cyanotic" TOF (Fig 11–5,B). In the extreme form of TOF, the pulmonary valve is atretic with the right-to-left shunting of the entire systemic venous return. In TOF, regardless of the direction of the ventricular shunt, the systolic pressure in the RV is equal to that of the LV and the aorta (see Fig 11–5). It should be noted that mere combination of a small VSD and a PS is not TOF; the size of the VSD must be nearly as large as the anulus of the aortic valve to equalize the pressure in the RV and LV.

In acyanotic TOF, a small-to-moderate left-to-right ventricular shunt is present, and the systolic pressures are equal in the RV, LV, and aorta (see Fig 11–5,A). The PA pressure is slightly elevated, with a moderate pressure gradient between the PA and the RV. Since the presence of the PS minimizes the magnitude of the left-to-right shunt, the heart size and the pulmonary vascularity are slightly to moderately increased, indistinguishable from those of small-to-moderate VSD. However, the ECG always shows RVH because of the high RV pressure, with occasional presence of LVH as well. The heart murmurs originate from the PS and in the VSD. Therefore, the murmur is a superimposition of a systolic ejection murmur (of PS) and a regurgitant systolic murmur (of VSD). The murmur is best audible along the LLSB and MLSB, sometimes extending to the ULSB. Therefore, in a child who has physical and x-ray findings similar to those of small VSD, the presence of RVH or CVH on ECG should raise the possibility of acyanotic TOF. (Small VSD is associated with LVH or normal ECG rather than with RVH or CVH.) Right aortic arch, if present, clinches the diagnosis. Infants with acyanotic TOF become cyanotic with time, usually by 1 or 2 years of age, and have clinical pictures of cyanotic TOF, including exertional dyspnea and squatting.

In infants with classic, cyanotic TOF, the presence of a severe PS produces a right-to-left shunt at the ventricular level (cyanosis) and a decrease in PBF (Fig 11–5,B). The pulmonary arteries are small, and the LA and LV may be slightly smaller than normal because of a reduction in the pulmonary venous return to the left side of the heart. Therefore, chest x-rays show normal heart size with decreased pulmonary vascularity. The systolic pressures are identical in the RV, LV and aorta. The ECG demonstrates RVH because of the pressure overload on the RV. It is important to remember that the right-to-left ventricular shunt is silent and that the heart murmur originates from the pulmonary stenosis (ejection type). The ejection murmur is best audible at the MLSB (over the infundibular stenosis) or occasionally at the ULSB (in cases with pulmonary valve stenosis). The intensity and the duration of the heart murmur are proportional to the amount of blood flow through the stenotic valve. When the PS is mild, a relatively large amount of blood goes through the stenotic valve (and relatively small right-to-left ventricular shunt), producing a loud, long systolic murmur. However, when the PS is severe, there is a relatively large right-to-left ventricular shunt (which is silent), and only a small amount of blood goes through the PS, producing a short, faint systolic murmur. In other words, the intensity and duration of the systolic murmur are *inversely* proportional to the severity of the PS. These findings are in contrast to those seen in isolated PS (Fig 11–6). Because of low pressure in the PA, the P2 is soft and often inaudible, resulting in a single S2. It is worth emphasizing that the heart size on x-rays is normal in TOF; if a cyanotic infant has a large heart on the chest x-rays, especially with an increase in pulmonary vascularity, TOF is very unlikely (unless the child has undergone a large systemic-pulmonary artery shunt operation). Another important point is that the infant with TOF does not develop

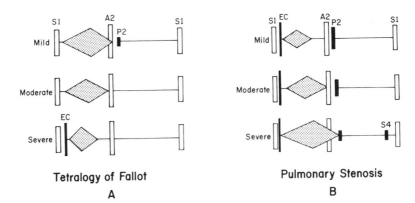

FIG 11–6.
Comparison of systolic ejection murmurs in tetralogy of Fallot **(A)** and isolated pulmonary valve stenosis **(B)** (see text).

CHF. This is because no cardiac chamber is under volume overload, and the pressure overwork placed on the RV is well tolerated, since the RV pressure does not exceed that of the aorta, which is under the baroreceptor control.

The extreme form of TOF is that associated with pulmonary atresia, in which the only source of PBF is through a constricting PDA. All systemic venous return is shunted right-to-left at the ventricular level, resulting in a marked systemic arterial desaturation. Probably the more important reason for such severe cyanosis is the markedly reduced pulmonary venous return to the left side of the heart, as the PBF is severely reduced in this condition. Unless the patency of the ductus is maintained, the infant will succumb. Infusion of prostaglandin E_1 has been successful in this and other forms of cyanotic CHDs that rely on the patency of the ductus arteriosus for PBF. Heart murmur is either absent or a faint murmur of PDA is present. RVH is present on the ECG as in other forms of TOF. Chest x-ray films show small heart (because of markedly reduced PBF).

It is important to understand what controls the degree of cyanosis and the amount of PBF, because this concept applies to understanding the mechanism and treatment of the "hypoxic" spell of TOF. Since the VSD of TOF is large enough to equalize systolic pressures in both ventricles, the RV and LV may be treated as a single chamber that ejects blood to the systemic and pulmonary circuits (Fig 11–7). The ratio of flows to the pulmonary and systemic circuits (Qp/Qs) is related to the ratio of resistance offered by the pulmonary stenosis (pulmonary resistance, PR) and that offered by the systemic vascular resistance (SVR). The degree of right-to-left shunt is increased by either an increase in PR or a decrease in SVR. By the same token, more blood passes through the pulmonary stenosis when SVR increases or PR decreases. Although controversies exist, we treat PR to be constant, since pulmonary valve stenosis has a fixed resistance, and infundibular stenosis consists of disorganized muscle fibers intermingled with fibrous tissue and is relatively nonreactive. Therefore, the degree of right-to-left shunt or the amount of PBF is controlled primarily by changes in SVR. A decrease in SVR will increase the right-to-left shunt and decrease the PBF, with a resulting increase in cyanosis. On the other hand, an increase in SVR lessens the right-to-left shunt and forces more blood through the stenotic RV outflow tract, resulting in improvement in arterial oxygen sat-

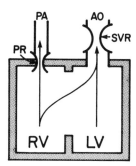

FIG 11–7.
Simplified concept of tetralogy of Fallot that demonstrates how a change in the systemic vascular resistance (SVR) or RV outflow obstruction (pulmonary resistance, *PR*) affects the direction and the magnitude of the ventricular shunt.

uration. Also, excessive tachycardia or hypovolemia will diminish RV filling and exaggerate the RV outflow obstruction, as in hypertrophic obstructive cardiomyopathy (or IHSS) for the LV. The concept discussed above is utilized in the treatment of hypoxic spells (see below).

The *hypoxic spell* (also called cyanotic spell or "tet" spell) occurs in young infants and consists of hyperpnea (*rapid* and *deep* respiration), worsening cyanosis, and disappearance of the heart murmur. This occasionally results in CNS complications and even death. Any event that suddenly lowers the SVR and produces a large right-to-left ventricular shunt (such as crying or defecation in infants or any increase in activity in toddlers) may precipitate the spell (Fig 11–8). The resulting fall in arterial Po_2, along with an increase in Pco_2 and a fall in pH, stimulates the respiratory center and produces hyperpnea. This, in turn, makes the negative thoracic pump more efficient, with the resulting increase in the systemic venous return. In the presence of a fixed opening or fixed resistance at the RV outflow tract (PR), the increased systemic venous return to the RV must go out the aorta, leading to a further decrease in the arterial O_2 saturation. A vicious cycle of hypoxic spells is established (see Fig 11–8).

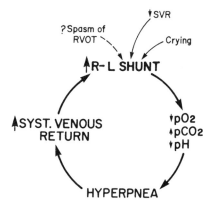

FIG 11–8.
Mechanism of hypoxic spell. A decrease in arterial Po_2 stimulates the respiratory center, and hyperventilation results. Hyperpnea increases systemic venous return. In the presence of a fixed RV outflow tract, the increased systemic venous return results in increased right-to-left shunt, worsening cyanosis. A vicious cycle is established.

Principles of treatment of hypoxic spells are aimed at breaking this vicious cycle by the use of one or more of the following maneuvers:

a. Knee-chest position and holding the baby will trap venous blood in the legs, decreasing the systemic venous return, and will help calm the baby. The knee-chest position might also increase SVR by reducing arterial blood flow through the femoral arteries.

b. Morphine sulfate suppresses the respiratory center and abolishes hyperpnea.

c. NaHCO$_3$ will correct acidosis and eliminate the respiratory center-stimulating effect of acidosis.

d. Oxygen may improve arterial oxygen saturation (but relatively little).

e. Vasoconstrictors such as phenylephrine raise SVR.

f. Propranolol has been used successfully in some cases. Its mechanism of action is not clear; it might reduce "spasm" of the RV outflow tract, but more likely acts peripherally, stabilizing vascular reactivity of the systemic arteries, thereby preventing a sudden decrease in SVR (see chap. 14 for more detailed discussion of treatment of hypoxic spells).

D. Tricuspid Atresia

In tricuspid atresia, the tricuspid valve and the inflow portion of the RV do not exist (Fig 11–9,A and B). Therefore, no direct communication exists between the RA and RV, and systemic venous return to the RA must be shunted to the LA through an ASD or a PFO. The pressure in the RA is elevated in excess of that in the LA and the RA chamber enlarges (RAH on the ECG and RA enlargement on x-rays). The LA and LV receive both the systemic and pulmonary venous returns and therefore dilate (enlargement of the LA and LV on the x-rays). The volume overload placed on the LV is unopposed by the hypoplastic RV, resulting in LVH on the ECG. Therefore, the ECG shows RAH and LVH, and the x-rays show enlargement of the RA, LA, and LV. In addition, left anterior hemiblock (or superior QRS axis) is a characteristic ECG finding in tricuspid atresia as in ECD. Embryologically, there is a similarity between these two defects, since tricuspid atresia results from an incomplete shift of the com-

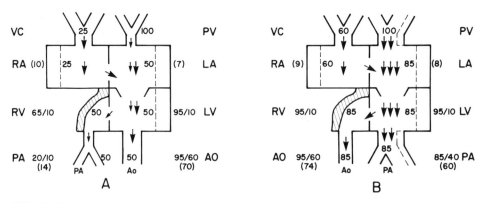

FIG 11–9.
Hemodynamics of tricuspid atresia with normally related **(A)** and transposed **(B)** great arteries. Numbers within the diagram denote O$_2$ saturations and those outside the diagram pressure values.

mon AV canal to the right; this may explain the similar QRS axis in both conditions.

Oxygen saturation values are equal in the aorta and the pulmonary artery, since there is a complete mixing of systemic and pulmonary venous blood in the LV from which both the systemic and pulmonary circuits receive blood. The level of arterial saturation is directly related to the magnitude of PBF. Anatomically, the great arteries are normally related in about 70% of the cases and transposed in about 30% of the cases. In patients with normally related great arteries (Fig 11–9,A), the PBF is in general reduced, since it comes through a small VSD, hypoplastic RV, and/or small pulmonary arteries. Therefore, the arterial O_2 saturation is low and the infant is notably cyanotic. In those infants with transposition of the great arteries (Fig 11–9,B), the PBF is usually greatly increased. Therefore, these infants are only minimally cyanotic, the heart size is large, and the pulmonary vascular markings are increased. However, because of an interplay of other factors, such as the size of VSD, the presence or absence of pulmonary stenosis or atresia, and the patency of the ductus arteriosus, some infants with normally related great arteries may have increased PBF, and some infants with transposed great arteries may have decreased PBF. In tricuspid atresia, the magnitude of PBF determines not only the level of arterial O_2 saturation, but also the degree of enlargement of the cardiac chambers.

No physical findings are characteristic of tricuspid atresia. These infants have varying degrees of cyanosis, and most have a heart murmur of VSD. Pulmonary stenosis murmur, if present, will be characteristic. In patients with increased PBF, increased amount of blood passing through the mitral valve may produce an apical diastolic rumble. The liver may be enlarged because of increased pressures in the RA, which may result from an inadequate interatrial communication or heart failure.

In summary, tricuspid atresia is the most likely diagnosis if a cyanotic infant shows a superiorly oriented QRS axis (left anterior hemiblock), RAH and LVH on the ECG, and an enlargement of the RA (with or without enlargement of the LA and LV), a concave MPA segment (due to hypoplasia of the PA), and decreased pulmonary vascular markings on chest x-rays.

E. Pulmonary Atresia

In pulmonary atresia, there is no direct communication between the RV cavity and the PA; the PDA is the major source of blood flow to the lungs. The systemic venous return to the RA must go to the LA through an ASD or a PFO. The RA enlarges and hypertrophies in order to maintain right-to-left atrial shunt (RA enlargement on x-rays and RAH on the ECG). The RV cavity is usually hypoplastic with a thick ventricular wall ("peach pit" RV, type I) but occasionally is of normal size (type II). Systemic and pulmonary venous returns mix in the LA and go to the LV to supply the body as well as the lungs (Fig 11–10). The volume load placed on the left side of the heart (LA and LV) is proportionally related to the magnitude of PBF. Since the PDA is the major source of PBF and it may close after birth, the PBF is usually decreased. Therefore, the infant is severely cyanotic, and the overall heart size is normal or only slightly increased. The hypoplasia of the RV (and possible volume overload to the LV) produces LVH on the ECG.

The infant is usually notably cyanotic, and the S2 is single because there is only one semilunar valve to close. A faint, continuous murmur of PDA may be present. Closure of the ductus results in a rapid deterioration of these infants.

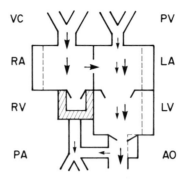

FIG 11–10.
Hemodynamics of pulmonary atresia. The chambers that enlarge are similar to those in tricuspid atresia; therefore, x-ray findings are similar in tricuspid atresia and pulmonary atresia. The ECG also shows LVH but without the characteristic left anterior hemiblock of tricuspid atresia. Because of the decreased PBF, the aortic saturation is low, and the infant is notably cyanotic.

Reopening or maintenance of the PDA with infusion of prostaglandin E_1 will increase PBF, improve cyanosis, and stabilize the infant's condition.

In summary, a severely cyanotic newborn infant, with decreased pulmonary vascularity and normal or slightly enlarged heart size on chest x-rays, and RAH or CAH and LVH on the ECG, may have pulmonary atresia. The QRS axis is usually normal, a finding in contrast to the superior QRS axis of tricuspid atresia. A faint, continuous murmur of PDA may be present.

F. Total Anomalous Pulmonary Venous Return (TAPVR)
In this condition, the pulmonary veins drain abnormally to the RA, either directly or indirectly through its venous tributaries. An ASD is almost always present. Depending on the site of the drainage, TAPVR may be divided into three types (see Fig 14–16).

a. Supracardiac: the common pulmonary vein drains to the SVC through the vertical vein and the left innominate vein.

b. Cardiac: the pulmonary veins empty into the RA directly or indirectly through the coronary sinus.

c. Infracardiac (or subdiaphragmatic): the common pulmonary vein traverses the diaphragm and drains into the portal or hepatic vein or the IVC.

Physiologically, however, TAPVR may be divided into two types: obstructive and nonobstructive, depending on the presence or absence of obstruction to the pulmonary venous return. The infracardiac type is almost always obstructive, and the majority of the cardiac and supracardiac types are nonobstructive.

Hemodynamics of *nonobstructive* types are similar to those of a large ASD. The ratio of the volume of blood shunted from the RA to the LA and the volume that enters the RV is determined by the size of the interatrial communication and the relative compliance of the ventricles. Since the RV compliance normally increases after birth with a rapid fall in the PVR, and the ASD may be of inadequate size, more blood enters the RV than the LA, with resulting volume overload of the right side of the heart and the pulmonary circulation. Therefore, the RA, RV, PA, and PV will be enlarged (Fig 11–11,A). This will be expressed in chest x-rays as an enlargement of the RA and RV, a prominent MPA segment, and increased pulmonary vascularity. The pressures in the RV and PA are slightly elevated. The ECG will show RBBB or RVH, as in secundum ASD, and occasional RAH. Since there is complete mixing of systemic and pulmonary venous return in the RA, oxygen saturation values are nearly identical in the aorta and the PA. Physical examination reveals a systolic ejection murmur at the ULSB owing to increased flow through the pulmonary valve and a diastolic flow rumble of relative tricuspid stenosis, as these valves handle three arrows (see Fig 11–11,A). The S2 splits widely (for reasons that are identical to ASD), and this contributes to the characteristic "quadruple" rhythm of TAPVR, which consists of S1, widely split S2, and S3 or S4. These children with a large PBF are only minimally desaturated, and cyanosis is often missed, as the arterial O_2 saturation is in the range of 85%–90% (see Fig 11–11,A).

If there is an *obstruction* to the pulmonary venous return, the hemodynamic consequences are notably different from those without pulmonary venous obstruction. The obstruction to the pulmonary venous return is almost always present in the infracardiac type and in some cases of supracardiac and cardiac types of TAPVR. The obstruction to the pulmonary venous return causes pulmonary venous hypertension and secondary pulmonary arterial and right ventricular hypertension (Fig 11–11,B) a situation similar to that seen in mitral stenosis (see chap. 10). Pulmonary edema results when the hydrostatic pressure in the capillaries exceeds the osmotic pressure of the blood. The RV cavity, however, remains relatively small (smaller than one arrow) because the RV hypertension prevents the RV compliance from increasing and because the PVR remains elevated. Therefore, chest x-rays will show a relatively small heart and characteristic patterns of pulmonary venous congestion or pulmonary edema ("ground-glass" appearance). The ECG will reflect the high pressure in the RV (RVH). The oxygen saturation values will be equal in the aorta and the PA because of complete mixing of systemic and pulmonary venous return at the RA level, and the arterial saturation will be much lower than that in patients without obstruction. The degree of arterial desaturation (or cyanosis) is inversely related to the amount of PBF. This concept is very important, and we will

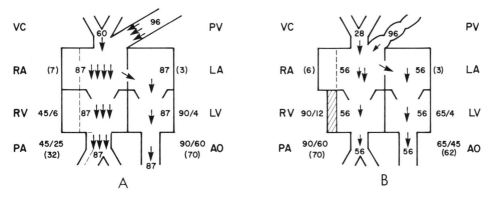

FIG 11–11.
Hemodynamics of TAPVR without **(A)** and with **(B)** obstruction to the pulmonary venous return. In nonobstructive type **(A)**, the hemodynamics are similar to those of a large ASD, with the exception of a mild systemic arterial desaturation. In obstructive type **(B)**, the hemodynamics are characterized by pulmonary venous hypertension, pulmonary edema, pulmonary arterial hypertension, and a marked arterial desaturation. The heart size is not enlarged on chest x-rays. Severe RVH is present on the ECG.

discuss it in detail with two extreme examples of TAPVR (see below). On physical examination, infants with obstruction will have severe cyanosis and respiratory distress. The latter is due to pulmonary edema and may be the cause of pulmonary rales on auscultation. The pulmonary valve closure sound (P2) is loud because of pulmonary hypertension, resulting in a single and loud S2. The heart murmur may be absent because of the lack of increased flow through the pulmonary or tricuspid valve (smaller than one arrow) (Fig 11–11,B).

Full comprehension of the relationship between the magnitude of PBF and the systemic arterial O_2 saturation is very important in the understanding and the management of most cyanotic CHDs. We will discuss this relationship using two extreme examples of TAPVR shown in Figure 11–11.

If the PBF is three times as great as the systemic cardiac output (or blood flow) ($\dot{Q}p/\dot{Q}s$ = 3:1), as in most nonobstructive cases, the arterial oxygen saturation will be close to 90%, and cyanosis will not be obvious (Fig 11–11,A). This figure is derived as follows: an assumed pulmonary venous saturation of 96% and a vena caval saturation of 60% will result in an average mixed venous saturation of 87%:

$$\frac{(96 \times 3) + (60 \times 1)}{4} = 87(\%)$$

The difference in the arterial and venous O_2 saturation is kept at 27% to indicate the absence of heart failure (Fig 11–11,A). If there is an obstruction to the pulmonary venous return and the PBF is small, a marked arterial desaturation will result based on the following calculation (Fig 11–11,B). We assume the PBF is 70% of the systemic flow (Qp/Qs = 0.7:1) and the PV saturation 96%:

$$\frac{(96 \times 0.7) + (28 \times 1)}{1.7} = 56(\%)$$

It is also assumed that the infant is not in heart failure; i.e., the systemic AV difference is 28% (see Fig 11–11,B). This relationship holds true for other forms of cyanotic CHD. *For a given defect, an increase in the magnitude of PBF results in a rise in systemic arterial oxygen saturation, and a decrease in PBF results in a greater arterial desaturation.* An improvement in cyanosis following a systemic-pulmonary artery shunt operation in an infant with decreased PBF is an example of this relationship. On the other hand, an infant with CHF from a single ventricle (in which a large PBF and pulmonary hypertension are present) may improve following a pulmonary artery banding (the procedure which decreases the PBF and lowers pulmonary artery pressure), but the arterial oxygen saturation usually decreases and cyanosis worsens.

PART IV

Specific Congenital Heart Defects

In the following three chapters common left-to-right shunt lesions, obstructive lesions, and cyanotic cardiac defects will be discussed. Aortic arch anomalies, primarily "vascular ring" and cardiac malposition, will be discussed in separate chapters. Miscellaneous rare anomalies that belong to none of the above categories will be grouped into one chapter for brief discussion. Emphasis is on brevity for a quick reference rather than lengthy, essay-type descriptions.

12 / Left-to-Right Shunt Lesions

In this chapter common left-to-right shunt lesions such as atrial septal defect (ASD), ventricular septal defect (VSD), patent ductus arteriosus (PDA), endocardial cushion defect (ECD), and partial anomalous pulmonary venous return (PAPVR) will be discussed.

I. ATRIAL SEPTAL DEFECT (OSTIUM SECUNDUM DEFECT)

Incidence
Five percent to 10% of all congenital heart disease (CHD).

Pathology

1. There is a defect in the atrial septum, at the site of fossa ovalis, allowing left-to-right shunting of blood from the left atrium (LA) to the right atrium (RA) (Fig 12–1). Anomalous pulmonary venous return is present in about 10% of the cases.

2. A defect in the posterosuperior portion of the septum immediately under the SVC is called sinus venosus defect and is often associated with PAPVR to the SVC. (This defect produces clinical manifestations indistinguishable from those of ostium secundum ASD.)

3. Mitral valve prolapse occurs in 20% of patients with either ostium secundum or sinus venosus defect.

Clinical Manifestations

History
Infants and children with ASD are usually asymptomatic.

PE (Figure 12–2 shows cardiac findings.)

a. Somewhat slender body build.

b. Widely split and fixed S2 is a characteristic finding. A grade 2–3/6 systolic ejection murmur is present at ULSB.

c. With a large left-to-right shunt, middiastolic rumble (owing to relative tricuspid stenosis) may be audible at the LLSB.

ECG (Fig 12–3)
Right axis deviation (RAD) ($+90°$ to $+180°$) and mild RVH or RBBB with rsR' pattern in V1.

X-Rays (Fig 12–4)

a. Cardiomegaly with enlargement of the RA and RV.

b. A prominent MPA segment.

c. Increased pulmonary vascular markings.

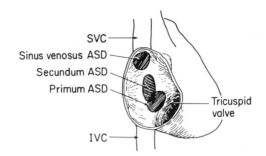

FIG 12–1.
Anatomical types of atrial septal defects, viewed with the right atrial wall removed.

ECHO

a. Two-dimensional echocardiography (2D ECHO) is diagnostic. It shows the position as well as the size of the defect, best seen in the subcostal four-chamber view. It also gives indirect assessment of the magnitude of the shunt.

b. M-mode ECHO may show increased RV dimension and paradoxical motion of the interventricular septum.

Natural History and Complications

a. Spontaneous closure of the defect has been reported in the first 5 years of life (up to 40% in some series). The defect may decrease in size in some children.

b. CHF and pulmonary hypertension may occur in adult life (3rd and 4th decades).

c. Atrial arrhythmias (flutter/fibrillation) may occur in adult life.

d. Infective endocarditis is almost never seen in ASD.

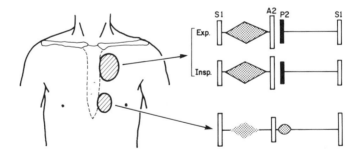

FIG 12–2.
Cardiac findings of atrial septal defect. Exp = expiration; Insp = inspiration; S1 = first heart sound; A2 and P2 = aortic and pulmonary components of the second heart sound, respectively. Throughout this book, heart murmurs *with solid borders* are the primary murmurs, and those *without solid borders* are transmitted murmurs or those occurring occasionally. Abnormalities in heart sounds are shown in *black*.

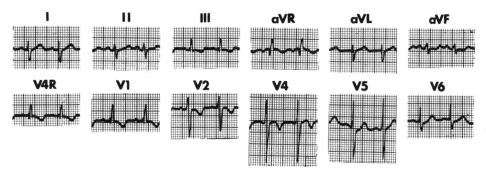

FIG 12–3.
Tracing from a 5-year-old girl with secundum-type ASD.

    e. Cerebrovascular accident due to paradoxical embolization through an ASD is extremely rare.

Management

  Medical

    a. Exercise restriction is not required.

    b. Infective endocarditis prophylaxis is not indicated, unless the patient has associated mitral valve prolapse or PAPVR.

    c. In rare cases of CHF that develop in infancy, medical management is recommended by some because of a possibility of spontaneous closure.

  Surgical

    a. Procedure: Open repair (simple suture or with a patch) under cardiopulmonary bypass.

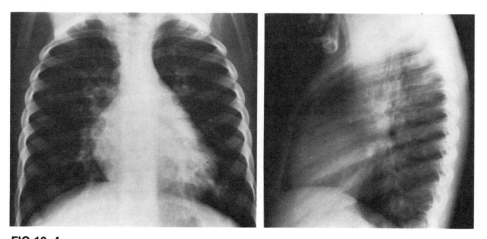

FIG 12–4.
PA and lateral views of chest roentgenogram from a 10-year-old child with ASD. The heart is mildly enlarged with involvement of the RA (best seen in PA view) and the RV (best seen in the lateral view with obliteration of the retrosternal space). Pulmonary vascularity is increased, and the MPA segment is slightly prominent.

b. Indications: A significant left-to-right shunt ($\dot{Q}p/\dot{Q}s > 2:1$).* Small defects do not require repair. High pulmonary vascular resistance (≥ 10 units/m^2) is a contraindication to surgery.

c. Timing: Usually performed in children 2–5 years of age. Delayed until 4–5 years of age by those who believe there is a high rate of spontaneous closure. Rarely performed during infancy; only if CHF not responding to medical management.

d. Mortality: Less than 1%. Higher risk in small infants and those with CHF or increased PVR.

e. Complications:

1) Postoperative arrhythmias, including atrial flutter/fibrillation, atrial tachycardia, and nodal rhythm, may develop in the immediate postoperative period or later.

2) Sick sinus syndrome is occasionally seen following ASD repair, particularly sinus venosus defect.

Follow-up

1. Heart size on x-rays may remain abnormal up to 1–2 years postoperatively, and wide splitting of the S2 may persist.

2. Some patients manifest mitral valve prolapse syndrome (MVPS).

Differential Diagnosis

The following conditions have some similarities with ASD and require differentiation from ASD. (Also refer to Table 2–5.)

a. Functional pulmonary ejection murmur (see chap. 2).

b. Mild pulmonary stenosis (see chap. 2). Pulmonary vascular marking is normal in this condition.

c. Ebstein's anomaly. Pulmonary vascularity is not increased.

d. Partial anomalous pulmonary venous return (PAPVR). This defect is often associated with ASD. Isolated PAPVR resembles findings of secundum ASD, with the exception of the S2, which is generally normally split.

II. VENTRICULAR SEPTAL DEFECT (VSD)

Incidence

The most common form of congenital heart disease (20%–25% of all CHD).

Pathology

1. The ventricular septum may be divided into a small membranous portion (black area in Fig 12–5) and a large muscular portion. The muscular septum has three components: inlet, trabecular, and infundibular (outlet) components (see Fig 12–5).

2. A VSD may be classified into perimembranous, muscular, and subarterial infundibular defects, with further subdivisions (see Fig 12–5):

---

*$\dot{Q}p/\dot{Q}s$ is the ratio of pulmonary to systemic blood flow (see chap. 7). In normal persons without a shunt lesion, the $\dot{Q}p/\dot{Q}s$ ratio is 1:1.

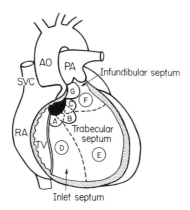

FIG 12–5.
Anatomical locations of various ventricular septal defects, viewed with the right ventricular free wall removed. A = perimembranous inlet ("AV canal-type") VSD; B = perimembranous trabecular (typical membranous) VSD; C = perimembranous infundibular ("tetralogy-type") VSD; D = Inlet muscular VSD; E = trabecular muscular VSD; F = infundibular (or outlet) muscular VSD; G = subarterial infundibular ("supracristal") VSD. *Black area* represents the membranous ventricular septum.

    a. Perimembranous VSD (70%) are those membranous VSDs that extend into adjacent inlet (AV canal-type), trabecular (typical membranous VSD), or infundibular (tetralogy-type) muscular septum. Isolated membranous VSD (black area) is extremely rare.

    b. Muscular VSD (25%) are those defects located entirely within the muscular septum such as inlet, trabecular, or infundibular septum.

    c. Subarterial infundibular defect (supracristal VSD) (5%) is located in the infundibular septum, and part of the rim is formed by the aortic and pulmonary valve anulus.

3. The defect varies in size, ranging from a tiny defect without hemodynamic significance to a large defect with pulmonary hypertension and CHF.

4. The AV conduction axis is always related to the posteroinferior quadrant of perimembranous defects and the superoanterior quadrant of the inlet muscular VSD. Defects in other parts of the septum are usually unrelated to the conduction tissue.

5. Frequently associated with PDA or COA.

6. In subarterial infundibular (or supracristal) VSD, the aortic valve may prolapse through the VSD because of the absence of support for the valve, with resulting aortic regurgitation (AR) (see VSD-AR Syndrome below).

Clinical Manifestations

History

    a. Small VSD: Normal growth and development without symptoms.

    b. Moderate to large VSD: Decreased exercise tolerance, repeated pulmonary infections, delayed growth and development, and CHF are relatively common in infancy.

    c. With long-standing pulmonary hypertension: History of cyanosis and decreased level of activity may be present.

PE (Figures 12–6 and 12–7 show cardiac findings.)

    a. Infants with small VSD are well developed and acyanotic. Infants with large VSD may have poor weight gain or signs of CHF (usually by 2–3 months of age). Cyanosis and clubbing may be present in PVOD or Eisenmenger's stage.

    b. A systolic thrill may be present at the LLSB. Precordial bulge and hyperactivity are present with a large-shunt VSD.

    c. A grade 2–5/6 regurgitant systolic murmur is present at the LLSB (see Figs 12–6 and 12–7). It may be holosystolic or early systolic.

    d. An apical diastolic rumble is present with a moderate to large shunt (see Fig 12–7).

    e. The intensity of the P2 is normal with a small shunt, moderately increased with a large shunt (see Fig 12–7), and loud (and single S2) in PVOD.

    f. With subarterial infundibular ("supracristal") VSD, a grade 1–3/6 early diastolic decrescendo murmur of AR may be audible.

ECG (see chap. 7)

    a. Small—normal.

    b. Moderate—LVH, LAH (±) (see Fig 3–15).

    c. Large—CVH, LAH (±) (Fig 12–8).

    d. PVOD—pure RVH.

X-Rays (Fig 12–9)

    a. Cardiomegaly of varying degrees involving the LA, LV, and possibly the RV is present. The degree of cardiomegaly and the increase in pulmonary vascularity are directly related to the magnitude of the left-to-right shunt.

    b. Pulmonary vascular markings (PVM) are increased.

    c. In PVOD, the MPA and the hilar pulmonary arteries are notably enlarged, but the peripheral lung fields are ischemic.

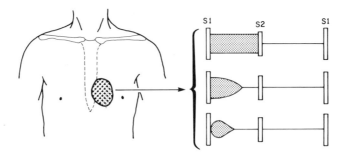

FIG 12–6.
Cardiac findings of a small VSD. A regurgitant systolic murmur is best audible at the LLSB; it may be holosystolic or less than holosystolic. Occasionally, the heart murmur is in early systole. A systolic thrill *(dots)* may be palpable at the LLSB. The S2 splits normally and the P2 is of normal intensity.

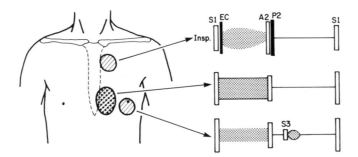

FIG 12–7.
Cardiac findings of a large VSD. A classic holosystolic regurgitant murmur is audible at the LLSB. A systolic thrill is also palpable at the same area *(dots)*. There is usually a middiastolic rumble (due to relative mitral stenosis) at the apex. The S2 is narrowly split and the P2 is accentuated in intensity. Occasionally an ejection click (EC) may be audible in the ULSB when associated with pulmonary hypertension. The heart murmurs shown without solid borders are those murmurs that are transmitted from other areas and are not characteristic of the defect. Abnormal sounds are shown in *black*.

ECHO (Fig 12–10)

   a. 2D ECHO provides accurate diagnosis of the position and the size of the VSD (Fig 12–10).

   b. LA and LV dimensions (by M-mode and 2D ECHO) provide indirect assessment of the magnitude of the shunt.

   c. M-mode ECHO of the pulmonary valve and Doppler studies of the pulmonary artery can be useful in indirect assessment of PA pressure and PVR.

Natural History and Complications

   a. Spontaneous closure occurs in 30%–40% of all VSDs. It occurs more frequently in small defects and more often in the first year of life than thereafter.

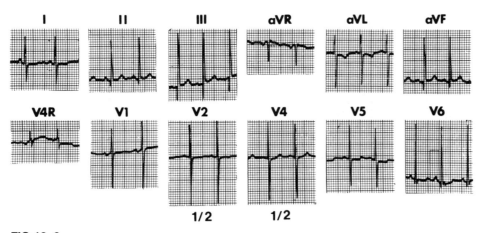

FIG 12–8.
Tracing from a 3-month-old infant with large VSD, PDA, and pulmonary hypertension. The tracing shows CVH with left dominance. Note that V2 and V4 are in 1/2 standardization.

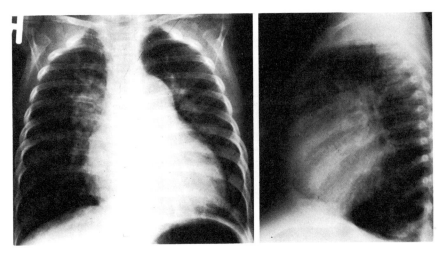

FIG 12–9.
PA and lateral views of chest roentgenogram in VSD with large shunt and pulmonary hypertension. The heart size is moderately increased, with enlargement on both sides. Pulmonary vascular markings are increased, with prominent MPA segment.

    b. Large defects tend to become smaller with age.

    c. Infundibular stenosis may develop in some infants with large defects, with resulting decrease in the magnitude of the left-to-right shunt (acyanotic TOF), and occasionally producing a right-to-left shunt.

    d. CHF develops in infants with large VSD but usually not until 6–8 weeks of age.

    e. Pulmonary vascular obstructive disease (PVOD) may begin to develop as early as 6–12 months of age in patients with untreated large VSD, but right-to-left shunt usually does not develop until the 2nd decade of life.

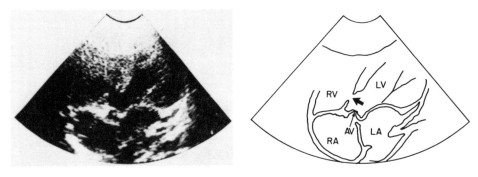

FIG 12–10.
Apical four-chamber view with LV outflow tract in a patient with perimembranous VSD (arrow). AV = aortic valve; LA = left atrium; LV = left ventricle; RA = right atrium; RV = right ventricle.

Management

Understanding of the natural history of VSD is important in planning its management (see above).

Medical

   a. Watch for signs of CHF (changes in feeding patterns and tachypnea are earliest signs of left heart failure).

   b. Treatment of CHF with digitalis and diuretics (see chap. 27).

   c. No exercise restriction is required in the absence of pulmonary hypertension.

   d. Maintenance of good dental hygiene and prophylaxis against infective endocarditis (see chap. 19).

Surgical

   a. Procedure:

      1) PA banding as a palliative procedure is rarely performed unless additional lesions make the complete repair difficult.

      2) Direct closure of the defect under cardiopulmonary bypass and/or deep hypothermia. Atrial approach is preferable to the right ventriculotomy.

   b. Indications and Timing:

      1) Significant left-to-right shunt with $\dot{Q}p/\dot{Q}s$ of greater than 2:1 is an indication for surgical closure. Surgery is not indicated for a small VSD with $\dot{Q}p/\dot{Q}s$ less than 1.5:1.

      2) Infants with CHF and growth retardation unresponsive to medical therapy should be operated on at any age, including infancy. Those infants who respond to medical therapy may be operated on by the age of 12–18 months.

      3) Infants with a large VSD and evidence of increasing PVR should be operated on as soon as possible.

      4) Asymptomatic children with a moderate shunt may be operated on between 2 and 4 years of age.

   c. Contraindications: PVR/SVR 0.5 or greater or PVOD with predominant right-to-left shunt.

   d. Mortality:

      1) Less than 5%.

      2) Mortality is higher in small infants, those with associated defects, or those with multiple VSDs.

   e. Complications:

      1) RBBB in most patients in whom the VSD is repaired via right ventriculotomy.

      2) RBBB + left anterior hemiblock (less than 10%) as a cause of sudden death is controversial.

3) Complete heart block is rare.

4) CVA is extremely rare.

5) Residual shunt, usually small.

f. Surgical Approaches for Special Situations:

1) VSD + PDA: If PDA is large, the ductus alone may be closed in the first 6–8 weeks, and the VSD may be closed at an appropriate time.

2) VSD + COA: Controversies exist. One approach is the repair of COA alone initially with or without PA banding. The VSD is closed later if indicated.

3) VSD-AR Syndrome: The prolapsed aortic cusp with resulting aortic regurgitation (AR) is usually associated with subarterial infundibular (or supracristal) VSD and occasionally with perimembranous VSD. It occurs in about 5% of patients with VSD (higher incidence among the Orientals, 15%–20%). Once AR appears, it gradually worsens. When AR is present, a prompt operation is usually performed, even if the Qp/Qs is less than 2:1, to abort progression of or to abolish AR. When AR is trivial or mild, the VSD alone is closed. When AR is moderate or severe, the aortic valve is repaired or replaced.

III. PATENT DUCTUS ARTERIOSUS (PDA)

Incidence
1. Five percent to 10% of all CHD, excluding premature infants.

2. Female-to-male ratio = 3:1

3. A common problem in premature infants (see chap. 26).

Pathology
Persistent patency of a normal fetal structure between the left PA and the descending aorta.

Clinical Manifestations

History

a. Asymptomatic when the ductus is small.

b. Hoarse cry or cough, as well as lower respiratory tract infection and atelectasis, may be frequent with large shunt.

c. When the defect is large, CHF (with dyspnea and poor weight gain) may develop.

PE (Fig 12–11 shows cardiac findings.)

a. Tachypnea and exertional dyspnea with a large-shunt PDA. Cyanosis in the lower half of the body (differential cyanosis) with PVOD.

b. Bounding peripheral pulses with wide pulse pressure.

c. Hyperactive precordium. A systolic thrill may be present at the ULSB.

d. The P2 is usually normal, but may be accentuated in intensity with pulmonary hypertension.

e. A grade 1–4/6 continuous ("machinery") murmur best audible at the ULSB or left infraclavicular area (see Fig 12–11). The heart murmur may be (crescendo) systolic at the ULSB in a small infant, or if there is pulmonary hypertension.

f. An apical diastolic rumble with a large-shunt PDA.

ECG (Findings similar to those of VSD.)

a. Normal or LVH in small-to-moderate-shunt PDA.

b. CVH in a large PDA.

c. RVH when PVOD develops.

X-Rays (Findings also similar to those of VSD.)

a. May be normal with a small-shunt PDA.

b. Cardiomegaly with an enlargement of the LA and LV (including an enlargement of the ascending aorta) of varying degrees, and an increase in pulmonary vascular markings.

c. With PVOD, the heart size is normal, with marked prominence of the MPA and hilar vessels.

ECHO

a. The PDA can be directly visualized by 2D ECHO in a parasternal short-axis view at the aortic valve level or in a suprasternal notch view (see Figs 6–2 and 26–4).

b. The Doppler examination in the PA or in the descending aorta confirms the ductal shunt.

c. LA and LV dimensions provide indirect assessment of the magnitude of left-to-right ductal shunt.

Natural History and Complications

a. CHF and/or recurrent pneumonia if the shunt is large.

b. PVOD may develop if a large PDA with pulmonary hypertension is left untreated.

c. Infective endocarditis, more frequently with small PDA than with large one.

d. Rarely, aneurysm of PDA with possible rupture.

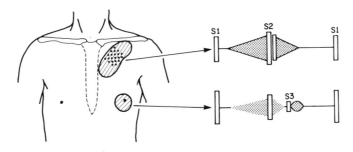

FIG 12–11.
Cardiac findings of patent ductus arteriosus. A systolic thrill may be present in the area shown by *dots.* Abbreviations are the same as in previous figures.

Management

Medical

a. No exercise restriction in the absence of pulmonary hypertension.

b. Precautions against infective endocarditis.

Surgical

a. Indications: Anatomical existence of a PDA regardless of the size.

b. Contraindications: The presence of PVOD.

c. Procedure: Ligation with or without division through left posterolateral thoracotomy (without cardiopulmonary bypass).

d. Timing:

1) Elective procedure any time between 1 and 2 years of age or whenever diagnosis is made in an older child.

2) Urgent operation in infants with CHF, pulmonary hypertension or recurrent pneumonia.

e. Mortality: Less than 1% (excluding premature infants).

f. Complications are rare:

1) Injury to the recurrent laryngeal nerve (hoarseness).

2) Injury to the left phrenic nerve (paralysis of the left hemidiaphragm).

3) Reopening of the ductus (after ligation alone without division); not if done correctly.

4) Chylothorax (injury to the thoracic duct).

Differential Diagnosis

The following are the conditions that may present with continuous murmurs.

1. Coronary AV fistula: The continuous murmur is audible over the precordium (usually along the right sternal border) but not maximally at the ULSB.

2. Systemic AV fistula: A wide pulse pressure with bounding pulse may be present. Heart failure may develop without continuous murmur over the precordium. A continuous murmur may be present over the fistula (head or liver).

3. Pulmonary AV fistula: A continuous murmur over the back, cyanosis, and clubbing in the absence of cardiomegaly are helpful clinical clues.

4. Venous hum: It disappears in a supine position (see Innocent Heart Murmurs in chap. 2).

5. Murmurs of collaterals in patients with COA or TOF: The murmur is audible in the intercostal spaces, usually bilaterally.

6. VSD with aortic regurgitation: The murmur is maximally audible at the MLSB or LLSB and is more to-and-fro than continuous.

7. Absence of pulmonary valve: A to-and-fro murmur ("sawing-wood sound") at the ULSB, large central pulmonary arteries on x-rays, and RVH on the ECG are characteristic. These infants are frequently cyanotic (as it is often asso-

ciated with TOF) (see chap. 17, Miscellaneous Congenital Cardiac Conditions).

8. Persistent truncus arteriosus: A continuous murmur may occasionally be audible in locations other than 2LICS, such as 2RICS and the back. Cyanosis is usually present.

9. Aortopulmonary septal defect (AP window): Peripheral pulses are bounding, but the heart murmur resembles that of VSD. CHF develops early in infancy.

10. Peripheral pulmonary artery stenosis: A continuous murmur may be audible all over the thorax. The ECG may show RVH if the stenosis is severe. This is often seen in children with rubella syndrome or Williams' syndrome.

11. Ruptured sinus of Valsalva aneurysm: Sudden onset of severe heart failure is characteristic.

12. TAPVR draining into the RA: The murmur is similar to venous hum and best audible along the right sternal border. Mild cyanosis may be present. ECG shows RVH.

13. Obstruction to pulmonary venous return following the Mustard operation for TGA: A soft, continuous murmur is audible along the MRSB or LRSB.

IV. COMPLETE ENDOCARDIAL CUSHION DEFECT:
(Complete AV Canal, AV Communis)

Incidence

Two percent of all congenital heart defects. 30% of the defects occur in children with Down's syndrome.

Pathology

1. This is the result of a developmental abnormality of the endocardial cushion, which normally contributes to the formation of the primum portion of the atrial septum, the inlet ventricular septum and the mitral and tricuspid valves.

2. The complete form of ECD consists of the following defects (Fig 12–12):

   a. Ostium primum ASD

   b. VSD in the inlet portion of the ventricular septum (see Fig 12–5).

   c. A cleft in the anterior mitral valve leaflet (with resulting mitral regurgitation), and

   d. A cleft in the septal leaflet of the tricuspid valve, together with the cleft mitral valve, forming common anterior and posterior cusps of the AV valve.

3. The combination of the above defects may result in interatrial and/or interventricular shunts, LV-RA shunt or AV valve regurgitation.

4. Two major associated cardiac anomalies are PDA (10%) and TOF (10%).

5. When the ventricular septum is intact, the defect is termed partial ECD or ostium primum ASD (see below).

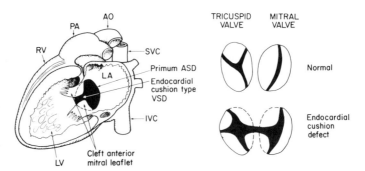

FIG 12–12.
Diagrammatic illustrations of complete endocardial cushion defect viewed with the LA and LV posterior wall removed. Cleft mitral and tricuspid valves with resulting common AV valve are compared with normal AV valves.

Clinical Manifestations

History

Failure to thrive, repeated respiratory infections, and signs of CHF are common.

PE (Fig 12–13 shows cardiac findings.)

a. An undernourished infant with tachycardia and tachypnea.

b. Hyperactive precordium with a systolic thrill at the LLSB (area with dots in Fig 12–13).

c. The S1 is accentuated. The S2 splits narrowly and the P2 is increased in intensity.

d. A grade 3–4/6 holosystolic regurgitant murmur is audible along the LLSB (see Fig 12–13). The systolic murmur may transmit well to the left back and may well be audible at the apex (mitral regurgitation).

e. A middiastolic rumble at the LLSB or at the apex (from relative stenosis of tricuspid and/or mitral valve).

f. Signs of CHF (such as hepatomegaly or gallop rhythm) may be present.

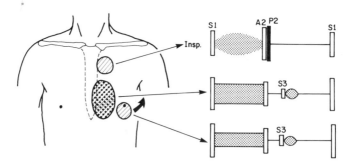

FIG 12–13.
Cardiac findings of complete endocardial cushion defect (ECD), which resemble those of large VSD. A systolic thrill may be present at the LLSB *(dotted area),* where the systolic murmur is loudest.

ECG

   a. Left anterior hemiblock ("superior" QRS axis) with the QRS axis between −40° and −150° is characteristic of the defect (Fig 12–14 shows the superior QRS axis with deep S waves in aVF).

   b. Prolonged PR interval (first-degree AV block) is common.

   c. RVH or RBBB is present in all, and many have LVH as well.

X-Rays (See Fig 9–10 for diagrammatic drawing.)

   a. Cardiomegaly is always present, involving all four chambers.

   b. Pulmonary vascular markings are increased and the MPA segment is prominent.

ECHO (Fig 12–15.)
2D ECHO allows visualization of all components of ECD as well as an assessment of the severity of these defects. In addition, it is an integral part of the study for evaluation of surgically important findings (such as the size of the AV valve orifices, chordal attachment, and relative and absolute size of the RV and LV).

Natural History and Complications

   a. Heart failure occurs 1–2 months after birth.

   b. Recurrent pneumonia is commonly seen.

   c. The majority of the patients without surgical intervention die in 2–3 years.

   d. The survivors develop PVOD and die in late childhood or as young adults.

Management

Medical

   a. All attempts should be made to treat infants with CHF medically, as surgical mortality is relatively high in this age group.

   b. Digitalis and diuretics for CHF.

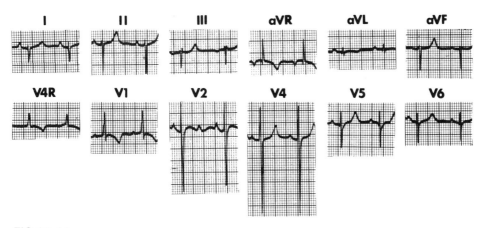

FIG 12–14.
Tracing from a 5-year-old boy with Down's syndrome and complete AV canal. Note superior QRS axis (−110°) and RVH.

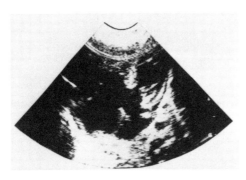
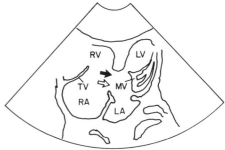

FIG 12–15.
Apical four-chamber view in a patient with complete endocardial cushion defect. The *closed arrow* points to the defect in the ventricular septum, and the *open arrow* points to the defect in the primum atrial septum. LA = left atrium; LV = left ventricle; MV = mitral valve; RA = right atrium; RV = right ventricle; TV = tricuspid valve.

    c. Antibiotics and other supportive measures for pneumonia.

    d. Prophylaxis against infective endocarditis, even on those who have had surgical repair.

Surgical

    a. Procedures:

        1) Palliative: Pulmonary artery banding may be carried out in small infants at a slightly higher mortality than that for other left-to-right shunt lesions, if significant mitral regurgitation is not present.

        2) Corrective: Closure of ASD and VSD and reconstruction of cleft AV valves under cardiopulmonary bypass and/or deep hypothermia. The repair is much more difficult technically than repairs of a secundum ASD and a perimembranous VSD. In a small number of patients, mitral valve replacement may become necessary.

    b. Indications:

        1) Heart failure unresponsive to aggressive medical therapy.

        2) Repeated pneumonia with failure to thrive.

        3) Large left-to-right shunt with pulmonary hypertension and increasing PVR.

    c. Timing: Varies with institutions and depends on the hemodynamics of the patients. Ranges from a few months to several years of age, but many centers perform the repair at 6–12 months of age.

    d. Mortality rate has been reduced to 5%–10% in recent years. Factors known to increase the surgical risk include (1) very young age, (2) severe AV valve incompetence, (3) hypoplastic LV, and (4) severe symptoms preoperatively. Mortality rate for PA banding may be as high as 15%.

    e. Complications:

        1) Persistence or worsening of mitral regurgitation (10%).

2) Complete heart block, especially with mitral valve replacement (up to 20%).

3) Postoperative arrhythmias (usually supraventricular).

V. PARTIAL ENDOCARDIAL CUSHION DEFECT
(Ostium Primum ASD)

Incidence
One percent to 2% of all congenital heart defects.

Pathology
A defect is present in the lower part of the atrial septum near the AV valves. Clefts of the mitral and occasionally of the tricuspid valve are present (see Figs 12–1 and 12–12).

Clinical Manifestations
History
Usually asymptomatic during childhood.

PE
Findings are identical to those of secundum ASD, with the exception of a regurgitant systolic murmur of mitral regurgitation, which may be present at the apex.

ECG

a. Left anterior hemiblock or superiorly oriented QRS axis, ranging from $-20°$ to $-150°$, is characteristic of this condition (see Fig 12–14).

b. RVH or RBBB (rsR′ pattern in V1) as in secundum ASD.

c. First-degree AV block (prolonged PR interval) is present in 50% of cases.

X-Rays
Identical to those of secundum ASD (see Fig 12–4) with the exception of enlargement of the LA and LV when mitral regurgitation is significant.

ECHO
2D ECHO allows accurate diagnosis of primum ASD by direct visualization of the defect, best from the subcostal position.

Natural History and Complications

a. CHF may develop in childhood (earlier than in secundum ASD).

b. Pulmonary hypertension in adulthood.

c. Infective endocarditis, usually of AV valves.

d. Arrhythmias (20%).

Management

Medical

a. No exercise restriction.

b. Precautions against infective endocarditis.

Surgical

   a. Indications:

      1) Significant left-to-right shunt ($\dot{Q}p/\dot{Q}s > 2{:}1$).

      2) Congestive heart failure.

   b. Procedure: Closure of the ASD and reconstruction of the cleft mitral and tricuspid valves under cardiopulmonary bypass.

   c. Timing:

      1) Electively at 2–4 years in children with no symptoms.

      2) Earlier in infants with severe CHF or mitral regurgitation who are unresponsive to medical management.

   d. Mortality: 1%–2%.

   e. Complications:

      1) Persistence or worsening of mitral regurgitation.

      2) Infective endocarditis (prophylaxis should be continued even after the surgery, unlike in secundum ASD).

      3) Atrial and nodal arrhythmias.

VI. PARTIAL ANOMALOUS PULMONARY VENOUS RETURN (PAPVR)

Incidence

Less than 1% of all congenital heart defects.

Pathology

1. One or more (but not all) pulmonary veins drain into the RA or its venous tributaries, such as the SVC, IVC, or left innominate vein.

2. The right pulmonary veins are involved twice as often as the left pulmonary veins.

3. The right PVs may drain into the SVC (associated with sinus venosus defect), the RA (associated with secundum ASD), or the IVC (the scimitar syndrome, in association with bronchopulmonary sequestration and intact atrial septum).

Pathophysiology

1. The fundamental hemodynamic alteration is similar to that in ASD; increased pulmonary blood flow as a consequence of recirculation through the lungs (see chap. 9 for pathophysiology of ASD).

2. The magnitude of the recirculation is determined by the number of anomalous pulmonary veins, the presence and the size of the ASD, and the pulmonary vascular resistance.

Clinical Manifestations

History

Children with PAPVR are usually asymptomatic.

PE

a. Physical findings are similar to those of ASD (see Fig 12–2).

b. When associated with ASD, the S2 is split widely and fixed. When the atrial septum is intact, the S2 is normal.

c. A grade 2–3/6 systolic ejection murmur (SEM) is present at the ULSB.

d. A middiastolic rumble (due to relative tricuspid stenosis) may be present.

ECG

Similar to that of ASD (showing RVH, RBBB or normal ECG)

X-Rays

a. Cardiomegaly with enlargement of the RA, RV, and MPA.

b. Increased pulmonary vascularity.

c. Occasionally, a dilated SVC, a crescent-shaped vertical shadow in the right lower lung, or a distended vertical vein may suggest the site of anomalous drainage.

ECHO

ECHO diagnosis of PAPVR is less reliable.

Natural History and Complications

a. Cyanosis and exertional dyspnea may develop during the 3rd and 4th decades owing to pulmonary hypertension and PVOD.

b. Pulmonary infections are common in patients with anomalous drainage of the right pulmonary veins to the IVC (the scimitar syndrome; see chap. 17).

Management

Medical

a. Exercise restriction is not required.

b. Infective endocarditis prophylaxis is probably not indicated.

Surgical

a. Procedures:
Surgical correction is carried out under cardiopulmonary bypass. The procedure to be performed depends on the site of anomalous drainage.

1) To the RA: The ASD is widened, and a patch is sewn in such a way that the anomalous pulmonary veins drain into the LA (similar to Figure 14–19,B).

2) To the SVC: A tunnel is created between the anomalous vein and the ASD, through the SVC and the RA, by the use of Teflon or pericardial patch. A plastic or pericardial gusset is placed in the SVC to prevent obstruction to the SVC.

3) To the IVC: In case of the scimitar syndrome, resection of the involved lobe(s) may be indicated without having to connect the anomalous vein to the heart. When the anomalous venous drainage is an isolated lesion, the vein is reimplanted to the RA, and an intra-atrial tunnel is created to drain into the LA.

b. Indications: Significant left-to-right shunt with $\dot{Q}p/\dot{Q}s$ greater than 1.5:1 or 2:1. Isolated single lobe anomaly is not ordinarily corrected.

c. Timing: 2–5 years of age.

d. Mortality: Less than 1%.

e. Complications:

1) Superior vena caval obstruction for those draining into the SVC.

2) Postoperative arrhythmias (supraventricular).

13 / Obstructive Lesions

In this chapter lesions that produce obstruction to ventricular outflow, such as pulmonary stenosis (PS), aortic stenosis (AS), and coarctation of the aorta (COA), will be briefly discussed.

I. PULMONARY STENOSIS

Incidence
Five percent to 8% of all congenital heart defects.

Pathology

1. Pulmonary stenosis may be valvular, subvalvular (infundibular), or supravalvular.

2. The valvular PS accounts for more than 90% of pulmonary stenosis. Dysplasia of the pulmonary valve is frequently seen with Noonan's syndrome.

3. Isolated infundibular PS is uncommon, usually associated with a large VSD (tetralogy of Fallot).

4. Supravalvular PS is also called stenosis of the pulmonary arteries and is often associated with rubella syndrome and Williams' syndrome (peculiar facies, mental retardation, hypercalcemia of infancy).

Clinical Manifestations

History

a. Patients may be completely asymptomatic with mild stenosis.

b. Exertional dyspnea and easy fatigability in moderately severe cases.

c. Heart failure may develop in severe cases.

PE (Figure 13–1 shows cardiac findings.)

a. Acyanotic (usually) and well developed.

b. Right ventricular tap may be present. A systolic thrill may be present at the ULSB and, rarely, in the suprasternal notch.

c. A systolic ejection click is present with valvular stenosis at the ULSB. The S2 may split widely, and the P2 may be diminished in intensity. A systolic ejection murmur (grade 2–5/6) is best audible at the ULSB and transmits fairly well to the back. The louder and longer the murmur, the more severe is the stenosis (see Fig 13–1).

d. Hepatomegaly may be present if CHF develops.

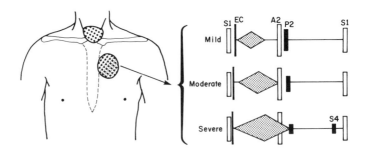

FIG 13–1.
Cardiac findings of pulmonary valve stenosis. EC = ejection click; S4 = fourth heart sound. Abnormal sounds are shown in *black. Dots* represent areas with systolic thrill.

ECG

a. Normal ECG in mild cases.

b. RAD and RVH in moderate PS. The degree of RVH on the ECG correlates fairly well with the severity of PS (R in V1 greater than 20 mm Hg is usually associated with systemic pressure in the RV).

c. RAH and RVH with "strain" in severe PS.

d. "Superior" QRS axis with dysplastic pulmonary valve (often seen with Noonan's syndrome).

X-Rays (See Figs 4–7 and 13–2.)

a. Heart size is normal, but the MPA segment is prominent (poststenotic dilatation).

b. Pulmonary vascular markings are usually normal but may be decreased in severe PS.

c. Cardiomegaly if CHF develops.

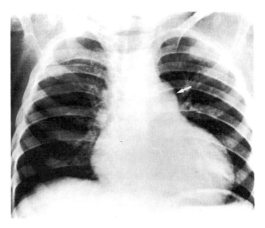

FIG 13–2.
A PA view of chest film in pulmonary valve stenosis. Note a marked poststenotic dilatation *(arrow)* and normal pulmonary vascularity. (Courtesy of Dr. Ewell Clarke, San Antonio, Texas).

ECHO

    a. 2D ECHO in the parasternal short-axis view may show thick pulmonary valve with restricted systolic motion (doming). Poststenotic dilatation of the MPA is often visualized.

    b. The Doppler study can estimate the pressure gradient.

Natural History and Complications

    a. The severity of the obstruction is less likely to progress with age than in aortic stenosis.

    b. CHF may develop in patients with more severe stenosis.

    c. Infective endocarditis.

    d. Possible sudden death in patients with severe stenosis.

Management

Medical

    a. Restriction of activity is usually not indicated except for severe PS.

    b. Precaution against infective endocarditis.

    c. Balloon valvuloplasty (performed at the time of cardiac catheterization) is the procedure of choice (over surgical repair) for significant pulmonary valve stenosis (with transpulmonary valve pressure gradient of 50 mm Hg or greater).

Surgical

    a. Procedures:

        1) Pulmonary valvotomy under cardiopulmonary bypass or deep hypothermia, preferably without right ventriculotomy. (Balloon valvuloplasty is preferred for valvular PS in children.) Neonates with critical PS may require a transventricular valvotomy while receiving PGE_1 infusion (and left Gore-Tex shunt, if severe infundibular hypoplasia is present).

        2) Complete excision of the dysplastic valve is required (seen in Noonan's syndrome).

        3) Stenoses at the PA level usually require patch widening of the narrowings.

        4) Infundibular stenosis requires resection of the muscle and patch widening.

    b. Indications and Timing:

        1) Children with RV pressure 80–100 mg Hg in whom balloon valvuloplasty is unsuccessful (such as seen with dysplastic pulmonary valve) or is not indicated (infundibular stenosis).

        2) Infants with critical PS and CHF on an urgent basis.

    c. Mortality: Less than 1% in older children. A higher mortality in critically ill infants.

II. AORTIC STENOSIS

Incidence

Five percent of all congenital heart defects. Male preponderance (M:F = 4:1).

Pathology

Stenosis may be at the valvular, subvalvular, or supravalvular levels (Fig 13–3).

1. Valvular stenosis: A bicuspid valve is more common than a unicuspid or tricuspid valve.

2. Supravalvular stenosis: An anular constriction above the aortic valve, at the upper margin of the sinus of Valsalva. This is often associated with Williams' syndrome (mental retardation, characteristic facies, and pulmonary artery stenosis).

3. Subvalvular stenosis may be due to a simple diaphragm (discrete) or a long, tunnel-like narrowing of the outflow tract. Another type of subvalvular stenosis is idiopathic hypertrophic subaortic stenosis (IHSS). This condition is a primary disorder of heart muscle and is discussed under cardiomyopathy in chap. 18.

Clinical Manifestations

History

a. Most children with mild to moderate AS are asymptomatic. Occasional patients will have exercise intolerance.

b. Exertional chest pain or syncope may occur with a more severe degree of obstruction.

c. CHF may occur within the first few months of life, with critical stenosis of the aortic valve.

PE (Figure 13–4 shows cardiac findings.)

a. Acyanotic, normally developed child.

b. Blood pressure is normal in the majority of patients, but:

1) A narrow pulse pressure is present in severe AS.

2) Higher systolic pressure in the right arm than in the left arm is seen in supravalvular AS.

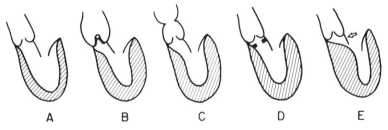

A   B   C   D   E

FIG 13–3.
Anatomical types of aortic stenosis. **A,** normal; **B,** valvular stenosis; **C,** supravalvular stenosis; **D,** discrete subaortic stenosis; and **E,** IHSS. IHSS is discussed under cardiomyopathy in chap. 18.

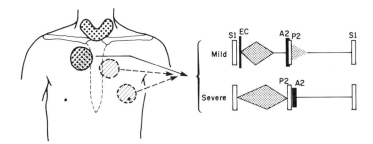

FIG 13–4.
Cardiac findings of aortic valve stenosis. Abbreviations are the same as in previous figures. Abnormal sounds are indicated in *black*. Systolic thrill may be present in areas with *dots*.

    c. A systolic thrill is present at the URSB, suprasternal notch, or over the carotid arteries.

    d. An ejection click may be audible with valvular AS. The S2 splits normally or slightly narrowly. The S2 may split paradoxically in severe AS (see Fig 13–4).

    e. A rough or harsh SEM (grade 2–4/6) is best audible at the 2RICS or 3LICS, with a good transmission to the neck and frequently to the apex (see Fig 13–4).

    f. A high-pitched, early diastolic decrescendo murmur (due to aortic insufficiency) may be audible in patients with bicuspid aortic valve and those with (discrete) subvalvular stenosis (see Fig 13–4).

    g. Peculiar "elfin facies" and mental retardation may be present in supravalvular AS (Williams' syndrome).

    h. Newborn infants with critical AS may develop CHF. The heart murmur may be absent or faint, and the peripheral pulses are weak and thready. The heart murmur becomes louder when CHF improves.

ECG

    a. Normal in mild cases.

    b. LVH with "strain" in more severe cases (Fig 13–5).

    c. Correlation of the severity of AS and the ECG abnormalities is relatively poor.

X-Rays

    a. Usually normal in children, but dilated ascending aorta or a prominent aortic knob may be seen occasionally in valvular AS (due to poststenotic dilatation).

    b. Significant cardiomegaly does not develop unless CHF develops later in life or unless aortic regurgitation is substantial.

ECHO

    a. An eccentric closure of the aortic valve on M-mode ECHO is suggestive of bicuspid aortic valve. Fluttering of the aortic valve during systole is seen with subaortic stenosis.

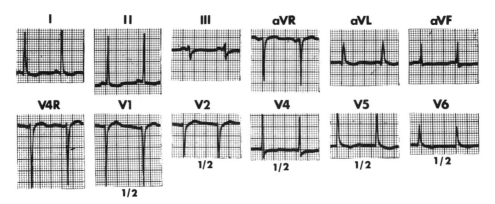

FIG 13–5.
Tracing from a 7-year-old boy with severe aortic stenosis. It shows LVH with probably "strain" pattern.

  b. 2D ECHO shows the anatomy of the aortic valve (bicuspid, tricuspid, or unicuspid) and that of subvalvular and supravalvular AS.

  c. Doppler examination can estimate pressure gradient in various forms of AS.

Natural History and Complications

  a. Chest pain, syncope, and even sudden death (1%–2%) may occur in children with severe AS.

  b. Heart failure during the newborn period or later in life with severe AS.

  c. Significant increase in the pressure gradient may occur with growth in some children.

  d. Worsening of the stenosis with aging (due to calcification of the valve cusps), requiring prosthetic valve replacement in a significant number of adult patients.

  e. Progressive worsening of aortic regurgitation is possible in the discrete subvalvular AS.

  f. Infective endocarditis is a rare complication.

Management

Medical

  a. Exercise restriction against sustained strenuous activity is recommended in children with moderate to severe AS.

  b. Maintenance of good oral hygiene and prophylaxis against bacterial endocarditis (see chap. 19, Infective Endocarditis).

  c. Anticongestive measures with digitalis and diuretics in infants with critical AS.

  d. Balloon valvuloplasty may be tried at the time of cardiac catheterization on selected patients. The results are not as promising as for PS.

  e. Prostaglandin E_1 infusion and oxygen in critically ill newborns.

Surgical

  a. Procedures:

    1) Closed aortic valvotomy using calibrated dilators without cardiopulmonary bypass may be the procedure of choice in sick infants.

    2) The following procedures may be performed under cardiopulmonary bypass:

      a) Aortic valve commissurotomy.

      b) Replacement with an artificial valve may be necessary if the valve is unicuspid. Replacement with aortic homograft is preferred.

      c) For severe anular narrowing or tunnel-like narrowing, valve replacement following aortic root enlargement (Konno procedure) may be indicated.

      d) Excision of the membrane for discrete subvalvular AS.

      e) Widening of the stenotic area using a diamond-shaped fabric patch for discrete supravalvular AS.

  b. Indications and Timing:

    1) At any age in infants with CHF from critical AS.

    2) Children with severe AS with peak systolic pressure gradient >80 mm Hg on an elective basis.

    3) Children with peak systolic pressure gradient of 50–80 mm Hg may be operated on on an individual basis. Asymptomatic children with a systolic pressure gradient less than 50 mm Hg usually do not require surgery.

    4) Symptoms (chest pain, syncope) related to AS with "strain" pattern on the ECG or abnormal exercise test (even with systolic gradient of 50 mm Hg).

    5) Earlier elective operation may be considered for subvalvular AS of moderate degree because of the progressive nature of aortic regurgitation.

    6) Valve replacement surgery should be delayed as long as possible, ideally until an adult-sized prosthetic valve can be used. Replacement with aortic homograft can be done at an earlier age.

  c. Mortality:

    1) The overall mortality for infants and small children is 15%–20%. Higher mortality in sick neonates (as high as 50%) and those with poor preoperative functional status.

    2) The hospital mortality in older children is 1%–2%.

  d. Complications:

    1) Significant aortic insufficiency may develop following aortic valvotomy.

    2) Residual or recurrent aortic pressure gradient.

III. COARCTATION OF THE AORTA (COA)

Incidence

8% of all congenital heart defects. More common in males (M : F = 2 : 1). 30% of patients with Turner's syndrome have COA.

Pathology

1. The coarctation occurs most commonly in the upper thoracic aorta.

2. Preductal COA is a narrowing of either a short or long segment of the aorta proximal to the ductus arteriosus and is frequently associated with other cardiac defects (40%), such as VSD, PDA, or TGA. Collateral circulation is poorly developed. These patients become symptomatic very early in life.

3. Postductal COA is usually a localized narrowing occurring distal to the ductus arteriosus. It is less frequently associated with other cardiac defects and usually does not produce symptoms in infancy.

4. Over 50% of the patients with COA, both preductal and postductal, have bicuspid aortic valve.

5. In infants with CHF from COA, necrosis of papillary muscles with mitral regurgitation may be present.

I. ASYMPTOMATIC CHILDREN

Clinical Manifestations

History

Most children are symptomatic.

PE (Figure 13–6 shows cardiac findings.)

   a. Normal growth and development.

   b. Absent or weak and delayed pulse in the leg. Hypertension in the arm or higher BP readings in the arm than the thigh.

   c. A systolic thrill may be present in the suprasternal notch.

   d. The S2 splits normally, and A2 is accentuated. An ejection click is frequently audible at the apex and/or at the base (due to frequently associated bicuspid aortic valve or systemic hypertension) (Fig 13–6).

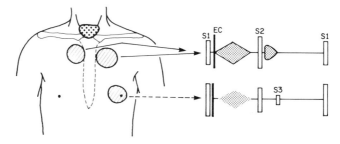

FIG 13–6.
Cardiac findings of coarctation of the aorta. A systolic thrill may be present in the SSN (area shown by *dots*).

e. A systolic ejection murmur, grade 2–3/6 at the URSB and MLSB or LLSB (see Fig 13–6). A similar murmur is also heard, well localized, in the left interscapular area in the back.

f. Occasionally, an early diastolic decrescendo murmur (of AR from the bicuspid aortic valve) may be audible in 3LICS (see Fig 13–6).

ECG

Leftward QRS axis and LVH are usually present, but the ECG is normal in 20%.

X-Rays

a. The heart size may be normal or slightly enlarged.

b. Dilatation of the ascending aorta may be visualized.

c. "E sign" on the barium-filled esophagus or "3 sign" on overpenetrated films (see Fig 4–8).

d. Rib notching between 4th and 8th ribs may be seen in older children (rarely under 5 years of age).

ECHO

a. A discrete shelflike membrane can be visualized in the posterolateral aspect of the descending aorta by 2D ECHO (suprasternal notch view).

b. Bicuspid aortic valve is frequently present.

c. Doppler examination reveals disturbed flow distal to the coarctation.

Natural History and Complications

a. Bicuspid aortic valve may cause stenosis and/or regurgitation.

b. LV failure may develop in adult life.

c. Infective endocarditis (on the bicuspid aortic valve or the coarctation.)

d. Intracranial bleeding, hypertensive encephalopathy, and hypertensive cardiovascular disease.

Management

Medical

a. Good dental hygiene and precaution against infective endocarditis.

b. Children with mild COA should be followed closely for hypertension in the arm or increasing pressure difference between the arm and leg.

c. Treatment of hypertensive crisis (see chap. 28).

Surgical

a. Procedures: Resection of the coarctation segment and end-to-end anastomosis (Fig 13–7,B) is the procedure of choice for discrete COA in children. Circular or patch grafts (Fig 13–7,C and D) or the use of the left subclavian artery as a patch (Fig 13–7,A) may also be used.

b. Indications and Timing:

1) COA with hypertension in the upper extremities or those with a large pressure gradient between the arms and the legs should be repaired electively, at age 3–4 years.

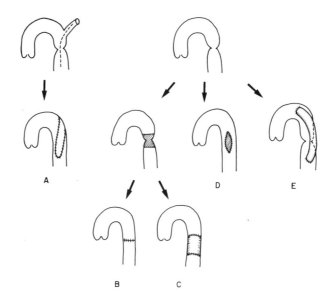

FIG 13–7.
Surgical correction of coarctation of the aorta. Subclavian artery angioplasty *(A)* can be done for both discrete COA and the long-segment preductal COA. Resection and primary end-to-end anastomosis *(B)* is possible in many older children. Other options include an interposition of Dacron graft *(C)*, a Dacron patch repair *(D)*, and a bypass tube graft *(E)* for long-segment COA or recoarctation.

2) Children with mild COA (20–30 mm Hg) may be considered for surgery if a prominent pressure gradient develops with exercise.

c. Mortality: Less than 1% in older children.

d. Complications:

1) Spinal cord ischemia producing paraplegia following cross-clamping of the aorta during the operation (less than 1%).

2) Postcoarctectomy syndrome (see chap. 32). (Necrotizing mesenteric arteritis manifested by abdominal pain and distention.)

3) Persistence of hypertension in the arms and legs in occasional patients (cause not clearly determined), particularly with exercise.

II. SYMPTOMATIC INFANTS

Clinical Manifestations

History

Signs of CHF (poor feeding, dyspnea, poor weight gain) in the first 2–6 weeks of life.

PE

a. Infants are pale, with varying degrees of respiratory distress. Oliguria or anuria with general circulatory shock and severe acidemia are not uncommon. Differential cyanosis may be present (only the lower half of the body may be cyanotic owing to a right-to-left ductal shunt).

b. Weak and thready pulses throughout owing to CHF. Blood pressure differential may become apparent after digitalization.

c. The S2 is often single and loud. A loud S3 gallop is usually present. A nonspecific systolic ejection murmur, poorly localized over the precordium, is present. No heart murmur is present in 50% of sick infants. The heart murmur may become louder after digitalization.

ECG

a. Normal or rightward QRS axis.

b. RVH or RBBB pattern is present in the majority of infant patients, rather than LVH seen in older children with COA (Fig 13–8).

X-Rays

Marked cardiomegaly, and pulmonary edema or pulmonary venous congestion.

ECHO

2D ECHO usually shows the site and extent of the coarctation clearly, and cardiac catheterization may not be necessary. Other associated defects are also well visualized.

Natural History and Complications

a. More than 80% of infants with preductal COA develop CHF by 3 months of age.

b. Early death from CHF and renal shutdown.

Management

Medical

a. Intensive anticongestive measures with inotropic agents (digitalis or dopamine), diuretics, and oxygen before cardiac catheterization and surgical treatment.

b. Prostaglandin E_1 infusion may be occasionally indicated to reopen the ductus arteriosus.

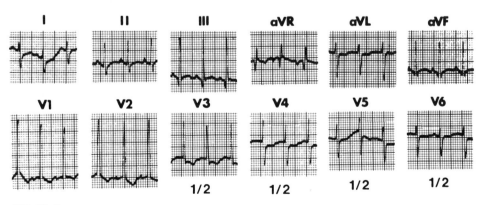

FIG 13–8.
Tracing from a 6-week-old infant with preductal type of coarctation of the aorta. Note a marked RVH.

Surgical

    a. Procedures:

        1) Subclavian flap aortoplasty is preferred by many centers (see Fig 13–7,A).

        2) Resection of the coarcted segment and end-to-end anastomosis, patch graft, bypass tube graft, or Dacron graft may also be used (see Fig 13–7).

    b. Indications and Timing:

        1) If CHf with/without circulatory shock develops, operation should be performed on an urgent basis.

        2) If there is a large associated VSD, one of the following procedures may be performed:

            a) PA banding at the time of COA repair. Later VSD repair and removal of the PA band at 6–24 months of age.

            b) No PA banding. If CHF persists after COA repair, either PA banding or VSD closure is indicated.

    c. Mortality: Less than 5%.

    d. Complications:

        1) Postoperative renal failure (the most common cause of death).

        2) Recoarctation rate is high in neonates.

14 / Cyanotic Congenital Heart Defects

In this chapter common and rare, but well-known, congenital heart defects that produce cyanosis will be discussed. Some of these defects have increased pulmonary blood flow (PBF) and some have decreased PBF. Defects discussed in this chapter include complete transposition of the great arteries (D-TGA), tetralogy of Fallot (TOF), total anomalous pulmonary venous return (TAPVR), tricuspid atresia, pulmonary atresia with intact ventricular septum, Ebstein's anomaly, persistent truncus arteriosus, single ventricle, and double-outlet right ventricle (DORV). Although uncomplicated cases of congenitally corrected transposition of the great arteries (L-TGA) do not produce cyanosis, they are included in this chapter, since the majority of the cases are associated with other cardiac defects resulting in cyanosis.

I. COMPLETE TRANSPOSITION OF THE GREAT ARTERIES (TGA)

(D-Transposition, or D-TGA)

Incidence

Five percent of all congenital heart defects. More common in males (M-to-F ratio = 3:1).

Pathology

1. The aorta arises anteriorly from the RV, carrying desaturated blood to the body, and the PA arises posteriorly from the LV, carrying oxygenated blood to the lungs. The end result is complete separation of the two circuits, with hypoxemic blood circulating in the body and hyperoxemic blood circulating in the pulmonary circuit (see Fig 11–1).

2. Defects that permit mixing of the two circulations, such as ASD, VSD, and PDA, are necessary for survival.

3. A VSD is present in 40% of the cases. Pulmonary stenosis (valvular or subvalvular) occurs in 30%–35% of the cases with VSD. Dynamic LV outflow tract obstruction occurs in 20% of the cases without VSD.

4. The classic complete TGA is called D-transposition, in which the aorta is located anteriorly and to the right of the PA; hence the prefix "D." When the transposed aorta is located to the left of the PA, it is called L-transposition (see Fig 16–4).

Clinical Manifestation

History

a. History of cyanosis from birth is always present.

b. Signs of CHF with dyspnea and feeding difficulties in the newborn period.

157

PE (Figure 14–1 shows cardiac findings.)

    a. Moderate to severe cyanosis, usually in a large male newborn infant. Tachypneic but without retraction (unless CHF supervenes).

    b. The S2 is single and loud. No heart murmur is audible in infants with intact ventricular septum. A systolic (regurgitant) murmur of VSD may be audible in less cyanotic infants with VSD. A soft systolic ejection murmur of PS may be present.

    c. Hepatomegaly and dyspnea develop, if CHF supervenes.

Laboratory

    a. Severe arterial hypoxemia and acidosis. Hypoxemia is unresponsive to oxygen inhalation.

    b. Hypoglycemia and hypocalcemia are occasionally present.

ECG

    a. Rightward QRS axis ($+90°$ to $+200°$ [or $-160°$]).

    b. RVH is almost always present after the first few days of life. An upright T wave in V1 after 3 days of life may be the only abnormality suggestive of RVH.

    c. CVH may be present in infants with large VSD, PDA, PS, or PVOD (as they produce an additional LVH).

    d. Occasional RAH may be present.

X-Rays

    a. Cardiomegaly with increased pulmonary vascularity is almost always present (Fig 14–2).

    b. An "egg-shaped" cardiac silhouette with a narrow superior mediastinum is characteristic.

In summary, TGA is presumed present until proved otherwise, when a large male newborn infant has intense cyanosis, increased pulmonary vascularity on chest x-rays, and RVH on the ECG. Auscultatory findings are nonspecific and not helpful in the diagnosis of this condition.

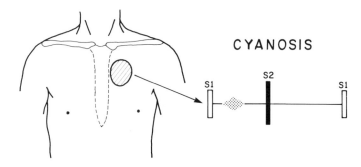

FIG 14–1.
Cardiac findings of transposition of the great arteries. Heart murmur is usually absent, and the S_2 is single in the majority of patients.

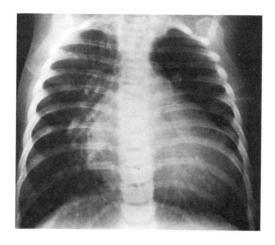

FIG 14–2.
A PA view of the chest roentgenogram from a 2-month-old infant with D-TGA. Note cardiomegaly (CT ratio of 0.7), "egg-shaped" heart with narrow waist, and increased pulmonary vascular markings, which are characteristic of this condition.

ECHO

    a. The subcostal views reveal a great artery (PA) arising from the LV, which courses posteriorly and immediately bifurcates (indicating it is the pulmonary artery).

    b. The parasternal short-axis view fails to show a "circle and sausage" of the normal great arteries (see Fig 6–2); instead, it shows two circular structures.

    c. Associated anomalies (VSD, LV outflow tract obstruction, PS, and ASD, PDA) can be visualized.

    d. Status of an interatrial communication, before and after the balloon septostomy can be evaluated.

Natural History and Complications

    a. Progressive hypoxia and acidosis resulting in death, unless the intracardiac mixing is improved. Death occurs in 90% of the patients before 6 months of age.

    b. CHF develops in the first weeks of life.

    c. Infants with intact ventricular septum are the sickest group, but demonstrate the most dramatic improvement following the Rashkind balloon atrial septostomy (see below). These infants have the best chance for complete surgical repair.

    d. Infants with VSD are the least cyanotic group but most likely to develop CHF and PVOD. Their surgical risk is greater than the group with intact ventricular septum.

    e. Infants with a significant PDA are similar to those with a large VSD because of early development of PVOD.

    f. Combination of VSD and PS allows considerably longer survival without surgery, but carries a high surgical risk for correction.

g. Cerebrovascular accident.

h. Progressive PVOD, particularly in infants with large VSD or PDA.

Management

Medical

a. The following measures should be carried out before an emergency cardiac catheterization:

1) Obtain arterial blood gases and pH, and carry out hyperoxitest to confirm the presence of a cyanotic CHD.

2) Correct metabolic acidosis and treat hypoglycemia and/or hypocalcemia.

3) Prostaglandin E_1 infusion to improve arterial PO_2 by reopening of PDA (see pulmonary atresia in this chapter for the dosage of prostaglandin E_1).

4) Oxygen for severe hypoxia. Oxygen may be helpful in lowering PVR and increasing PBF with resulting increase in the systemic arterial saturation.

b. An emergency cardiac catheterization and therapeutic balloon atrial septostomy (BAS) (Rashkind procedure) should be carried out. In this procedure, a balloon-tipped catheter is advanced into the LA through the PFO. The balloon is inflated with diluted radiopaque dye and rapidly and forcefully withdrawn to the RA under fluoroscopic monitoring. This procedure creates a large defect in the atrial septum. It carries a minimal complication rate and often dramatically improves the aortic oxygen saturation.

c. Blade atrial septostomy: In older infants and those in whom the initial balloon atrial septostomy was only temporarily successful, the interatrial communication may be widened by the use of a catheter with a built-in surgical blade.

d. Treatment of heart failure with digitalis and diuretics.

Surgical

1. Palliative Procedures:
If the Rashkind procedure (and blade atrial septostomy in some institutions) and prostaglandin E_1 infusion are unsuccessful or only temporarily successful in increasing arterial O_2 saturation, a surgical excision of the posterior aspect of the atrial septum (the Blalock-Hanlon operation) without cardiopulmonary bypass may be performed. Mortality rate of this procedure is fairly high (10%–25%).

2. Definitive Repairs:
Definitive surgeries consist of switching the right- and left-sided structures either at the atrial level (Senning's or Mustard's operation), at the ventricular level (Rastelli's operation), or at the great artery level (Jatene procedure). The intra-atrial switch operations have had extensive experiences with their complications well defined, but the arterial switch operation (Jatene operation) is gaining popularity and appears promising with fewer complications.

a. Procedures:

1) Intra-atrial repair operations:

a) The Mustard operation: The oldest form of surgical technique redirects the pulmonary and systemic venous return at the atrial level by the use of a pericardial or prosthetic baffle (Fig 14–3 shows schematic drawing of the procedure).

　b) The Senning operation: This is a modification of the Mustard operation. It utilizes the atrial septal flap and the RA free wall to redirect the pulmonary and systemic venous return (Fig 14–4 shows schematic drawings of the procedure).

　2) The Rastelli operation:
　　The redirection of the pulmonary and systemic venous blood is carried out at the ventricular level in patients with VSD and severe PS. The LV is directed to the aorta by placing an intraventricular tunnel between the VSD and the aortic valve. A conduit is placed between the RV and the PA (Fig 14–5 shows schematic drawing of the procedure).

　3) The Jatene operation (arterial switch operation):
　　This is the newest of the definitive surgeries for TGA (Fig 14–6). It is indicated in patients with systemic pressures in the LV (those with large VSD or PDA, those who received PA banding for VSD, and selected newborn infants). This procedure minimizes many complications associated with the intra-atrial repair operations such as arrhythmias, obstruction to systemic or pulmonary venous return, RV dysfunction, etc.

　b. Complications:

　　1) Intra-atrial repair surgeries, especially the Mustard operation:

　　　a) Residual atrial shunt.

　　　b) Obstruction to the pulmonary venous return (<5%).

　　　c) Obstruction to the systemic venous return (<5%).

　　　d) Depressed RV (systemic ventricular) function during exercise.

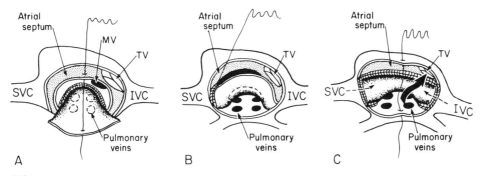

FIG 14–3.
The Mustard operation viewed through an incision made on the RA free wall. **A,** atrial septum *(dotted area)* has been excised at the site of ASD. A pericardial patch is placed in the LA in such a way to redirect pulmonary venous blood to the RA. The pulmonary veins *(four broken circles)* are seen under the baffle. The mitral valve *(MV)* and tricuspid valve *(TV)* are seen. **B,** the remaining edge of the pericardial baffle is reflected and sewn along the right margin of the openings of the SVC and IVC and to the anterior edge of the ASD. **C,** atrial incision is closed. When completed, systemic venous blood from the SVC and IVC is directed to the anatomical LA and the mitral valve. Pulmonary venous blood *(heavy arrow)* is directed to the tricuspid valve.

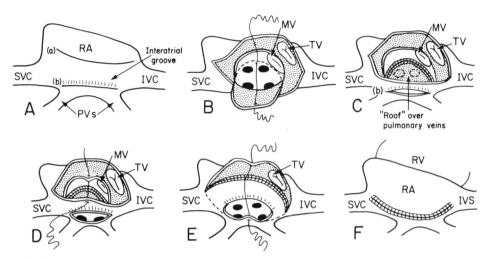

FIG 14–4.
The Senning operation. **A,** this procedure requires two incisions, *(a)* and *(b)*. The incision *(b)* is made along the left side of the interatrial groove. **B,** an atrial septal flap is made. A patch closure of the ASD or alternative measures to augment the atrial septal flap is sometimes required. **C,** the atrial septal flap is sewn in the LA in such a way to direct pulmonary venous blood to the RA through an opening created by the incision *(b)*. **D,** the posterior right atrial flap is then sewn to the atrial septum and the anterior margin of the ASD in such a way to direct blood from the SVC and IVC to the anatomical LA. **E** and **F,** the anterior atrial flap is sewn to the RA free wall *(dotted lines)* and to the LA flap created by the incision *(b)*.

      e) Tricuspid regurgitation (rare).

      f) Arrhythmias, early or late and transient or permanent, are common (50% or more). Arrhythmias include ectopic atrial tachycardia, sick sinus syndrome with slow nodal rate, and AV conduction disturbances.

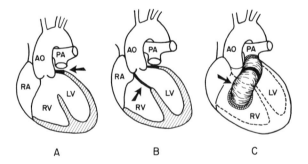

FIG 14–5.
The Rastelli operation. This procedure consists of the following steps: **A,** the PA is divided from the LV and the cardiac end is oversewn *(arrow)*. **B,** an intracardiac tunnel *(arrow)* is placed between the large VSD and the aorta so that the LV communicates with the aorta. **C,** the RV is connected to the divided PA by an aortic homograft or a valve-bearing prosthetic conduit.

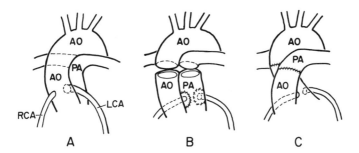

FIG 14–6.
The Jatene operation. **A,** anatomy of D-transposition of the great arteries. **B,** excision of the two coronary arteries from the aorta *(AO)* and their implantation to the pulmonary artery *(PA)* and transection of the aorta and the PA. **C,** anastomoses between the proximal end of the PA and the distal end of the ascending aorta and between the proximal end of the aorta and the distal end of the PA.

    g) Sudden death attributable to arrhythmias (3% of survivors).

    h) Pulmonary vascular obstructive disease.

  2) Rastelli operation:

    a) Conduit obstruction, especially with those containing porcine heterograft valves.

    b) Complete heart block (rare).

  3) Jatene operation:
    Complications are much fewer than with the intra-atrial repair surgeries. Arrhythmias are extremely rare. The LV function is normal. Pulmonary artery stenosis (up to 15%) is the only major complication which requires reoperation.

  c. Indication, Timing, and Mortality:
    The indication, timing, and mortality vary greatly from institution to institution, and are subject to change with the development of new information and new procedures. Figure 14–7 is a partial listing of many approaches used now.

    1) Infants with simple TGA (intact ventricular septum) who have had good results from the balloon atrial septostomy (BAS) receive an intra-atrial repair (either the Senning or Mustard procedure) at 6–12 months of age (because of their tendency to develop PVOD at an earlier age than with other forms of CHD). An increase in systemic arterial oxygen saturation of 10% or more and a minimal interatrial pressure difference are considered as a good result from the BAS.

    2) Infants who have had poor results from BAS should receive the Senning procedure at 1–3 months of age. Some centers prefer the Jatene operation during the neonatal period (mortality rate 0%–15%). Rarely, the Blalock-Hanlon operation (mortality 5%–25%) or blade atrial septostomy followed by the Senning operation (at 6–18 months) is recommended by some centers.

TRANSPOSITION OF THE GREAT ARTERIES

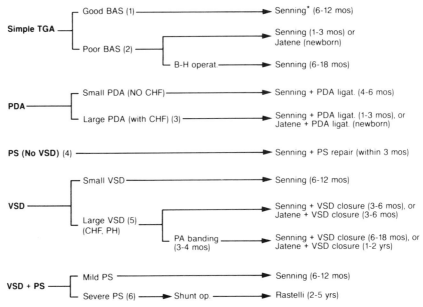

FIG 14–7.
Management flow diagram for TGA (see text for discussion). BAS = balloon atrial septos-tomy; B-H operat. = Blalock-Hanlon operation; CHF = congestive heart failure; PS = pulmonary stenosis. *Senning** is used to represent an intra-atrial repair, either the Senning operation or the Mustard operation.

3) Infants with a large PDA carry the worst prognosis, and, therefore, require an early surgical intervention. If CHF develops because of large PDA, the ligation of the PDA and the Senning operation are usually mandatory in early infancy (1–3 months). Some recommend ligation of the PDA and the Jatene operation during the neonatal period. If the PDA is small without CHF, the ligation of PDA and the Senning operation should be undertaken at 4–6 months of age.

4) Infants with discrete pulmonary stenosis (without VSD) should have the Senning operation and relief of PS within the first 3 months of life.

5) Infants with a large VSD receive a palliative procedure such as PA banding at 3–4 months of age. Senning's operation and closure of VSD are performed at 6–18 months of age (mortality 5%–10%). Alternatively, the Jatene operation and VSD closure may be performed at 1–2 years of age (mortality rate 10%–15%). Some centers advocate early repairs without PA banding; the Jatene operation + VSD closure at 3–6 months of age (mortality 25%–40%) or the Senning procedure + VSD closure at 3–6 months of age. Infants with a small VSD may be handled the same way as infants with simple TGA.

6) Infants with a VSD and severe PS may need a systemic-pulmonary artery shunt surgery (see Fig 14–14) during infancy. Rastelli's opera-

tion is carried out later at 2–5 years of age (mortality 5%–30%). Infants with a VSD and mild PS may receive the Senning operation at 6–12 months of age.

II. CONGENITALLY CORRECTED TRANSPOSITION OF THE GREAT ARTERIES
(L-Transposition, L-TGA, Ventricular Inversion)

Incidence
Much less than 1% of all congenital heart disease.

Pathology

1. Visceroatrial relationship is normal (the RA on the right of the LA).

2. The RA empties into the anatomical LV through the mitral valve, and the LA empties into the RV through the tricuspid valve. For this to occur, the RV is located to the left of the LV, and the LV is located to the right of the RV ("ventricular inversion") (Fig 14–8).

3. The great vessels are transposed, with the aorta arising from the RV and the PA arising from the LV. The aorta is located to the left of and anteriorly to the PA (see Fig 16–4,D).

4. The final result is functional correction: oxygenated blood coming into the LA goes to the anatomical RV and out the aorta. This is why the term "corrected" has been used for this condition.

5. Theoretically, no functional abnormalities exist, but, unfortunately, most cases are complicated by associated intracardiac defects, AV conduction disturbances, and arrhythmias.

   a. VSD is a common associated cardiac lesion occurring in 80% of the patients. Pulmonary stenosis (valvular or subvalvular) occurs in 50% of the patients and is usually associated with VSD.

   b. Systemic AV valve (tricuspid) regurgitation occurs in 30% of the patients.

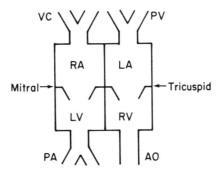

FIG 14–8.
Diagrammatic drawing of congenitally corrected transposition of the great arteries. There is an inversion of ventricular chambers with their corresponding AV valves. The great arteries are transposed, but functional *correction* results, with oxygenated blood going to the aorta. Unfortunately, however, a high percentage of the patients with L-TGA have associated defects with resulting cyanosis.

      c. Varying degrees of, and sometimes progressive, AV block and paroxysmal supraventricular tachycardia are frequently found.

    6. The cardiac apex is in the right chest (dextrocardia) in about 50% of the cases.

Clinical Manifestations

History

    a. Most patients become symptomatic during first few months of life with cyanosis (VSD + PS) or CHF (large VSD).

    b. Exertional dyspnea and easy fatigability (with systemic AV regurgitation).

    c. Asymptomatic when not associated with other defects.

PE

    a. Cyanosis if PS is present.

    b. Hyperactive precordium if a large VSD is present.

    c. The S2 is single and loud at the ULSB.

    d. A grade 2–4/6 harsh, holosystolic murmur along the LLSB may indicate VSD or systemic AV valve (tricuspid) regurgitation. A grade 2–3/6 systolic ejection murmur at the ULSB or URSB may indicate the presence of PS.

    e. An apical diastolic rumble may be present (large VSD or significant tricuspid valve regurgitation).

ECG (Fig 14–9)

    a. Absence of Q waves in I, V5, and V6 and/or the presence of Q waves in V4R or V1 is characteristic (this is because the direction of ventricular septal depolarization is from embryonic LV to RV).

    b. Varying degrees of AV block; first-degree AV block (50%) and second-degree AV block may progress to complete heart block.

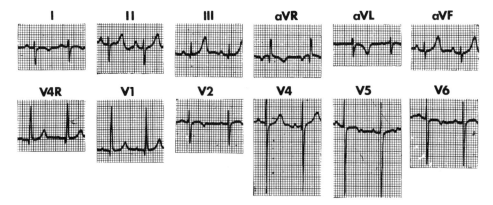

FIG 14–9.
Tracing from an 8-year-old girl with L-TGA, VSD, and PS. Note that no Q waves are seen in leads I, V5, and V6. Instead, the Q waves are seen in V4R and V1. This suggests ventricular inversion. The ECG also suggests hypertrophy of the right-sided ventricle (anatomical LV).

c. Atrial arrhythmias and WPW syndrome are occasionally present.

d. Atrial and/or ventricular hypertrophy may be present in complicated cases.

X-Rays

a. Straight left upper cardiac border (formed by the ascending aorta) is a characteristic finding (Fig 14–10).

b. Cardiomegaly and increased pulmonary vascular markings (with VSD).

c. Pulmonary venous congestion and LA enlargement (with severe AV valve regurgitation).

d. Occasional positional abnormalities (dextrocardia, mesocardia, etc.).

ECHO

By the use of segmental approach (see chap. 16), 2D ECHO can demonstrate that the RA is connected to the LV, and the LV gives rise to the PA (posterior course and immediate branching), and/or that the LA is connected to the RV (with the AV valve attached more toward the apex) and the aorta arises from the RV. Associated cardiac defects can also be identified.

Natural History and Complications

Clinical course is determined by the presence or absence of associated defects and complications.

a. Some palliative surgeries are usually required in infancy when L-TGA is associated with other defects; PA banding for large VSD and systemic-pulmonary artery shunt for PS.

b. Twenty percent to 30% of the patients die in the first year, CHF being the most common cause of death.

c. Progressive AV conduction disturbance, including complete heart block, may occur. (This may occur following a successful cardiac repair.)

d. Occasional adult patients are asymptomatic.

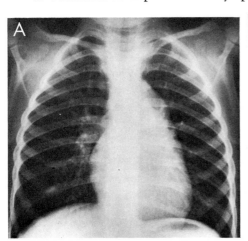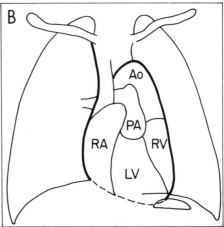

FIG 14–10.
A PA view of actual **(A)** and a diagram **(B)** of chest roentgenogram from a 10-year-old child with L-TGA. Note the straight left cardiac border formed by the ascending aorta.

Management

Medical

a. Treatment of CHF with anticongestive drugs.

b. Antiarrhythmic drugs for arrhythmias.

c. Prophylaxis against infective endocarditis.

Surgical

a. Palliative Procedures:

    1) Pulmonary artery banding for uncontrollable CHF.

    2) Systemic-pulmonary artery shunt for patients with severe PS (usually with VSD).

b. Corrective Procedures:

    1) Closure of VSD: Complete heart block is a frequent complication of the surgery (10%–20%), and mortality rate is 5%–10%.

    2) Corrective surgery for VSD + PS is more difficult with a higher mortality rate (10%–15%) than closure of VSD alone.

    3) Valve replacement for significant tricuspid regurgitation.

c. Pacemaker implantation for complete heart block, either spontaneous or surgically induced.

III. TETRALOGY OF FALLOT

Incidence

Ten percent of all congenital heart defects. The most common cyanotic cardiac defect beyond infancy.

Pathology

1. The original description of tetralogy of Fallot (TOF) included four abnormalities: a large VSD, RV outflow tract obstruction, right ventricular hypertrophy, and an overriding of the aorta. However, only two abnormalities are required: a VSD large enough to equalize systolic pressures in both ventricles and an RV outflow tract obstruction. The RV hypertrophy is secondary to the RV outflow tract obstruction and the overriding of the aorta is not a requirement.

2. In most cases of TOF, the VSD is a perimembranous infundibular defect.

3. The RV outflow tract obstruction is most frequently in the form of infundibular stenosis (50%). Rarely, the obstruction may be at the pulmonary valve level (10%) or a combination of the two (30%). In the most severe form of the anomaly, the pulmonary valve is atretic (10%). Right aortic arch is present in 25% of the cases.

Clinical Manifestations

History

a. Most of the patients are symptomatic with cyanosis, dyspnea on exertion, squatting, or hypoxic spells.

b. Patients with "acyanotic" tetralogy are usually asymptomatic.

c. Severe cyanosis immediately after birth is seen in patients with TOF and pulmonary atresia.

PE (Figure 14–11 shows cardiac findings.)

a. Varying degree of cyanosis and clubbing.

b. Right ventricular tap (along the LLSB). A systolic thrill at the lower and middle LSB (50%).

c. An ejection click (aortic) may be audible. The S2 is usually single (aortic component only) (see Fig 14–11).

d. A long, loud (grade 3–5/6) SEM at the middle and upper LSB (see Fig 14–11). This murmur may easily be confused with the holosystolic regurgitant murmur of a VSD. The more severe the obstruction of the RV outflow tract, the shorter the systolic murmur.

e. Occasionally, a continuous murmur representing PDA shunt may be audible in a deeply cyanotic neonate (TOF with pulmonary atresia).

f. In "acyanotic" form, a long systolic murmur resulting from VSD and infundibular stenosis is audible along the entire LSB, and cyanosis is absent. (Thus, findings resemble those of small-shunt VSD, but the ECG shows RVH or CVH.)

ECG

a. RAD (+120° to +150°) in cyanotic TOF. In acyanotic TOF, the QRS axis may be normal.

b. RVH is almost always present, but the "strain" pattern is unusual. CVH may be seen in acyanotic form.

c. RAH is occasionally present.

X-Rays

a. Cyanotic TOF:

1) No cardiomegaly (or even smaller than normal heart).

2) Decreased pulmonary vascular markings, or "black" lung fields in TOF with pulmonary atresia.

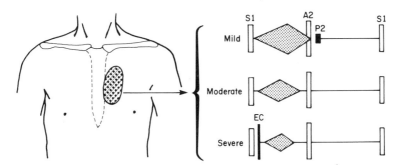

FIG 14–11.
Cardiac findings in cyanotic tetralogy of Fallot. A long SEM at the middle and upper LSB and a loud, single S2 are characteristic auscultatory findings of TOF.

3) Concave MPA segment with upturned apex ("boot-shaped" heart, or coeur en sabot) (Fig 14–12).

4) RA enlargement is occasionally present.

5) Right aortic arch in 25% of the cases.

   b. Acyanotic TOF: The x-ray findings of acyanotic TOF are indistinguishable from those of a small to moderate VSD (but they have RVH or CVH on the ECG, rather than LVH).

ECHO

2D ECHO shows a large VSD and overriding of the aorta (Fig 14–13). Anatomy of the RV outflow tract and pulmonary valve can usually be imaged.

Natural History and Complications

   a. Children with the acyanotic form of TOF gradually develop the cyanotic form by 1–3 years of age.

   b. Symptoms tend to progress because of increasing severity of the infundibular stenosis.

   c. Hypoxic spells in infants (see below and chap. 11).

   d. Growth retardation with severe cyanosis.

   e. Brain abscess and CVA (see chap. 11).

   f. Infective endocarditis.

   g. Polycythemia.

   h. Relative iron-deficiency anemia (hypochromic) (see chap. 11).

   i. Coagulopathies are a late complication of long-standing severe cyanosis.

Complications *d* through *i* are common to all types of cyanotic CHD.

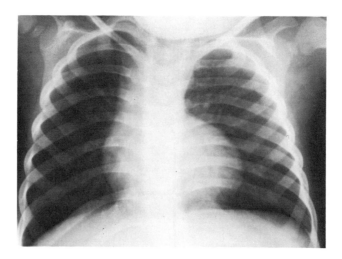

FIG 14–12.
A PA view of chest roentgenogram in TOF. The heart size is normal, and pulmonary vascular markings are decreased. A hypoplastic MPA segment contributes to the formation of the "boot-shaped" heart.

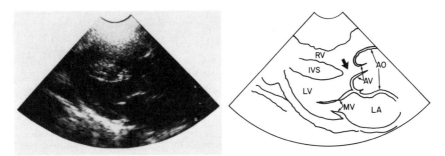

FIG 14–13.
Parasternal long-axis view in a patient with tetralogy of Fallot. Note a large subaortic VSD *(arrow)* and a relatively large aorta *(AO)* overriding the interventricular septum *(IVS).* AV = aortic valve; LA = left atrium; LV = left ventricle; MV = mitral valve; RV = right ventricle.

Hypoxic Spell

Hypoxic spell (cyanotic spell, "tet" spell) of TOF requires immediate recognition of the condition and appropriate therapy, as it can lead to serious CNS complications. Since primary care physicians are likely to take care of these infants initially, a special section is included in this chapter.

Hypoxic spells occur in young infants, with peak incidence between 2 and 4 months of age. The spells usually occur in the morning, following defecation, crying, or feeding. It is characterized by:

1) A paroxysm of hyperpnea (*rapid* and *deep* respiration).

2) Irritability and prolonged cry.

3) Increasing cyanosis.

4) Decreased intensity of the heart murmur.

A severe spell may lead to limpness, convulsion, CVA, or even death. There appears to be no relationship between the degree of cyanosis at rest and the likelihood of having hypoxic spells.

Pathophysiology of the spell has been discussed in detail in chapter 11, but a brief review may be in order. In TOF, the RV and LV can be considered as a single pumping chamber, since there is a large VSD equalizing pressures in both ventricles (see Fig 11–7). Lowering of the systemic vascular resistance (SVR) or increasing resistance at the RV outflow tract can increase right-to-left shunting, and this in turn stimulates the respiratory center to produce hyperpnea. Hyperpnea results in an increase in systemic venous return which, in turn, increases the right-to-left shunt through the VSD, because of the presence of pulmonary stenosis. A vicious cycle becomes established (see Fig 11–8).

Treatment of the hypoxic spell is aimed at breaking the vicious cycle. One or more of the following may be employed, in decreasing order of preference, in treating the spell.

1) Pick up and hold the infant over the shoulder and place in a knee-chest position. Picking him up helps calm down the infant, and the knee-chest position traps venous blood in the legs, decreasing systemic venous return, at least temporarily. The knee-chest position might also increase SVR by blocking blood flow to the legs.

2) Morphine sulfate, 0.1–0.2 mg/kg, SC, or IM, suppresses the respiratory center and abolishes hyperpnea. Rarely, general anesthesia may be required.

3) Treat acidosis with $NaHCO_3$, usually at the dose of 1 mEq/kg IV. In severe cases, the same dose may be repeated in 10–15 minutes. $NaHCO_3$ reduces the respiratory center-stimulating effect of acidosis.

4) Oxygen inhalation may help to improve oxygenation but has only limited value, since the problem is a reduced pulmonary blood flow, not the ability to oxygenate.

With the above treatment, the infant usually becomes less cyanotic and the heart murmur becomes louder, indicating improved pulmonary blood flow. If not fully responsive with the above measures:

5) Vasoconstrictors, such as phenylephrine (Neo-Synephrine) 0.02 mg/kg IV, may be effective. This raises the systemic vascular resistance and forces more blood to the lungs.

6) Oral propranolol therapy (2–6 mg/kg/day) may be used to prevent the recurrence of hypoxic spells and to delay corrective surgical procedures. The beneficial effect of propranolol may be related to its stabilizing action on peripheral vascular reactivity.

Management

Medical

a. Maintain good dental hygiene.

b. Antibiotic prophylaxis against infective endocarditis on indications (see Infective Endocarditis, chap. 19).

c. Detect and treat relative iron-deficiency anemia. Normal hemoglobin or hematocrit values or decreased red cell indices in a patient with arterial desaturation is an indication of iron-deficiency anemia. Anemic children are more prone to CVA.

d. Recognize and treat hypoxic spells (see above and chap. 11).

e. Oral propranolol therapy may prevent hypoxic spells and allow infants to grow to a more acceptable size for corrective surgeries.

Surgical

1. Palliative procedures are to increase pulmonary blood flow.

a. Indications:

1) Neonates with TOF and pulmonary atresia.

2) Severely cyanotic infants less than 6 months of age.

3) Infants with medically unmanageable hypoxic spells.

4) Infants with hypoplastic pulmonary anulus which requires transanular patch for complete repair.

5) Children with hypoplastic PA in whom the corrective surgery is technically difficult.

b. Procedures, Complications, and Mortality:

1) The Blalock-Taussig shunt (anastomosis between the subclavian artery and the ipsilateral PA) is the procedure of choice in infants older than

3 months (Fig 14–14). A right-sided shunt is performed in patients with left aortic arch and a left-sided shunt for right aortic arch. Thrombosis and closure of the shunt are the main problems when performed in younger infants. Mortality is low.

2) Waterston's shunt (anastomosis between the ascending aorta and the right PA) is no longer popular because of many complications following the operation (see Fig 14–14). Complications of this procedure include (a) too large a shunt, resulting in CHF and/or pulmonary hypertension; and (b) narrowing and kinking of the right PA at the site of anastomosis. At the time of corrective surgery, difficult problems may arise in closing the shunt and reconstructing the right pulmonary artery. Mortality is relatively low.

3) Potts' operation (anastomosis between the descending aorta and the left PA) is rarely performed and is important only from a historical point of view (see Fig 14–14). It may result in heart failure or pulmonary hypertension as in the Waterston operation. A separate incision (left thoracotomy) is required to close the shunt at the time of corrective surgery, which is usually done through a midsternal incision. Mortality rate is relatively low.

4) Gore-Tex interposition shunt between the subclavian artery and the ipsilateral PA is the procedure of choice in small infants younger than 3 months (see Fig 14–14). A left-sided shunt is performed in patients with left aortic arch and a right-sided shunt in patients with right-sided aortic arch.

2. Conventional Repair Surgery:

   a. Indications and Timing:

      1) Symptomatic infants or those with hematocrit 60% or higher who have had no previous shunt procedure and who have favorable anatomy of

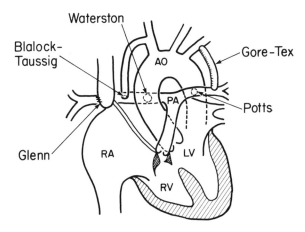

FIG 14–14.
Palliative procedures that can be used in patients with cyanotic cardiac defects with decreased PBF. The Glenn procedure (anastomosis between the SVC and the right PA) may be performed in older infants with hypoplastic RV, such as is seen with tricuspid atresia.

the RV outflow tract and pulmonary arteries may have primary repair at any time after 6 months of age.

2) Asymptomatic and minimally cyanotic children who have had previous shunt surgery may have total repair at 2–4 years of age.

3) Asymptomatic and acyanotic children ("pink tet") may be operated on at 2–4 years of age.

b. Procedure: Total repair of the defect is carried out under cardiopulmonary bypass. The procedure includes patch closure of the VSD and the widening of the RV outflow tract by resection of the infundibular tissue and usually placement of a fabric patch (Fig 14–15).

c. Mortality: Mortality rate is 5%–10% in the first two years for uncomplicated TOF. For complicated TOF, the mortality is higher.

d. Complications:

1) Bleeding problem in the postoperative period, particularly in older polycythemic patients.

2) Pulmonary valve regurgitation (well tolerated).

3) Congestive heart failure, usually transient.

4) RBBB on the ECG (due to right ventriculotomy).

5) Complete heart block; rare.

6) Ventricular arrhythmias which can lead to sudden death (2%–5%), primarily related to persistent RV hypertrophy and residual VSD.

7) Infective endocarditis is rare.

3. Rastelli's Operation:

a. Indications: Cases with severe hypoplasia or atresia of the RV outflow tract.

b. Procedure: See Figure 14–5 for schematic drawings of the procedure.

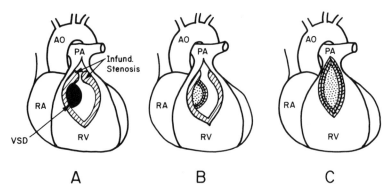

FIG 14–15.
Total correction of tetralogy of Fallot. **A,** anatomy of tetralogy of Fallot showing a large VSD, infundibular stenosis, and hypoplasia of the pulmonary valve anulus. **B,** patch closure of the VSD and resection of the infundibular stenosis. **C,** placement of a fabric patch on the outflow tract of the RV.

    c. Timing: Around 5 years of age (when adult-sized homograft-valved conduit can be used).

    d. Mortality: 10%.

IV. TOTAL ANOMALOUS PULMONARY VENOUS RETURN (TAPVR)

Incidence

One percent of all congenital heart defects. Marked male preponderance in infracardiac type (M:F = 4:1).

Pathology

1. There is no direct communication between the pulmonary veins and the LA. Depending on the site of the drainage of the pulmonary veins, it may be divided into the following four types (Fig 14–16).

    a. Supracardiac (50%): The common pulmonary vein drains into the SVC, via the left superior vena cava (vertical vein) and the left innominate vein (Fig 14–16,A).

    b. Cardiac (20%): The common pulmonary vein drains into the coronary sinus (Fig 14–16,C), or the pulmonary veins enter the RA separately through four openings (note that only two openings are illustrated in Figure 14–16,B).

    c. Infracardiac (subdiaphragmatic) (20%): The common pulmonary vein drains to the portal vein, ductus venosus, hepatic vein, or the IVC. The common pulmonary vein penetrates the diaphragm through the esophageal hiatus (Fig 14–16,D).

    d. Mixed type (10%): A combination of the above types.

2. An interatrial communication, either in the form of an ASD or patent foramen ovale, is necessary for survival.

3. The left side of the heart is relatively small.

4. A sizable number of patients with supracardiac and cardiac types, and almost all patients with the infracardiac type, have pulmonary hypertension secondary to the obstruction to the pulmonary venous return.

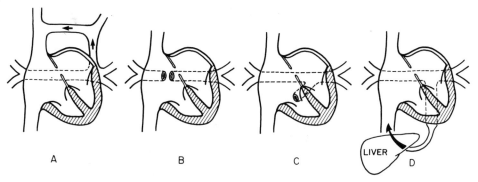

FIG 14–16.
Anatomical classification of TAPVR. **A,** supracardiac. **B** and **C,** cardiac. **D,** infracardiac.

Clinical Manifestations *(Without Pulmonary Venous Obstruction)*

History

 a. CHF with growth retardation in infancy.

 b. Frequent pulmonary infections.

 c. Mild cyanosis from birth.

PE (Figure 14–17 shows cardiac findings.)

 a. Mild to moderate growth retardation, and mild cyanosis.

 b. Signs of CHF (tachypnea, dyspnea, tachycardia, and hepatomegaly).

 c. Precordial bulge with hyperactive RV impulse (cardiac impulse is maximal at the xyphoid process and the LLSB).

 d. Characteristic quadruple or quintuple rhythm (see Fig 14–17). The S2 is widely split and fixed, and P2 may be accentuated. A grade 2–3/6 SEM at the ULSB is usually present.

 e. A middiastolic rumble at the LLSB is always present.

ECG

RAD, RVH of so-called "volume overload" type (rsR′ pattern in V1), and occasional RAH are present.

X-Rays

 a. Moderate to marked cardiomegaly (involving RA and RV).

 b. Increased pulmonary vascular markings.

 c. "Snowman" sign or figure-of-8 configuration in the supracardiac type (seen rarely before 4 months of age) (Fig 14–18).

ECHO

 a. M-mode ECHO may show signs of RV volume overload (abnormal motion of the interventricular septum) or a linear echo posterior to the LA.

 b. 2D ECHO may visualize the pulmonary veins draining into a common chamber posterior to the LA, not directly into the LA. A markedly dilated coronary sinus protruding into the LA (in TAPVR to the coronary sinus) or dilated left innominate vein and SVC (in the supracardiac type) may be vi-

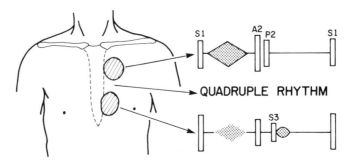

FIG 14–17.
Cardiac findings of TAPVR without obstruction to pulmonary venous return.

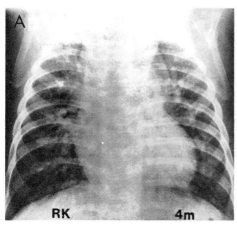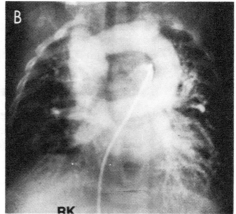

FIG 14–18.
A PA view of plain chest film demonstrating "snowman" sign **(A)** and an angiocardiogram demonstrating anatomical structures that participate in the formation of the "snowman" sign **(B)**; the vertical vein (left SVC), the left innominate vein, and the (right) SVC.

sualized. The obligatory ASD and relatively small LA and LV are usually visualized.

Natural History and Complications

a. CHF by 6 months of age with growth retardation.

b. Repeated pneumonias.

c. Without surgical repair, two-thirds of the infants die by 1 year of age.

Clinical Manifestations *(With Pulmonary Venous Obstruction)*

History

a. Marked cyanosis and respiratory distress in the neonatal period.

b. Growth failure.

c. Worsening of cyanosis with feeding, particularly in infants with infracardiac type (owing to compression of the common pulmonary vein by the food-filled esophagus).

PE

a. Moderate to marked cyanosis and tachypnea with retraction (in an under-nourished infant).

b. Cardiac findings may be minimal. Loud and single S2 and gallop rhythm are present. Heart murmur is usually absent. If present, it is usually a faint systolic ejection murmur at the ULSB.

c. Pulmonary rales may be audible.

d. Hepatomegaly is usually present.

ECG

RAD for age and RVH, usually in the form of tall R waves in the RPLs, are invariably present.

X-Rays

a. The heart size is usually normal.

b. The lung fields reveal findings of pulmonary edema (diffuse reticular pattern and Kerley's B lines). These findings may be confused with pneumonia or hyaline membrane disease.

ECHO

2D ECHO shows relatively hypoplastic LA and LV. Anomalous pulmonary venous return below the diaphragm can also be directly visualized and the venous flow pattern in the vessel can be tested by Doppler ECHO.

Natural History and Complications

a. Pneumonia may supervene, and most patients die by 2 months of age.

b. Patients with the infracardiac type rarely survive more than a few weeks without surgery.

Management *(With/Without PV Obstruction)*

Medical

a. Intensive anticongestive measures with digitalis and diuretics.

b. Oxygen and diuretics for pulmonary edema.

c. Intubation and respiratory therapy with oxygen and positive end-expiratory pressure (PEEP) may be necessary in infants with severe pulmonary edema (infracardiac type).

d. Balloon atrial septostomy at the time of cardiac catheterization to enlarge the interatrial communication. Blade atrial septostomy may be indicated in older infants with a thick interatrial septum.

Surgical

a. Indications and Timing:
Corrective surgery is indicated in all patients with this condition, since there is no palliative procedure.

    1) All infants with pulmonary venous obstruction, even in the newborn period.

    2) Infants without pulmonary venous obstruction, but with heart failure that is difficult to control, usually by 12 months of age.

b. Procedures:
Procedures vary with the site of the anomalous drainage, but all are performed under cardiopulmonary bypass.

    1. Supracardiac type: A side-to-side anastomosis is made between the common pulmonary vein and the LA, and the vertical vein is ligated. The ASD is closed with a cloth patch (Fig 14–19,A).

    2. TAPVR to the RA: The atrial septum is excised and a patch is sewn in such a way that the pulmonary venous return is diverted to the LA (Fig 14–19,B).

    3. TAPVR to coronary sinus: An incision is made in the anterior wall of the coronary sinus to make a communication between the coronary sinus and

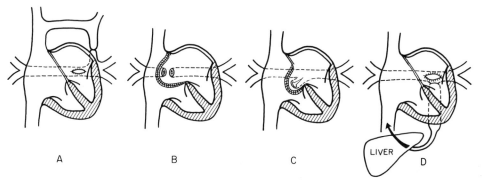

FIG 14–19.
Surgical approaches to various types of TAPVR (see text).

the LA. The original ASD and the ostium of the coronary sinus are closed by a single patch. This makes the coronary sinus blood and pulmonary venous blood drain into the LA (Fig 14–19,C).

4. Infracardiac type: An anastomosis is made between the common pulmonary vein and the LA, and the common pulmonary vein that descends vertically to the abdominal cavity is ligated at the upper end (Fig 14–19,D).

c. Mortality: Although the mortality rate is high, surgical management is superior to medical management. Mortality is 10%–25% in infants younger than 12 months. It is higher in infants with the infracardiac type than in those with other types.

d. Complications:

1) Small and poorly compliant left heart may cause pulmonary edema, requiring prolonged respiratory support.

2) Obstruction at the site of anastomosis, which may require additional surgery later.

3) Postoperative atrial arrhythmias, including "sick sinus syndrome."

V. TRICUSPID ATRESIA

Incidence

One percent to 2% of all congenital heart disease in infancy.

Pathology

1. The tricuspid valve is absent and the RV is hypoplastic, with absence of the inflow portion of the RV.

2. The pulmonary artery is usually hypoplastic and PBF is decreased.

3. The great arteries are transposed in 30% of the cases.

4. Associated defects, such as ASD and VSD or PDA, are necessary for survival.

5. Other commonly associated anomalies include persistent left SVC (20%) and COA (more commonly seen in tricuspid atresia with TGA).

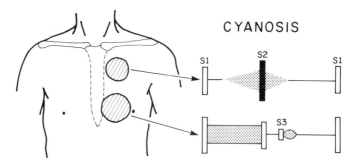

FIG 14–20.
Cardiac findings of tricuspid atresia, suggesting PDA and VSD. Left anterior hemiblock and cyanosis are characteristic of the defect.

Clinical Manifestations

History

    a. Cyanosis, usually severe, from birth.

    b. Poor feeding and tachypnea.

    c. History of hypoxic spell may be present.

PE (Figure 14–20 shows cardiac findings.)

    a. Cyanosis with or without clubbing is always present.

    b. A systolic thrill is rarely present, but is usually associated with PS.

    c. The S2 is single. A grade 2–3/6 systolic regurgitant murmur (of VSD) at the LLSB is usually present. A continuous murmur (of PDA) is occasionally present.

    d. An apical diastolic murmur may be rarely present with large PBF.

    e. Hepatomegaly is present when there is an inadequate interatrial communication or CHF.

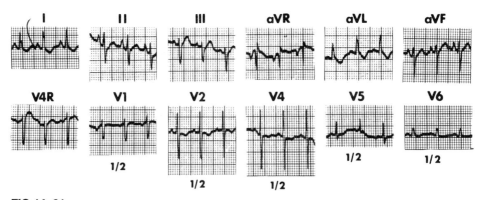

FIG 14–21.
Tracing from a 6-month-old girl with tricuspid atresia showing left anterior hemiblock (−30°), RAH, and LVH.

ECG (Fig 14-21)

a. "Superior" QRS axis (left anterior hemiblock), usually between 0° and −90°, is characteristic. It is present in the majority of the patients without TGA and 50% of the patients with TGA.

b. RAH or CAH in the majority of the cases.

c. LVH is almost always present.

X-Rays (Fig 14-22)

a. The heart size is normal or slightly increased (involving the RA and LV).

b. Pulmonary vascularity is decreased in most patients, although it may be increased in infants with TGA.

c. The concave MPA segment may produce a "boot-shaped" heart (coeur en sabot).

ECHO
2D ECHO shows absence of a functioning tricuspid valve, large LV and diminutive RV, presence or absence of TGA, VSD, or COA, and contractility of the LV.

Natural History and Complications

a. Few infants survive beyond 6 months of life without surgical palliation.

b. Occasional patients with increased PBF develop CHF.

c. Hypoxic spell is seen rarely.

Management

Medical

a. Treatment of CHF, if present.

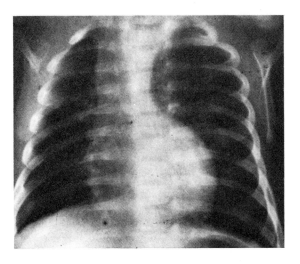

FIG 14–22.
A PA view of chest roentgenogram in an infant with tricuspid atresia with normally related great arteries. The heart is minimally enlarged. The pulmonary vascular markings are decreased, and the MPA segment is somewhat concave.

b. The Rashkind procedure (balloon atrial septostomy) in small infants as a part of the initial cardiac catheterization to improve the right-to-left atrial shunt.

c. Infective endocarditis prophylaxis on indications.

Surgical

1. Palliative Surgery: Most patients with tricuspid atresia require a palliative procedure to survive. It is to increase PBF when this is deficient and to diminish PBF when it is excessive.

    a. Systemic-pulmonary artery shunt:

      1) Indications: Inadequate PBF or hypoxic spells.

      2) Procedures, timing and mortality:

         a) The Blalock-Taussig or Gore-Tex shunt (see Fig 14–14) at any age, including newborn period. The Blalock-Hanlon operation (surgical creation of atrial septal defect) may be performed at the same time if the interatrial communication is small. Mortality rate is about 5%.

         b) Glenn's procedure (anastomosis between the SVC and the right PA) (see Fig 14–14) is recommended by some centers in older infants and children, but it is more clearly indicated when the Fontan procedure results in an inadequate RA to PA pathway. Mortality rate is 15%–20%.

    b. Pulmonary artery banding:

      1) Indications: Infants with increased PBF and CHF.

      2) Timing: Any time, including infancy.

      3) Mortality: Less than 5%.

2. Definitive Surgery (Fontan-type operation)

    a. Procedure (see Fig 14–23 for schematic drawings):

      1) Direct connection of the RA to the PA.

      2) Placement of a conduit (with/without valve) between the RA and PA (Fig 14–23,A).

      3) Conduit anastomosis of the RA to the RV outflow chamber with or without valve (Fig 14–23,B).

    b. Indications and Timing:
    Infants 4 years of age or older with normal PVR and PA pressure (mean pressure <20 mm Hg), adequate PA size, and normal LV function should have Fontan-type operation. More recently, some centers report good results in children younger than 4 years of age. Contraindications for the procedure include (1) small or stenotic pulmonary arteries (the combined diameter of the right and left PAs should be at least twice as large as that of the descending aorta), (2) elevated PVR (greater than 4 units/m^2), (3) elevated LA pressure (secondary to LV dysfunction or mitral valve abnormalities), and (4) chronic atrial fibrillation.

    c. Mortality rate: About 10%–15%.

    d. Complications:

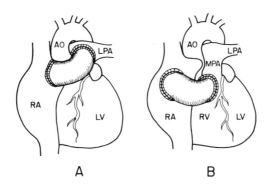

FIG 14–23.
Diagrammatic illustration of the Fontan-type operation in which a conduit with or without valve is placed between the dilated RA and the PA **(A)** or between the RA and the RV outflow chamber **(B)**.

1) Transient superior vena cava syndrome (distention of neck veins, edema of the face and arm, and headache).

2) Transient right heart failure (edema, ascites, and hepatomegaly).

3) Pleural effusion, more often on the right, is commonly seen.

4) Stenosis and fibrosis of the conduit valve (porcine heterograft) or obstruction of the Dacron conduit may occur, requiring reoperation. Homograft valves are preferred.

5) Protein-losing enteropathy (secondary to elevated central venous pressure).

6) Arrhythmias (usually supraventricular).

VI. PULMONARY ATRESIA

Incidence
Less than 1% of all congenital heart diseases.

Pathology

1. In the majority of patients, the valve is atretic with diaphragm-like membrane. Infundibular atresia (20%) or atresia of the pulmonary trunk may also be present. The interventricular septum is intact.

2. The RV cavity is usually hypoplastic, with a thick ventricular wall ("peach pit" RV, type I) occurring in about 85% of all cases. Occasionally, the RV is of normal size with significant tricuspid regurgitation (type II) occurring in about 15% of the cases.

3. Other defects, such as an interatrial communication (either ASD or PFO) and PDA, are necessary for survival.

Clinical Manifestations

History
Severe and progressive cyanosis from birth.

PE (Figure 14–24 shows cardiac findings.)

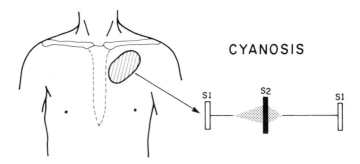

FIG 14–24.
Cardiac findings of pulmonary atresia. These are nonspecific for the defect and may be found in TOF with pulmonary atresia as well.

   a. Severe cyanosis and tachypnea in a neonate.

   b. The S2 is single. No heart murmur is present in many patients. A soft, continuous murmur of PDA may be audible at the ULSB (see Fig 14–24).

   c. Hepatomegaly is present if the interatrial communication is inadequate.

ECG

   a. Normal QRS axis ($+60°$ to $+140°$, in contrast to a superiorly oriented QRS axis of tricuspid atresia).

   b. LVH is usually present (type I), but occasional RVH is seen (in type II).

   c. RAH is present in 70% of the cases.

X-Rays

   a. The heart size may be normal or large (involving RA), and the MPA segment is concave (indistinguishable from x-ray findings of tricuspid atresia).

   b. Progressive decrease in pulmonary vascularity may occur.

ECHO
2D ECHO usually demonstrates the atretic pulmonary valve and hypoplastic RV cavity and tricuspid valve. The atrial communication can also be visualized and its size estimated.

Natural History and Complications
Exceedingly poor prognosis without appropriate medical management with prostaglandin E_1 and surgery. Without surgery, about 50% of the patients die by the end of the first month and about 85% by 6 months of age.

Management

Medical:

   a. Prostaglandin E_1 (Prostin VR pediatric solution) infusion as soon as the diagnosis is suspected to maintain patency of the ductus arteriosus during cardiac catheterization and surgery. Starting dose of Prostin is 0.1 μg/kg/minute; when the desired effect is achieved, reduce the dosage step-by-step, down to 0.01 μg/kg/minute.

   b. A balloon atrial septostomy as part of cardiac catheterization to improve right-to-left atrial shunt.

c. Prophylaxis against infective endocarditis for survivors.

Surgical:

a. Indications: All infants with the diagnosis.

b. Urgent Procedures:

1) Systemic-pulmonary artery shunt (Gore-Tex shunt between the left sub-clavian artery and the left PA, or the Blalock-Taussig operation) is usually required, especially for type I.

2) Blind pulmonary valvotomy (Brock's procedure) or transpulmonary val-votomy without cardiopulmonary bypass is recommended by some at the time of the shunt operation.

3) Mortality of these procedures is moderately high (10%–25%).

c. Follow-up Procedures:

1) If the first shunt is inadequate, a repeated systemic-pulmonary artery shunt may be performed at a different location.

2) If an adequate forward flow from the RV following the Brock procedure (or transpulmonary valvotomy) is confirmed, the shunt may be taken down a year or two later.

3) Right ventricular outflow tract reconstruction (placement of patch across the pulmonary annulus) under cardiopulmonary bypass is carried out when the size of the RV is reasonable. Mortality rate is about 25%.

4) For those with hypoplastic RV (type I), the Fontan-type operation (see Fig 14–23) may be performed during late childhood. Mortality rate may be as high as 40%.

VII. EBSTEIN'S ANOMALY

Incidence
Less than 1% of all congenital heart defects.

Pathology

1. The leaflets of the tricuspid valve are displaced into the RV cavity, so that a portion of the RV is incorporated into the RA ("atrialized RV") and functional hypoplasia of the RV results. At the same time, tricuspid valve regurgitation results.

2. An interatrial communication is present in the majority of the patients (80%), with resulting right-to-left atrial shunt.

Clinical Manifestations

History

a. Cyanosis and CHF in the first few days of life, with some subsequent im-provement.

b. In milder cases, dyspnea, fatigue, and cyanosis on exertion in childhood.

c. Paroxysmal atrial tachycardia (PAT) may occur.

PE (Figure 14–25 shows cardiac findings.)

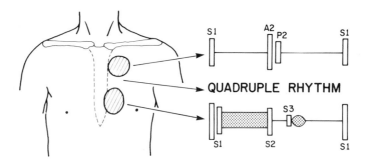

FIG 14–25.
Cardiac findings of Ebstein's anomaly. Quadruple rhythm and a soft, regurgitant systolic murmur are characteristic of the defect.

    a. Mild to severe cyanosis.

    b. The S2 is widely split. Characteristic triple or quadruple rhythm is present (consisting of split S1, split S2, S3, or S4).

    c. A soft systolic regurgitant murmur (of tricuspid regurgitation) is usually audible at the LLSB (see Fig 14–25).

    d. A soft, scratchy middiastolic murmur at the LLSB.

    e. Hepatomegaly is usually present.

ECG

    a. Characteristic ECG findings are RBBB and RAH (Fig 14–26).

    b. WPW syndrome is present in 20% of the patients.

    c. Occasional PAT and first-degree AV block are seen.

X-Rays (Fig 14–27)

    a. Extreme cardiomegaly (involving principally the RA).

    b. Diminished pulmonary vascular markings.

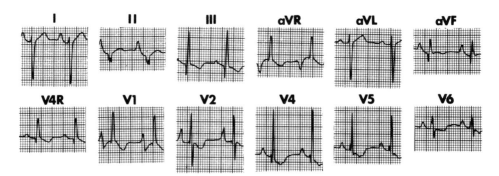

FIG 14–26.
Tracing from a 5-year-old child with Ebstein's anomaly. The tracing shows RAH (or possible CAH), RBBB, and first-degree AV block.

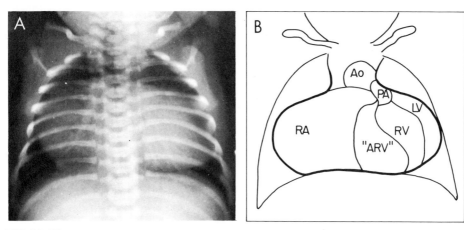

FIG 14–27.
A PA view **(A)** and a diagram **(B)** of chest roentgenogram from a 2-week-old infant with
severe Ebstein's anomaly. Note extreme cardiomegaly involving primarily the RA and diminished pulmonary vascularity.

ECHO

Characteristic 2D ECHO findings include (a) the apically displaced septal leaflet, and (b) the elongated, somewhat redundant anterior leaflet of the tricuspid
valve.

Natural History and Complications

a. Cyanosis tends to improve as the PVR falls in the newborn period, although
cyanosis may reappear later.

b. Patients with a less severe anomaly may be mildly symptomatic or asymptomatic.

c. 30% die before age of 10 years (a median age at death is about 20 years).

d. Attacks of PAT are common.

e. Other possible complications include CHF, brain abscess and/or CVA, and
infective endocarditis.

Management

Medical

a. Anticongestive measures, with digitalis and diuretics if CHF develops.

b. Varying degree of restriction of activity.

c. Prevention against infective endocarditis (good dental hygiene and preop-
erative use of antibiotics for dental and surgical procedures).

d. Treatment of PAT with digoxin alone or in combination with quinidine or
propranolol.

Surgical

a. Procedures:
There is controversy concerning the surgical procedure.

1) Tricuspid valve replacement with a prosthetic or tissue valve and closure of ASD are the most commonly used surgical approach. Mortality rate ranges from 5% to 20%. When possible the procedure should be delayed until 15 years.

2) Tricuspid annuloplasty is most desirable, although frequently limited by anatomy. Mortality is lower than with the valve replacement.

3) Glenn's procedure is performed by some centers, but gives at best mediocre long-term results. A systemic-pulmonary artery shunt procedure is very rarely performed.

4) The Fontan procedure is advocated in patients with severe hypoplasia of the functioning RV.

5) For those patients with WPW syndrome and severe PAT, surgical interruption of the accessory pathway is recommended at the time of surgery.

b. Indications:

1) Severe limitations in activity, moderate to severe cyanosis, and CHF.

2) Repeated life-threatening arrhythmias in patients with WPW syndrome.

c. Complications:

1) Complete heart block, rare.

2) Persistence of supraventricular arrhythmias following surgery (10%–20%).

VIII. PERSISTENT TRUNCUS ARTERIOSUS

Incidence

Less than 1% of all congenital heart disease.

Pathology (Fig 14–28)

1. Only a single arterial trunk (with a truncal valve) leaves the heart and gives rise to the pulmonary, systemic, and coronary circulations.

2. A large ventricular septal defect is always present.

3. The truncal valve may have 3 or 4 leaflets.

4. A right aortic arch is present in 50% of the patients.

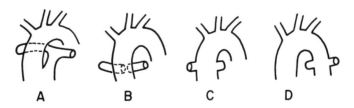

A   B   C   D

FIG 14–28.
Anatomical types of persistent truncus arteriosus **A,** type I, the MPA arises from the truncus and then divides into the right and left pulmonary arteries. **B,** type II, the pulmonary arteries arise from the posterior aspect of the truncus. **C,** type III, the pulmonary arteries arise from the lateral aspects of the truncus. **D,** type IV, or pseudotruncus arteriosus, bronchial arteries arising from the descending aorta and supplying the lungs.

5. Anatomically, this anomaly is divided into four types (Collett and Edwards' classification) (see Fig 12–28): type I (60%), type II (20%), type III (10%), and type IV (10%). Type IV is not a true persistent truncus arteriosus, but a severe form of TOF with pulmonary atresia (pseudotruncus arteriosus) with bronchial arteries supplying the lungs.

6. The magnitude of PBF is usually increased in type I, normal in types II and III, and decreased in type IV.

Clinical Manifestations

History

a. Cyanosis of varying degree may be noted immediately after birth.

b. Signs of CHF develop within several weeks.

c. Dyspnea with feeding, failure to thrive, and frequent respiratory infections are usually present in infants.

PE

a. Varying degree of cyanosis and signs of CHF with tachypnea and dyspnea.

b. Wide pulse pressure and bounding arterial pulses may be present.

c. A systolic click at the apex and ULSB is frequently present. A harsh (grade 2–4/6) systolic regurgitant murmur (suggestive of VSD) is usually present along the left sternal border.

d. An apical rumble with or without gallop rhythm may be present when PBF is increased.

e. Rarely, a continuous murmur may be heard over either side of the chest. A high-pitched, early diastolic decrescendo murmur may be audible if truncal valve insufficiency coexists.

ECG

a. Normal QRS axis ($+50°$ to $+120°$).

b. CVH is commonly present (70%); RVH or LVH is less common.

c. Occasionally LAH is present.

X-Rays

a. Marked cardiomegaly (biventricular and LA enlargement) and an increased pulmonary vascularity are usually present.

b. A right aortic arch is seen in 50% of the cases.

ECHO

2D ECHO demonstrates the following:

a. A large single great artery arising from the heart (truncus); the posterior branching of the pulmonary artery may be seen.

b. A large VSD directly under the truncal valve (similar to TOF).

c. Inability to show the pulmonary valve.

Natural History and Complications

a. Most infants die of CHF within 6–12 months.

b. Clinical improvement if the infant develops PVOD as in large VSDs.

c. Truncal valve insufficiency worsens with time.

d. Longer survival is seen in types with normal PBF.

Management

Medical

a. Vigorous anticongestive measures with digitalis and diuretics.

b. Prophylaxis against infective endocarditis.

Surgical

a. Palliative Procedure:
   Pulmonary artery banding may be indicated in small infants with large PBF
   and CHF. Mortality rate of this procedure may be as high as 30% in early
   infancy.

b. More Definitive Procedure:

   1) Rastelli's procedure may be performed for type I or II (see Fig 14–15).
      The VSD is closed in such a way that the LV ejects into the truncus, and
      a valved, preferably aortic homograft, conduit is placed between the RV
      and the PA.

   2) Optimal age: Nearly always during infancy (since only 10% of patients
      survive beyond infancy). Those infants who have received PA banding
      may be operated on at a slightly older age.

   3) Mortality: Varies widely (20%–60%).

   4) Complications: Calcification of the valve may occur in 5–10 years. The
      size of the conduit may be inadequate for somatic growth, requiring re-
      operation later.

IX. SINGLE VENTRICLE

(Common Ventricle, Univentricular Heart)

Incidence
Less than 1% of all congenital heart defects.

Pathology (Fig 14–29)

1. Both AV valves empty into a common ventricular chamber. The ventricular
   chamber has anatomical characteristics of the LV (double-inlet LV), occurring
   in 80% of the cases (see Fig 14–29). Occasionally, the common chamber has
   anatomical characteristics of the RV (double-inset RV). Rarely, there is a true
   common ventricle with normal components of RV and LV but absent septum.
   A rudimentary infundibular chamber is usually present and communicates
   with the common ventricular chamber (through the bulboventricular foramen).

2. A great artery arises from the common chamber and the other great artery
   arises from the infundibular chamber (single ventricle). Occasionally, no infundibular chamber is present, and two great arteries originate closely from the
   common outflow region (common ventricle).

3. Transposition of the great arteries (either D- or L-form in equal frequency) is
   present in 85% of the cases. The aorta usually arises from the infundibular

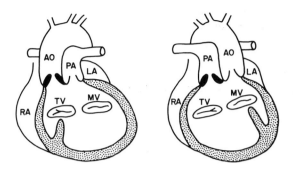

FIG 14–29.
Diagrammatic illustration of two more common forms of single ventricle; there are other, less common forms of single ventricle that are not shown in this figure. **A,** the single ventricle is anatomical LV. D-TGA and stenosis of the aortic valve are present. **B,** the single ventricle is anatomical LV also. L-TGA with pulmonary stenosis is present.

chamber and the PA from the main chamber. Aortic stenosis is commonly present in D-TGA (Fig 14–29,A) and pulmonary stenosis in L-TGA (Fig 14–29,B).

4. High incidence of asplenia or polysplenia syndrome (see chap. 17).

Clinical Manifestations

History

    a. Cyanosis of varying degree from birth.

    b. Symptoms and signs of CHF.

    c. Failure to thrive or bouts of pneumonia.

PE

Physical findings are dependent on the magnitude of PBF.

    a. With *increased PBF,* physical findings resemble those of TGA and VSD or persistent truncus arteriosus, or even large VSD:

        1) Mild cyanosis and CHF with growth retardation in early infancy.

        2) The S2 is single or narrowly split with loud P2. A grade 3–4/6 long systolic murmur is widely audible along the LSB.

        3) A diastolic murmur of pulmonary regurgitation may be present along the ULSB (due to pulmonary hypertension).

        4) A loud S3 or an apical diastolic rumble may be present.

    b. With *decreased PBF,* physical findings resemble those of TOF:

        1) Moderate to severe cyanosis (no CHF). Clubbing may be seen in older infants and children.

        2) The S2 is loud and single. A grade 2–4/6 SEM at the URSB (or ULSB).

ECG

    a. Unusual ventricular hypertrophy pattern with similar QRS complexes across most or all precordial leads (RS, rS or QR pattern).

    b. Abnormal Q waves (abnormalities in septal depolarization) are also common and take one of the following forms:

        1) Q waves in the RPLs,

        2) No Q waves in any precordial leads, or

        3) Q waves in both the RPLs and LPLs.

    c. AV block, either first- or second-degree.

    d. Arrhythmias (PAT, wandering pacemaker, etc.).

X-Rays

    a. When PBF is increased, the heart size is enlarged, and the pulmonary vascularity is increased.

    b. When PBF is normal or decreased, the heart size is normal, and the pulmonary vascularity is normal or decreased.

    c. Narrow waist suggestive of TGA may be present.

ECHO

    a. M-mode ECHO detects a single ventricular chamber without an intervening interventricular septum.

    b. 2D ECHO may show (1) two distinct AV valves emptying into a single ventricular chamber, (2) a rudimentary chamber that is not related to an AV valve, and (3) relationship of two great arteries to each other and to the ventricular chamber and the rudimentary chamber.

Natural History and Complications

    a. CHF and growth failure in early infancy.

    b. Clinical improvement occurs if PVOD develops.

    c. Cyanosis increases, if there is reduction in the size of the communication between the common and rudimentary chambers or if there is worsening of subpulmonary stenosis.

    d. 50% of the patients die by 1 year of age.

    e. Infective endocarditis or cerebral complications may develop as in TOF.

Management

Medical

    a. Anticongestive measures with digitalis and diuretics.

    b. Prophylaxis against infective endocarditis.

Surgical

    a. Palliative Procedures:

        1) Systemic-pulmonary artery shunt (for infants) or Glenn's procedure (for children older than 2 years) may be required for patients with PS and severe cyanosis (see Fig 14–14 for schematic drawings of the procedures).

        2) PA banding for patients without PS and uncontrollable CHF. Later, these patients may develop cyanosis and require a shunt procedure.

b. More Definitive Procedures:

1) The Fontan procedure: By closing the tricuspid valve, a situation similar to tricuspid atresia is created, and then, the Fontan procedure is performed at 4–6 years of age as in tricuspid atresia (see Fig 14–23). This procedure cannot be performed if the PVR is high. The mortality and morbidity are higher than those for patients with tricuspid atresia (20%–30%). For patients who have had a prior Glenn's shunt, the Fontan anastomosis is between the RA and the main or left PA.

2) Attempts at partitioning the single ventricle with a Dacron patch or Teflon patch are usually not successful.

X. DOUBLE-OUTLET RIGHT VENTRICLE (DORV)

Incidence

Less than 1% of all congenital heart disease.

Pathology (Fig 14–30)

1. Both the aorta and PA arise side-by-side from the RV, and the aortic and pulmonary valves are at the same level.

2. The only outlet from the LV is a large VSD.

3. The presence or absence of pulmonary stenosis (PS) and location of the VSD (whether it is close to the aorta or the pulmonary artery) influence hemodynamic alterations as well as clinical manifestations.

4. DORV may be subdivided depending on the position of the VSD (and further by the presence of PS).

   a. Subaortic VSD (see Fig 14–30,A and C). This is the most frequently encountered type (60%–70%). The VSD is close to the aortic valve. Pulmonary stenosis (mostly infundibular PS) is common (about 50%) in this type of DORV (Fallot type).

   b. Subpulmonary VSD (Taussig-Bing anomaly) (Fig 14–30,B). The VSD is closer to the pulmonary valve than to the aortic valve.

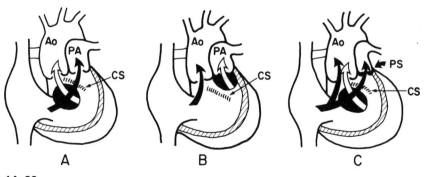

FIG 14–30.
Diagrammatic drawing of three representative types of DORV, viewed with the RV free wall removed. Doubly committed and remote VSDs are not shown. Ao = aorta; PA = pulmonary artery; CS = crista supraventricularis; PS = pulmonary stenosis.

c. Doubly committed VSD. The VSD is closely related to both semilunar valves.

d. Remote VSD: The VSD is clearly away from the semilunar valves.

Pathophysiology

Pathophysiology of DORV is determined primarily by the position of the VSD and the presence or absence of PS (see Fig 14–30).

1. When the VSD is close to the aortic valve (subaortic VSD), oxygenated blood *(open arrow)* from the LV is directed to the aorta (Ao) and desaturated systemic venous blood *(solid arrow)* is directed to the pulmonary artery (PA), producing mild or no cyanosis (see Fig 14–30,A). The PBF is increased in the absence of PS or PVOD, resulting in CHF. Therefore, clinical pictures of this type resemble those of a large VSD with pulmonary hypertension and CHF.

2. When the VSD is just beneath the pulmonary valve (subpulmonary VSD, Taussig-Bing anomaly), oxygenated blood from the LV is directed to the PA, and desaturated blood from the systemic vein is directed to the aorta, producing severe cyanosis (see Fig 14–30,B). The PBF is increased with the fall of PVR. Clinical pictures, therefore, resemble those of TGA.

3. In the presence of pulmonary stenosis (Fallot type), even though the VSD is subaortic, some desaturated blood goes to the aorta producing cyanosis, and the PBF is decreased. Thus, clinical pictures resemble those of TOF (see Fig 14–30,C).

4. With the VSD close to both semilunar valves (doubly committed VSD) or remotely located from these valves (remote VSD), cyanosis of mild degree is present and the PBF is increased.

Clinical Manifestations

Clinical manifestations vary greatly depending on the location of the VSD and the presence or absence of PS. Therefore, the clinical pictures of three representative types will be presented separately.

A. Subaortic VSD without PS:

The patient is not cyanotic, and the clinical picture resembles that of a large VSD with pulmonary hypertension and CHF.

PE

a. Growth retardation, tachypnea, and other signs of CHF are usually present.

b. An overactive precordium with loud S2. A VSD-type holosystolic regurgitant murmur is present at the LLSB.

c. An apical diastolic rumble may be present.

ECG: Often resembles that of complete ECD.

a. A superiorly oriented QRS axis ($-30°$ to $-170°$) may be present in this subtype.

b. LAH and RVH or CVH.

c. Occasionally, first-degree AV block is present.

X-Rays: Cardiomegaly with increased PVM and prominent MPA segment.

B. Subpulmonary VSD (Taussig-Bing malformation):

The clinical picture resembles that of TGA in newborn infants.

PE

  a. Growth retardation and severe cyanosis with/without clubbing.

  b. The S2 is loud, and a grade 2–3/6 systolic murmur is audible at the ULSB.

  c. An ejection click and occasional pulmonary regurgitation murmur (due to pulmonary hypertension) may be present.

ECG: RAD ($+90°$ to $+160°$), RAH, and RVH (or LVH during infancy).

X-Rays: Cardiomegaly with increased PVM and prominent MPA segment.

C. Fallot-type DORV (with PS):

The clinical picture is similar to that seen in cyanotic TOF.

PE

  a. Growth retardation, cyanosis, and clubbing.

  b. A systolic thrill may be present.

  c. The S2 is loud and single. A grade 2–3/6 systolic ejection murmur along the LSB is present.

ECG: RAD, RAH, RVH or RBBB, and first-degree AV block are frequently present.

X-Rays: The heart size is normal (with upturned apex). Pulmonary vascularity is decreased.

ECHO (for all types):

2D ECHO reveals (1) both great arteries arising from the RV and running a parallel course in their origin. (2) Absence of the LV outflow tract and the demonstration of a VSD. (3) Mitral-semilunar discontinuity.

Natural History and Complications (for all types):

  a. Children without PS may develop severe CHF in infancy and PVOD later.

  b. When PS is present, complications common to cyanotic CHD (polycythemia or CVA) may occur.

Management

Medical

  a. Medical treatment of CHF.

  b. Good dental hygiene and prophylaxis against infective endocarditis.

Surgical

  a. Palliative Procedures:

   1) PA banding for symptomatic infants with increased PBF and CHF (subaortic and subpulmonary VSD).

   2) For infants with Taussig-Bing type, the Blalock-Hanlon operation (atrial septectomy) is essential for better mixing of pulmonary and systemic venous blood.

3) Systemic-pulmonary artery shunt procedures in small infants with PS and cyanosis (Fallot type). Mortality is less than 5%.

b. Corrective Surgeries:

1) Subaortic VSD and doubly committed VSD: Creation of an intraventricular tunnel between the VSD and the root of the aorta. When carried out at 6 months to 2 years of age, the mortality is about 10%–20%.

2) Taussig-Bing anomaly (subpulmonary VSD): There are three possible surgical approaches, which should be carried out at 1–2 years of age.

   a) An intraventricular tunnel between the subpulmonary VSD and the aorta is most desirable if technically feasible. The mortality rate is relatively low.

   b) An intraventricular tunnel between the VSD and the PA, plus the arterial switch (the Jatene) operation. The mortality rate is 10%–20%.

   c) An intraventricular tunnel between the VSD and the PA, plus the Senning or the Mustard operation. Mortality rate is high (40%–50%).

3) Fallot type: An intraventricular tunnel procedure (VSD-Ao) plus relief of PS by a patch graft is carried out between 1 and 2 years of age. Mortality rate is about 10%–15%.

4) Remote VSD: The surgery may be delayed until 2–3 years of age. When possible, an intraventricular tunnel procedure (VSD-Ao) is preferred. If not possible, a Fontan-type operation is carried out. The mortality is high.

15 / Vascular Ring

Incidence

Rare, but the true incidence may be underestimated.

Pathology

Vascular ring refers to a group of anomalies of the aortic arch that cause respiratory symptoms or feeding problems. The vascular ring may be divided into two groups, complete and incomplete.

1. True or complete vascular ring refers to conditions in which the abnormal vascular structures form a complete circle around the trachea and esophagus. They are:

   a. Double aortic arch.

   b. Right aortic arch with left ligamentum arteriosum.

2. Incomplete vascular ring refers to vascular anomalies that do not form a complete circle around the trachea and esophagus but compress the trachea or esophagus. They include:

   a. Anomalous innominate artery.

   b. Aberrant right subclavian artery.

   c. Aberrant left pulmonary artery ("vascular sling").

A brief discussion of the pathology of each condition is presented (see Fig 15–1).

1. Double aortic arch is the most common vascular ring (40%). Both right and left fourth branchial arches persist, with resulting right and left aortic arches, respectively. These two aortic arches completely encircle the trachea and esophagus, producing respiratory distress and feeding problems in early infancy. The right aortic arch is usually larger than the left arch.

2. Right aortic arch with left ligamentum arteriosum is the second most common vascular ring (30%). This results from persistence of the right fourth branchial arch (forming the right aortic arch). When this structure is combined with the left-sided ligamentum arteriosum or patent ductus arteriosus, a constricting ring results and compresses the trachea and esophagus.

3. Anomalous innominate artery (10%). If the innominate artery takes off too far to the left from the aortic arch or has a more posterior take-off, it may compress the trachea, producing mild respiratory symptoms.

4. Aberrant right subclavian artery (20%). When the right subclavian artery arises independently from the descending aorta, it courses behind the esophagus, compressing the posterior aspect of the esophagus. This produces mild feeding problems.

197

	Anatomy	Ba-Esophagogram	Other X-ray Findings	Symptoms	Treatment
Double Aortic Arch	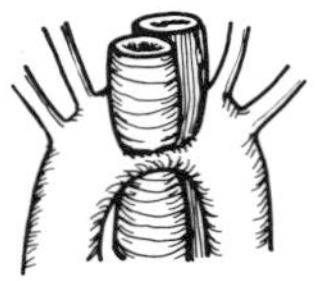	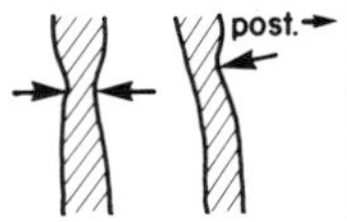	Anterior compression of trachea	Respiratory difficulty (onset < 3 mos.) Swallowing dysfunction	Surgical division of a smaller arch
Right Aortic Arch with Left Lig. Arteriosum	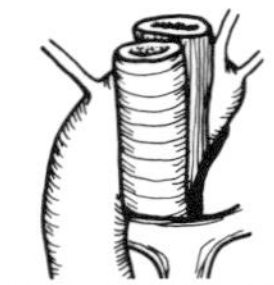	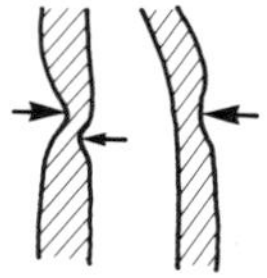		Mild respiratory difficulty (onset > 1 year) Swallowing dysfunction	Surgical division of the lig. arteriosum
Anomalous Innominate Artery	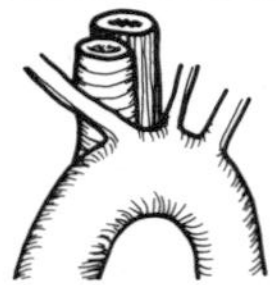	Normal	Anterior compression of trachea	Stridor and/or cough in infancy	Conservative management, or Surgical suturing of the artery to the sternum
Aberrant Right Subclavian Artery	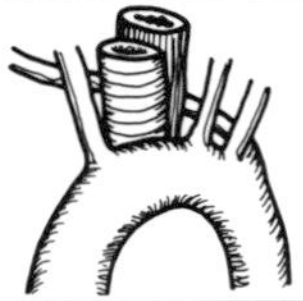	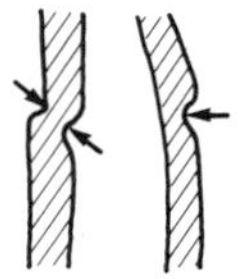		Occasional swallowing dysfunction	Usually no treatment is necessary
"Vascular Sling"	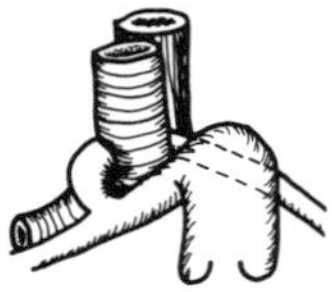	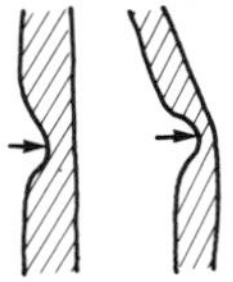	Right-sided emphysema or atelectasis. Posterior compression of trachea or Rt. main-stem bronchus	Wheezing and cyanotic episodes since birth	Surgical division of the anomal. LPA (from the RPA) and anastomosis to the MPA

FIG 15–1.
Summary and clinical features of vascular ring. P-A = posteroanterior view; Lat. = lateral view.

5. Anomalous left pulmonary artery ("vascular sling"). In this rare anomaly, the left PA arises from the right PA. To reach the left lung, it courses over the proximal portion of the right main-stem bronchus, then behind the trachea and in front of the esophagus to the hilum of the left lung, producing both respiratory and feeding problems.

Clinical Manifestations

History

a. Respiratory distress and feeding problems of varying severity and varying age of onset. In double aortic arch, symptoms tend to appear in early infancy (less than 3 months of age), and they are more severe than in right aortic arch with left ligamentum arteriosum.

b. Milder respiratory symptoms or feeding problems with incomplete forms of vascular ring.

c. History of pneumonia is frequently elicited.

d. Atelectasis, emphysema, or pneumonias of the right lung with vascular sling.

PE

a. Not revealing except for varying degrees of rhonchi.

b. Cardiac examination is normal.

ECG: Normal.

X-Rays (See Fig 15–1.)

a. Compression of the air-filled trachea may be visible on PA and lateral chest x-ray films. Aspiration pneumonia or atelectasis may be present.

b. Barium esophagogram is usually diagnostic, except in anomalous innominate artery (see Fig 15–1):

1) In double aortic arch, two large indentations are present on both sides (with the right one usually larger) in the PA view, and a posterior indentation on the lateral view.

2) In right aortic arch with left ligamentum arteriosum, a large right-sided indentation and a much smaller left-sided indentation are present. A posterior indentation is also present on the lateral view.

3) Barium esophagogram is normal in anomalous left innominate artery.

4) In aberrant right subclavian artery, there is a small oblique indentation extending toward the right shoulder on the PA view. There is a small posterior indentation on the lateral view.

5) In vascular sling, an anterior indentation of esophagus on the lateral view at the level of the carina is characteristic. A right-sided indentation is usually seen on the PA view.

Diagnosis

1. Vascular ring is suspected based on clinical symptoms.

2. Barium esophagogram is the most useful diagnostic tool.

3. Angiography is usually indicated to confirm the diagnosis and to prepare for surgery.

Management (See Fig 15–1.)

1. Medical management for infants with mild symptoms.

2. Surgical approach is indicated in infants with more severe symptoms or complications such as aspiration pneumonia. In infants who have had surgery for severe respiratory symptoms (such as seen in double aortic arch or right aortic arch with left ligamentum arteriosum), airway obstruction may persist for weeks or months, requiring careful respiratory management in the postoperative period. This is because of hypoplasia and deformity of the underlying tracheal cartilages.

16 / Chamber Localization and Cardiac Malposition

In this chapter clinical methods of locating cardiac chambers using simple laboratory tests (ECG and chest x-rays) and physical examination will be briefly discussed. This will be followed by application of the principle which may aid in anatomical diagnosis of the heart in the right chest (dextrocardia) or in the midline (mesocardia). Although these methods are valid, there are many exceptions, with both false positive and false negative results possible. 2D ECHO usually reveals the correct diagnosis, but occasionally cardiac catheterization and angiography may be needed.

I. CHAMBER LOCALIZATION

The heart and the great arteries can be viewed as three separate segments; i.e., the atria, the ventricles, and the great arteries. These three segments can vary from their normal positions either independently or together, resulting in many possible sets of abnormalities. The *segmental approach* of Van Praagh is very useful in determining the relationship at each segment. This approach also simplifies description of complex cardiac defects and abnormal position of the heart (dextrocardia, levocardia, mesocardia, etc.).

I. **Localization of the Atria**

The type of atrial situs almost always is the same as the type of visceral situs; the RA is on the same side as the liver or on the opposite side of the stomach bubble. This principle is used to localize the atria. Localization of the atria can be accomplished accurately by two noninvasive methods—chest x-rays and ECG:

A. **Chest x-rays**

Find the location of the liver shadow and the stomach bubble.

a. Right-sided liver shadow and left-sided stomach bubble (situs solitus, S) indicate situs solitus of the atria (the RA on the right of the LA as in normal) (Fig 16–1,A). Left-sided liver shadow and right-sided stomach bubble (situs inversus, I) indicate situs inversus of the atria (the RA on the left side of the LA) (Fig 16–1,B).

b. A midline (symmetric) liver shadow with variable location of stomach bubble suggests splenic abnormalities in which either two RA or two LA (situs ambiguus, A) and other complex cardiac anomalies are present (Fig 16–1,C) (see also asplenia and polysplenia syndromes in chap. 17).

B. **ECG**

The SA node is always located in the RA. Therefore, the P axis of the ECG can be used to locate the atria.

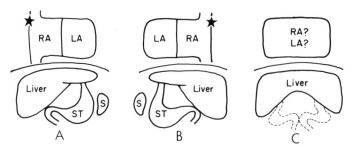

FIG 16–1.
The visceroatrial relationship. The RA is on the same side as the liver or on the opposite side of the stomach. The SA node *(star)* is always in the RA.

a. When the P axis is in the left lower quadrant of the hexaxial reference system (0 to +90°), situs solitus of the atria (the RA to the right of the LA) is present (Fig 16–2).

b. When the P axis is in the right lower quadrant (+90° to 180°), situs inversus of the atria (the RA on the left of the LA) is present (see Fig 16–2).

c. With splenic abnormalities, the P axis may be superiorly directed (polysplenia syndrome) or may change between the left lower quadrant and the right lower quadrant from time to time (asplenia syndrome).

Identification of the IVC or pulmonary veins by 2D ECHO, angiocardiogram, surgical inspection, or autopsy findings aid further the diagnosis of atrial situs.

II. Localization of the Ventricles
During embryogenesis, the straight cardiac tube normally bends to the right, forming a *D-loop.* If it bends to the left, it is called an *L-loop.* D-loop formation places the anatomical RV to the right of the LV, and the L-loop formation places the anatomical RV to the left of the LV. Ventricular localization can be accomplished by ECG and 2D ECHO (noninvasive) or ventriculography (invasive). 2D ECHO is helpful in identifying the AV valves (apical four-chamber

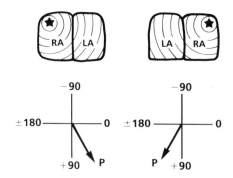

FIG 16–2.
Locating the atria by the use of the P axis. When the RA is on the right side, the P axis is in the left lower quadrant (0 to +90°). When the RA is on the left side, the P axis is in the right lower quadrant (+90 to +180°). (From Park MK, Guntheroth WG: *How to Read Pediatric ECGs,* ed 2. Chicago, Year Book Medical Publishers, 1987. Used by permission.)

view); the tricuspid septal leaflet usually inserts on the interventricular septum in a more apical position than does the mitral septal leaflet. The LV is invariably attached to the mitral valve and the RV to the tricuspid valve. On ventriculograms, the anatomical RV is coarsely trabeculated and triangular, while the anatomical LV is finely trabeculated and ellipsoidal.

The ECG method of localizing the ventricles is based on the fact that the depolarization of the ventricular septum takes place from the embryonic LV to the RV. This produces Q waves in the precordial leads that lie over the anatomical LV.

   a. If Q waves are present in V5 and V6 (as well as lead I) but not in V1, D-loop of the ventricle as in normal is likely (Fig 16–3,A).

   b. If Q waves are present in V4R, V1, and V2, but not in V5 and V6, L-loop of the ventricle is likely (ventricular inversion) (Fig 16–3,B).

III. Localization of the Great Arteries

Accurate determination of the relationship between the two great arteries can be accomplished by angiocardiography. ECHO can be equally accurate in identifying the relationship between the great arteries and the ventricles as well as between the two great arteries. The ECG is not helpful. In many cases, however, the relationship between the aorta and the pulmonary artery can be deduced by the *loop rule* (of Van Praagh). The loop rule states that D-loop of the ventricle is usually associated with normally related great arteries (S, Fig 16–4,A) or with D-transposition of the great arteries (D, Fig 14–4,C), and L-loop of the ventricle is usually associated with the mirror image of normally related great arteries (I, Fig 16–4,B) or with L-transposition of the great arteries (L, Fig 16–4,D).

One of the following relationships exists between the aorta and the pulmonary artery (see Fig 16–4):

1. Solitus (S): The aortic valve is posterior and rightward to the pulmonary valve as in the normal heart (normally related great arteries in situs solitus).

2. Inversus (I): The aortic valve is posterior and leftward to the pulmonary valve (mirror image of normal).

3. D-Transposition (D): The aortic valve is located anteriorly and to the right of the pulmonary valve.

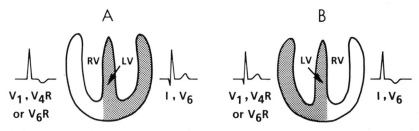

FIG 16–3.
Locating the ventricles from the ECG. The LV is usually located on the same side as the precordial leads that show Q waves. If V6 shows a Q wave, the LV is on the left side. If V4R and V1 shows a Q wave, the LV is to the right of the anatomical RV. Note that Q waves are also present in V1 in severe RVH. (From Park MK, Guntheroth WG: *How to Read Pediatric ECGs,* ed 2. Chicago, Year Book Medical Publishers, 1987. Used by permission.)

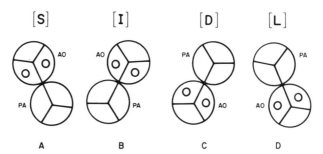

FIG 16–4.
Relationship between the great arteries. **A,** solitus. **B,** inversus. **C,** D-transposition. **D,** L-transposition.

4. L-Transposition (L): The aortic valve is located anteriorly and to the left of the pulmonary valve.

In summary, the following symbols may be used in describing segmental relationship.

Visceroatrial: S = solitus, I = inversus, A = ambiguus.

Ventricular loop: D = D-loop, L = L-loop, X = uncertain or intermediate.

Great arteries: S = solitus, I = inversus, D = D-transposition, L = L-transposition.

Using these symbols, segmental relationship of the heart can be expressed by three letters; the first letter signifies the visceroatrial relationship, the second letter the ventricular loop, and the third letter the relationship of the great arteries. A few examples of normal and well-known abnormal segmental relationships may be expressed as follows:

Normal heart with situs solitus—(S, D, S)
Normal heart with situs inversus (mirror image of normal)—(I, L, I)
Complete transposition of the great arteries (D-TGA)—(S, D, D)
D-TGA with situs inversus—(I, L, L)
Corrected transposition of the great arteries (L-TGA) with situs solitus—(S, L, L)
Normally formed heart that is displaced to the right side of the chest secondary to hypoplasia of the right lung (dextroversion)—(S, D, S)

II. DEXTROCARDIA AND MESOCARDIA

Dextrocardia refers to a condition in which the heart is located in the right side of the chest. Mesocardia indicates that the heart is located in approximately midline of the thorax; i.e., the heart lies predominantly neither to the right nor to the left on the PA chest x-ray film. The terms "dextrocardia" and "mesocardia" express the position of the heart as a whole, but do not specify the segmental relationship of the heart.

The four most common types of heart in the right chest (dextrocardia) are classic mirror-image dextrocardia (Fig 16–5,A), normal heart displaced to the right side of the chest (Fig 16–5,B), congenitally corrected TGA (Fig 16–5,C), and single ventricle. Less commonly, asplenia and polysplenia syndromes with situs ambiguus and

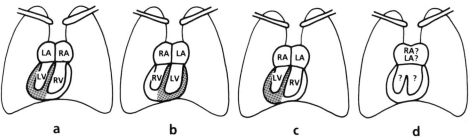

FIG 16–5.
Examples of common conditions when the apex of the heart is in the right chest. (From Park MK, Guntheroth WG: *How to Read Pediatric ECGs,* ed 2. Chicago, Year Book Medical Publishers, 1987. Used by permission.)

complicated cardiac defects cause dextrocardia (Fig 16–5,D). All of these abnormalities may result in mesocardia.

With chest x-rays and the ECG, the segmental approach discussed above can be used to deduce the nature of segmental relationship in dextrocardia (as well as in mesocardia). More conclusive diagnosis of the segmental relationship is accomplished by 2D ECHO and angiocardiography.

A. Classic mirror-image dextrocardia (I, L, I) (see Fig 16–5,A) will show:

    a. The liver shadow on the left and the stomach bubble on the right on x-rays and the P axis between +90° and +180° on the ECG (situs inversus).

    b. Q waves in V5R and V6R (V5R and V6R are right-sided precordial leads, mirror-image positions of V5 and V6, respectively).

B. Normal heart shifted toward the right side of the chest with the normal right-to-left relationship maintained (dextroversion) (S, D, S) (see Fig 16–5,B) will show:

    a. The liver shadow on the right and the stomach bubble on the left on x-rays and the P axis between 0° and +90° on the ECG (situs solitus).

    b. Q waves in V5 and V6.

C. Congenitally corrected transposition of the great arteries (L-TGA) with situs solitus (S, L, L) (see Fig 16–5,C) will show:

    a. Situs solitus of abdominal viscera on x-rays and the P axis in the normal quadrant (0° to +90°) on the ECG.

    b. Q waves in V5R and V6R.

D. Undifferentiated cardiac chambers (see Fig 16–5,D) are often associated with complicated cardiac defects and may show:

    a. Midline liver on the x-ray film and shifting P axis or superiorly oriented P axis on the ECG.

    b. Abnormal Q waves in the precordial leads (similar to those described for single ventricle; see chap. 14).

17 / Miscellaneous Congenital Cardiac Conditions

In this chapter congenital heart defects with relatively low incidence that have not been discussed will be presented briefly in alphabetical order.

Absence of the Pulmonary Valve

This anomaly is most often associated with tetralogy of Fallot. The pulmonary valve leaflets are absent, the anulus of the valve is stenotic, and there is a massive aneurysmal dilatation of the pulmonary arteries. The massive aneurysm (Fig 17–1,B) compresses anteriorly both bronchi and produces signs of airway obstruction (hyperinflated areas seen in Figure 17–1,A) and respiratory distress in early infancy.

A to-and-fro murmur ("sawing-wood sound") at the upper and middle LSB (due to free pulmonary regurgitation) and RVH on the ECG in a mildly cyanotic newborn infant are almost diagnostic. Cardiac catheterization and angiocardiography confirm the diagnosis.

Pulmonary complications rather than the intracardiac defect are the usual cause of death. Those infants who survive infancy usually have fewer respiratory symptoms and may have successful surgery later. The surgical approach during infancy is often unsatisfactory.

Aneurysm of the Sinus of Valsalva
(Congenital aortic sinus aneurysm)

There is a gradual downward bulge of a sinus of Valsalva, usually the right coronary sinus, herniating into the RA or RV. Associated congenital heart disease is not uncommon and includes VSD, bicuspid aortic valve, and coarctation of the aorta.

Unruptured aneurysm produces no symptoms or signs. The rupture of the aneurysm occurs during the 3rd and 4th decade, usually into the RA or RV. The rupture is characterized by sudden onset of chest pain, dyspnea, a continuous heart murmur over the right or left sternal border, and bounding peripheral pulses. Frank CHF eventually develops. Chest x-rays show cardiomegaly and increased pulmonary vascularity. ECG may show CVH, first- or second-degree AV block, or AV nodal rhythm.

Corrective surgery under cardiopulmonary bypass must be performed as soon as the diagnosis is made.

Anomalous Muscle Bundle of the Right Ventricle
(Double-chambered right ventricle)

This condition is characterized by aberrant hypertrophied muscle bands that divide the RV cavity into a proximal high-pressure chamber and a distal low-pressure chamber. In the majority of the patients, VSD or pulmonary valve stenosis is also present.

Clinical manifestations closely resemble those of pulmonary valvular or infun-

206

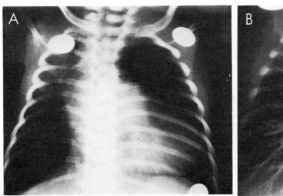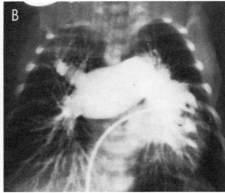

FIG 17–1.
A PA view of plain chest film **(A)** showing hyperinflated areas in the left upper lobe and right lower portion of the chest in a 1-month-old infant with absence of the pulmonary valve. An anteroposterior view of pulmonary arteriogram **(B)** showing massive aneurysmal dilatation of both right and left pulmonary arteries.

dibular stenosis: a loud systolic ejection murmur along the upper and middle LSB is present. Surgical resection of the bundle, as well as repair of other anomalies, is usually indicated.

Anomalous Origin of the Left Coronary Artery from the Pulmonary Artery
(Bland-White-Garland syndrome)
The left coronary artery arises abnormally from the PA. The patients are usually asymptomatic until the PA pressure falls to a critical level after birth. The direction of blood flow is from the right coronary artery, through intercoronary collaterals, to the left coronary artery, and into the PA. This results in left ventricular insufficiency or infarction.

Symptoms appear at 2–3 months of age and consist of recurring episodes of distress (anginal pain), marked cardiomegaly, and CHF. Significant heart murmur is usually absent. The ECG shows anterolateral myocardial infarction pattern consisting of abnormally deep and wide Q waves, inverted T waves, and ST segment shift in I, aVL, and left precordial leads (see Fig 24–4).

The optimal operation in infancy remains controversial. In the critically ill infant, simple ligation of the anomalous left coronary artery close to its origin from the PA may be carried out to prevent steal into the PA. This should be followed by an elective bypass procedure later. The tunnel operation can be performed in infants who are not critically ill or in those beyond infancy. The tunnel operation consists of creating a 5–6-mm aortopulmonary (AP) window and connecting the opening of the AP window and that of the anomalous coronary artery across the back of the MPA. The mortality rate is high (40%–50%) in infancy but is relatively low beyond the age of infancy.

Aortopulmonary Septal Defect
(Aortopulmonary window, AP window, aortopulmonary fenestration)
A large defect is present between the ascending aorta and the main pulmonary artery (Fig 17–2). This condition results from the failure of the spiral septum to divide completely the embryonic truncus arteriosus.

Hemodynamic abnormalities are similar to those of persistent truncus arterio-

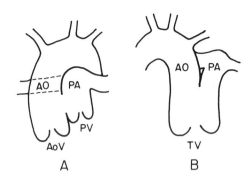

FIG 17–2.
Diagrammatic drawing of aortopulmonary window **(A)** and persistent truncus arteriosus **(B)**. These two conditions are similar from a hemodynamic point of view. Anatomically, however, there are two separate semilunar valves *(AoV, PV)* in AP window, whereas there is only one truncal valve *(TV)* with associated VSD in persistent truncus arteriosus.

sus and are more severe than those of patent ductus arteriosus. CHF and pulmonary hypertension appear in early infancy. Peripheral pulses are bounding, but the heart murmur is usually of the systolic ejection type (rather than continuous murmur) at the base. Surgical closure of the defect, preferably under cardiopulmonary bypass, is indicated.

Arteriovenous Fistula, Coronary

There is an abnormal channel connecting a coronary artery and a cardiac chamber or the pulmonary artery. It may be single or multiple. The right coronary artery is involved more often than the left coronary artery. Over 90% of the fistulas open into the right heart chambers or their connecting vessels. The most common site of drainage is the RV (40%), followed by the RA (25%) and the pulmonary artery (20%).

The patients are usually asymptomatic. A continuous murmur is audible over the precordium, similar to the murmur of PDA except for the location. Congestive heart failure is rare. Chest x-rays usually show normal heart size. The ECG may be normal or may show RVH or LVH. Ligation of the vessel may be indicated, especially in those patients with symptoms or cardiac enlargement, avoiding infarcting normal myocardium.

Arteriovenous Fistula, Pulmonary

There are direct communications between the pulmonary arteries and pulmonary veins without the interposition of the pulmonary capillaries. They may be single or multiple, unilateral or bilateral, and may involve vessels of different sizes. About 60% of patients with pulmonary AV fistulas have Osler-Weber-Rendu syndrome (see Table 1–2). Desaturated systemic venous blood from the pulmonary arteries reaches the pulmonary veins, bypassing the lung tissue, resulting in systemic arterial desaturation and cyanosis. The pulmonary blood flow and pressure remain unchanged, and there is no volume overload to the heart.

Physical examination may reveal cyanosis and clubbing. The peripheral pulses are normal (not bounding). A faint systolic or continuous murmur may be audible over the affected area in about 50% of the patients. Polycythemia is usually present, and arterial saturation runs between 50% and 85%. Chest x-rays show normal heart size. One or more rounded opacities of variable size may be present in the lung fields. The ECG is usually normal. Occasional complications include brain abscess, rupture of the fistula with hemoptysis or hemothorax, and infective endocarditis.

Surgical removal of the lesions, with preservation of as much healthy lung tissue as possible, may be attempted in symptomatic children, but the progressive character of the disorder calls for a conservative approach.

Arteriovenous Fistula, Systemic

There is a direct communication (either a vascular channel or angiomas) between the artery and a vein without the interposition of the capillary bed. The two most common sites of systemic AV fistulas are the brain and liver. Because of decreased peripheral vascular resistance, increased stroke volume (with a wide pulse pressure) and tachycardia result, leading to increased cardiac output, volume overload to the heart, and even CHF.

Physical examination reveals a systolic or continuous murmur over the affected organ. A systolic ejection murmur may be present over the precordium owing to increased blood flow through the semilunar valves. The peripheral pulses may be bounding during the high-output state, but weak when CHF develops. A gallop rhythm may be present with CHF. Chest x-rays show cardiomegaly and increased pulmonary vascular markings. The ECG may show hypertrophy of either or both ventricles.

Most patients with large cerebral AV fistulas and CHF die in the neonatal period, and surgical ligation of the affected artery is rarely possible without infarcting the brain. Surgical treatment of hepatic fistulas is often impossible because they are widespread throughout the liver. Corticosteroids or radiotherapy may prove to be effective.

Asplenia (Ivemark's) Syndrome

In this condition the spleen is absent. The spleen being a left-sided organ, bilateral right-sidedness characterizes this condition. Cardiac malformations are always present and are so severe that surgical correction is usually impossible. Other malformations include two right lungs (three-lobed), midline liver with two gallbladders, malrotation of the gut, and right- or left-sided stomach.

Cardiac malformations include most or some of the following: bilateral SVC, bilateral right atria (with two SA nodes), TAPVR, TGA, pulmonary stenosis or atresia, large ASD or single atrium, endocardial cushion defect, and large VSD or single ventricle. The IVC is commonly on the left side, and azygous continuation is extremely rare.

This syndrome is suggested by midline liver, superiorly oriented QRS axis in the ECG, varying degree of cyanosis, and the presence of Howell-Jolly and Heinz bodies on blood smear. It is confirmed by a negative radioactive spleen scan. ECHO is important in demonstrating various intracardiac anomalies.

The risk of fulminating infection, especially by pneumococcus, is high. Continuous antibiotic therapy is indicated in infants up to 2 years of age. Immunization of the patient with polyvalent pneumococcal vaccine is indicated in children 2 years and older. In patients with decreased PBF, a systemic-pulmonary artery shunt procedure is indicated. Without a surgical procedure, most patients with asplenia syndrome die in the first year of life (see also polysplenia syndrome in this chapter).

Cervical Aortic Arch

In this rare anomaly the aortic arch is elongated, usually into the neck just above the clavicle. The aortic arch is almost always right-sided. A pulsating mass with associated thrill is present in the right supraclavicular fossa. An aortogram may assist in making an accurate diagnosis.

Common Atrium

(Single atrium, cor triloculare biventriculare)

Either the atrial septum is completely absent or only the vestigial element of poorly developed atrial septum is present. This is a form of endocardial cushion defect with cleft mitral valve, producing a superiorly oriented QRS axis (left anterior hemiblock) on the ECG. An rsR' pattern is present in the right precordial leads as in ASD. This condition is most commonly seen with Ellis-van Creveld syndrome (see Table 1–2). Successful creation of polyvinyl septum has been reported.

Cor Triatriatum

This is a rare congenital cardiac anomaly in which the LA is divided into two compartments by an abnormal fibromuscular septum with a small opening (Fig 17–3), producing obstruction of pulmonary venous return. Pulmonary venous and arterial hypertension result. Embryologically, this condition results from the failure of incorporation of the embryonic common pulmonary vein into the LA. Therefore, the upper compartment (accessory LA) is a dilated common pulmonary vein and the lower compartment the true left atrium. Hemodynamic abnormalities of this condition are similar to those of mitral stenosis in that both conditions produce pulmonary venous and arterial hypertension (see chap. 10).

Important physical findings include dyspnea, basal pulmonary rales, loud P2, and a nonspecific systolic murmur. The ECG shows RAD and severe RVH and occasional RAH. Chest x-rays show evidence of pulmonary venous congestion or pulmonary edema, prominent MPA segment, and right-sided heart enlargement. ECHO demonstrates a linear structure within the LA cavity. Surgical correction is always indicated. Pulmonary hypertension regresses rapidly in survivors if the correction is made early.

Hemitruncus Arteriosus

(Origin of one pulmonary artery from the ascending aorta)

One of the pulmonary arteries, usually the right, arises from the ascending aorta. Associated defects such as PDA, VSD, and TOF are occasionally present. Hemodynamically, one lung receives blood directly from the aorta, as in PDA, with resulting volume and/or pressure overload, and the other lung receives the entire RV output, resulting in volume overload of that lung. Therefore, pulmonary hypertension of both lungs develops. CHF develops early in infancy, with respiratory distress and poor weight gain. A continuous murmur and bounding pulses

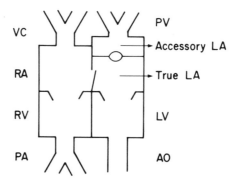

FIG 17–3.
Diagrammatic drawing of cor triatriatum.

may be present. The ECG shows CVH, and chest x-ray films show cardiomegaly and increased pulmonary vascular markings. Early surgical correction (anastomosis of the anomalous PA to the MPA) is indicated.

Idiopathic Dilatation of the Pulmonary Artery
(Congenital pulmonary insufficiency)
In this condition pulmonary regurgitation is present in the absence of pulmonary hypertension in asymptomatic children or adolescents. Many regard this as a mild pulmonary valve stenosis with resulting poststenotic dilatation and subsequent decrease in the murmur of PS.

A characteristic auscultatory finding is a grade 1–3/6 low-frequency, decrescendo diastolic murmur at the upper and middle LSB. The S2 is normal. The ECG is usually normal, but occasional RBBB is present. Chest x-rays show a prominent MPA segment with normal peripheral pulmonary vascularity. The prognosis is generally good, but right-sided heart failure may occur in adult life.

Interruption of the Aortic Arch
A segment of the aortic arch is entirely absent, an extremely severe form of coarctation of the aorta. It occurs commonly either between the left carotid artery and left subclavian artery or distal to the left subclavian artery, about 50% of the time each. It is almost always associated with PDA (producing differential cyanosis of the lower half of the body) and VSD. Severe CHF develops early in life, requiring early surgical intervention. Surgical mortality rate is high.

Kartagener's Syndrome
This syndrome consists of the triad of situs inversus totalis, paranasal sinusitis, and bronchiectasis. The dextrocardia is a mirror image of normal and is functionally normal. Bronchiectasis is believed to be due to functional defect of the mucociliary epithelium with immotility of the cilia.

Lutembacher's Syndrome
Lutembacher's syndrome is a rare combination of atrial septal defect and mitral stenosis. The mitral stenosis is usually of rheumatic origin. It becomes manifest in adults, often with CHF and atrial fibrillation.

Mitral Regurgitation, Congenital
This condition is extremely rare as an isolated defect. It is most frequently found in association with other congenital heart defects. A regurgitant holosystolic murmur is audible at the apex with radiation to the left axilla and left back. An apical rumble and a loud S3 may be present. The ECG and chest x-rays may show hypertrophy and enlargement of the LA and LV. Medical management is initially tried. In those unresponsive to medical management, mitral valvuloplasty or anuloplasty should be initially attempted to preserve the valve. If not possible, valve replacement is performed.

Mitral Stenosis, Congenital
The onset of symptoms or signs depends on the severity of the stenosis: neonatal onset with severe stenosis and later onset with less severe stenosis. Symptoms and signs are related to pulmonary venous congestion or pulmonary edema, eventually leading to pulmonary hypertension and right heart failure (see chap. 10). COA and AS are commonly associated anomalies, and LV endocardial sclerosis is also common.

Physical examination reveals an increased RV impulse and an apical middiastolic murmur. Other findings may include presystolic accentuation, loud S1, and opening snap. The ECG shows RVH and CAH, and chest x-rays show enlargement of the LA, MPA, and RV. Kerley's B lines may be present in severe cases. ECHO is diagnostic of the condition.

Conservative management with diuretics and digitalis is recommended. For severe obstruction, surgical relief by closed or open valvotomy or placement of a prosthetic valve may be indicated.

Parachute Mitral Valve is characterized by insertion of all the chordae tendineae into a single papillary muscle group, producing mitral stenosis. This can be suspected by 2D ECHO on the parasternal short-axis view. Commonly associated conditions include supramitral ring, subvalvular and/or valvular AS, and COA; all are components of the "Shone complex."

Pericardial Defect, Congenital

Congenital pericardial defect may be partial or complete. The majority of these cases occur on the left side (85%), and they are more often complete (65%) than partial. Pleural defect is almost always present.

Most patients are asymptomatic. Occasionally, partial defect may produce chest pain, syncope, or systemic embolism, secondary to herniation and strangulation of the left atrial appendage. A complete defect may produce vague positional discomfort in the supine or left lateral positions.

The appearance of pneumopericardium following the introduction of air into the left pleural cavity is diagnostic. Symptomatic patients require surgical procedures.

Polysplenia Syndrome

Multiple splenic tissues are present in this condition. The spleen is a left-sided organ; therefore, bilateral left-sidedness characterizes this syndrome. In addition to cardiac malformations, two left lungs (two-lobed), midline liver, and a right- or left-sided stomach are present.

Cardiac malformations are similar to but less severe than those found in asplenia syndrome. Normal heart is found in occasional patients. Common cardiac malformations include bilateral left atria (with absence of the sinus node), endocardial cushion defect, anomalous pulmonary venous return, and bilateral SVC. The absence of IVC with azygous continuation is characteristic, seen rarely in asplenia syndrome. Transposition of the great arteries and double-outlet RV are occasional anomalies. Unlike asplenia syndrome, pulmonary stenosis is uncommon, and two ventricles are almost always present.

This condition can be suspected by varying degrees of cyanosis, midline liver, and superiorly oriented P axis (owing to absence of the sinus node) and superiorly oriented QRS axis (reflecting ECD) on the ECG. The radioactive spleen scan may show multiple splenic tissue.

Although the prognosis is better than that for the asplenia syndrome, most of the infants with severe cardiac malformations die within the first few years of life. A systemic-pulmonary artery shunt is indicated in those patients with decreased PBF. A greater portion of polysplenia syndrome cases are operable than are asplenia syndrome cases.

Pseudocoarctation of the Aorta

Pseudocoarctation of the aorta is a condition in which the distal portion of the aortic arch and the proximal portion of the descending aorta are abnormally elongated and tortuous, giving the x-ray appearance of COA. Physical examination results are normal, and the ECG is normal early, but some might progress to show substantial pressure difference between the arms and legs.

Pulmonary Artery Stenosis

Stenosis of the pulmonary artery may be central (extraparenchymal) or peripheral (intraparenchymal) and single or multiple. It may be seen in rubella syndrome and Williams' syndrome. In two-thirds of the cases, other congenital heart defects, such as VSD and pulmonary valve stenosis, are found. It is also seen occasionally as an isolated lesion. It should be differentiated from peripheral narrowing of pulmonary artery branches normally seen in newborn infants, which produces innocent pulmonary flow murmur of the newborn.

A systolic ejection murmur is present at the ULSB, with good transmission to both axillae and the back. Occasionally, a continuous murmur is audible. The ECG shows RVH if the obstruction is severe. The central (extraparenchymal) type is surgically correctable, but the multiple peripheral (intraparenchymal) type is not amenable to surgery.

Rubella Syndrome

Rubella syndrome is caused by intrauterine infection of the fetus by rubella virus during the first trimester of pregnancy. The triad of this syndrome is deafness, cataracts, and cardiac defects. Other malformations include intrauterine growth retardation, microcephaly, microphthalmia, hepatitis, and neonatal thrombocytopenic purpura. The most common cardiac malformations are PDA and stenoses of the pulmonary arteries. Other intracardiac defects such as TOF, VSD, ASD, or TGA are found in 5%–10% of the cases.

Scimitar Syndrome

Partial anomalous pulmonary venous return from the lower lobe, and sometimes the middle lobe, of the right lung drains into the IVC, making a vertical (scimitar-shaped) shadow along the right lower cardiac border. Pulmonary parenchymal disease with anomalous systemic arterial supply from the descending aorta (bronchopulmonary sequestration) is frequently found. Hypoplasia of the right lung and dextroversion may also be present.

Systemic Veins, Anomalies of

Three well-established anomalies of systemic veins are: (1) persistence of the left superior vena cava, (2) systemic veins draining into the left atrium, and (3) absence of the inferior vena cava with azygous continuation.

Persistence of left SVC occurs in 3%–5% of children with CHD. In the most commonly encountered type, the left SVC is connected to the coronary sinus. Rarely the right SVC is absent. Persistence of the left SVC alone does not produce symptoms or signs. A much less common form is the connection of the left SVC to the LA, resulting in systemic arterial desaturation. In the majority of the patients, no treatment is necessary.

Systemic veins draining into the LA is a rare anomaly. Systemic veins, either the IVC, right SVC, or left SVC, can be connected to the LA. Clinical manifestations include cyanosis and clubbing in the absence of significant heart murmur. Chest x-ray films are usually normal, but the ECG may show LVH. Surgical correction is usually possible.

In absence of the IVC with azygous continuation, the upper part of the IVC does not connect to the RA but becomes continuous with the azygous vein, eventually draining into the SVC. The hepatic veins enter separately into the RA. In about 50% of cases, it occurs in association with a severely malformed heart, most commonly polysplenia syndrome. There is no specific treatment; the prognosis depends on the associated anomalies.

Taussig-Bing Malformation

Taussig-Bing malformation is a form of double-outlet RV (see chap. 14) in which the VSD is subpulmonic and pulmonary stenosis is absent. Because the VSD is closely related to the PA, oxygenated blood from the LV goes to the lungs and desaturated blood from the venae cavae to the aorta, producing marked cyanosis. Since there is no PS, early CHF develops in these infants. Therefore, clinical pictures resemble those of D-TGA with VSD. 2D ECHO, cardiac catheterization, and angiocardiography are required for diagnosis.

PART V

Acquired Heart Disease

Among acquired heart diseases, emphasis will be placed on the more common pediatric diseases, such as primary myocardial disease; cardiovascular infections, including myocarditis and infective endocarditis; acute rheumatic fever; and valvular heart disease. Although the etiology of Kawasaki's disease is not entirely clear at this time, it will be discussed in cardiovascular infection, and mitral valve prolapse in valvular heart disease. A brief listing of cardiac involvement in some systemic diseases is presented.

18 / Primary Myocardial Disease

Primary myocardial disease is characterized by myocardial insufficiency not associated with any other structural heart disease. Clinically, the majority of these patients have cardiomegaly, signs of CHF, and abnormal ECG. Representative entities include endocardial fibroelastosis of the infant and cardiomyopathy of adult patients. Cardiac tumors are included in this chapter, since they can produce cardiomegaly, although arrhythmias and conduction disturbances are more frequent presenting signs. Myocarditis produces a similar clinical picture, but it will be discussed in chapter 19, Cardiovascular Infections.

I. ENDOCARDIAL FIBROELASTOSIS (EFE)

Incidence
The incidence of nonfamilial form of EFE declined in the past decade for unknown reasons. It was as frequent as 4% of cardiac autopsy cases in children.

Etiology
Etiology is not known, but many favor the theory of intrauterine or extrauterine viral (such as coxsackievirus B) infection with pancarditis.

Pathology
EFE is a nonobstructive form of primary cardiomyopathy seen in infants and children.

1. The condition is characterized by diffuse changes in the endocardium, with a white, opaque, glistening appearance.

2. The heart chambers, primarily the LA and LV, are notably dilated and hypertrophied. Involvement of the right heart chambers is rare.

3. Deformities and shortening of the papillary muscles and chordae tendineae (resulting in mitral regurgitation) are often present late in the course.

4. Similar pathology appears secondary to severe obstructive CHD of the left heart (AS, COA, HLHS).

Clinical Manifestations
History
Symptoms and signs of CHF (feeding difficulties, tachypnea, sweating, irritability, pallor, failure to thrive) developing in the first 10 months of life.

PE

a. Tachycardia and tachypnea.

b. No heart murmur is audible in the majority of patients, although gallop rhythm is usually present. Occasionally, a heart murmur of mitral regurgitation is audible.

c. Hepatomegaly.

ECG
LVH with "strain" is typical of the condition. Occasionally, myocardial infarction patterns, arrhythmias, and varying degrees of AV block may be seen.

X-Rays
Marked generalized cardiomegaly with normal or congested pulmonary vascularity.

ECHO
A markedly dilated and poorly contracting LV in the absence of structural heart defects is characteristic. The LA is also markedly dilated.

Treatment

a. Early and long-term (for years) treatment with digoxin, diuretics, and afterload reducing agents during active phase.

b. Operative procedures are not recommended.

Differential Diagnosis
Infants with cardiomegaly and no heart murmur often present a diagnostic challenge. It may be due to diseases that primarily affect myocardium or coronary arteries, congenital heart defects with severe CHF, respiratory diseases or other miscellaneous conditions. Table 18–1 lists differential diagnosis of cardiomegaly without heart murmur in infants and young children. All of these conditions show cardiomegaly on chest roentgenograms, usually with, but occasionally without, signs of CHF. Conditions listed under myocardial diseases and coronary artery diseases (see Table 18–1) will be briefly discussed in this chapter.

A. Myocarditis
Viral myocarditis caused by coxsackievirus B carries a high mortality (70%) in the newborn period. Myocarditis caused by other viruses occurs more frequently in infants older than 1 year.

Acute myocarditis may manifest with history of a recent upper respiratory infection and signs of CHF (tachycardia, dyspnea, wheezing, pulmonary edema, cardiomegaly, gallop rhythm, etc.). Significant heart murmur is usually absent. The ECG often shows low QRS voltages (rather than LVH as in EFE) and prolongation of PR interval, QRS duration, or QT interval. Flat or inverted T waves may be present in leads representing the left ventricle.

Clinical manifestations may vary with the stage of the disease. Subacute or chronic myocarditis is characterized by persistent cardiomegaly, with or without signs of CHF, and the ECG findings of LVH or CVH with "strain" pattern. Therefore, clinical pictures of subacute or chronic myocarditis are indistinguishable from those of EFE.

Treatment consists of anticongestive and supportive measures (see also chap. 19 under Myocarditis).

B. Glycogen Storage Disease
The classic glycogen storage disease that causes heart failure in infancy is Pompe's disease (Cori's type II) due to deficiency of α-1,4-glycosidase. This is

TABLE 18–1.
Differential Diagnosis of Cardiomegaly Without Heart Murmur
in Pediatric Patients

Myocardial diseases
    Endocardial fibroelastosis
    Myocarditis (viral or idiopathic)
    Glycogen storage disease
Coronary artery diseases resulting in myocardial insufficiency
    Anomalous origin of the left coronary artery from the pulmonary artery
    Collagen disease (periarteritis nodosa)
    Kawasaki's disease (mucocutaneous lymph node syndrome)
Congenital heart disease with severe heart failure
    Coarctation of the aorta in infants
    Ebstein's anomaly (a soft tricuspid regurgitation murmur is frequently present)
Miscellaneous conditions
    CHF secondary to respiratory disease (upper airway obstruction, chronic
        alveolar hypoxia such as seen with bronchopulmonary dysplasia, extensive
        pneumonia)
    Supraventricular tachycardia with CHF
    Pericardial effusion
    Severe anemia
    Tumors of the heart
    Neonatal thyrotoxicosis
    Malnutrition (infantile beriberi, protein calorie malnutrition)
    Toxicity (drugs, such as Adriamycin, or radiation)

a familial disease characterized by generalized muscle weakness, macroglossia, hepatomegaly, and signs of CHF or severe arrhythmias. The onset of CHF is around 2–3 months of age, with fatal outcome usually during infancy. The ECG may show a short PR interval, LVH in the majority of the patients, occasional CVH, and ST-T changes in the left precordial leads. Excessive glycogen deposits in a skeletal muscle biopsy specimen are diagnostic. No treatment is available, but genetic counseling should be provided for the family.

C. Anomalous Left Coronary Artery From the Pulmonary Artery

In this condition, signs and symptoms of myocardial infarction and CHF may be manifested around 2–3 months of age. About 65% of the patients die during the first year of life. The ECG typically shows evidence of anterolateral myocardial infarction (see also chapters 17 and 24).

D. Kawasaki's Disease

Mucocutaneous lymph node syndrome of Kawasaki may present with evidence of coronary insufficiency and heart failure during the subacute phase of the disease. It usually involves children younger than 4 years. Signs of CHF or other cardiac involvement are preceded by characteristic clinical pictures of the disease by a week or two (see also chap. 19).

Other rare conditions which involve coronary arteries include periarteritis nodosa, calcification of coronary arteries, and medial necrosis of coronary arteries. It seems likely that there are overlaps, if not identity, among the four arterial disorders.

II. PRIMARY CARDIOMYOPATHY

Primary cardiomyopathy is a disease of the heart muscle itself, not associated with congenital, valvular, or coronary heart diseases or systemic disorders, and is distinct from the specific heart muscle diseases of known cause. The condition has been classified into three types based on pathophysiology: (a) hypertrophic, (b) dilated, and (c) restrictive. In hypertrophic cardiomyopathy, there is massive ventricular hypertrophy, accompanied early by enhanced contractile function in the absence of cavity dilatation. The hallmark of hypertrophic cardiomyopathy is impaired filling due to relaxation abnormalities. Dilated (or congestive) cardiomyopathy is characterized by a weakness of systolic contraction of the ventricle associated with ventricular dilatation. Restrictive cardiomyopathy denotes a restriction to diastolic filling of the ventricles caused by endocardial or myocardial disease, and contractile function may be normal. The three types of cardiomyopathies are functionally different from one another, and the demands of therapy are different.

A. Hypertrophic Cardiomyopathy (Formerly Idiopathic Hypertrophic Subaortic Stenosis [IHSS], Muscular Subaortic Stenosis)

Pathology and Pathophysiology

1. Massive ventricular hypertrophy of symmetric or asymmetric nature, particularly involving the interventricular septum, is present. Extensive disarray of hypertrophied myocardial cells is characteristic. Although asymmetric septal hypertrophy (ASH), a condition formerly known as idiopathic hypertrophic subaortic stenosis (IHSS) (Fig 18–1), is most common, concentric hypertrophy with symmetric thickening of the LV rarely occurs.

2. In some, but not all, patients, an intracavitary pressure gradient develops during systole partly because of systolic anterior motion of the mitral valve (SAM) against the hypertrophied septum (hypertrophic obstructive cardiomyopathy, HOCM) (see Fig 18–1).

3. The myocardium itself has an enhanced contractile state, but diastolic ventricular filling is impaired because of abnormal stiffness of the LV, which may lead to left atrial enlargement and pulmonary venous congestion.

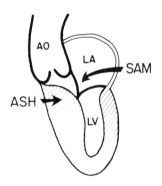

FIG 18–1.
Diagrammatic representation of the mechanism of systolic obstruction in HOCM (or IHSS). ASH = asymmetric septal hypertrophy; SAM = systolic anterior motion (of the mitral valve).

4. These patients are prone to develop arrhythmias, which may lead to a sudden death.

5. It appears to be genetically transmitted as an autosomal dominant trait, although sporadic cases occur.

6. A unique aspect of HOCM is the variability of the degree of obstruction from moment to moment. Since the LV outflow tract obstruction occurs as a result of systolic anterior motion (SAM) of the mitral valve against the hypertrophied ventricular septum, any influence that reduces the LV systolic volume (positive inotropic agents, reduced blood volume, lowering of SVR) will increase the obstruction, and any influence that increases the systolic volume (negative inotropic agents such as β-adrenergic blockers, leg raising, blood transfusion, increasing SVR) lessens the obstruction.

7. A large portion of the stroke volume (about 80%) is ejected during the early part of systole, when there is little or no obstruction. This produces a sharp upstroke of the arterial pressure, a characteristic finding of HOCM. The obstruction occurs late in systole, producing a late systolic murmur. Because of the variable degree of obstruction, the intensity of the heart murmur varies from time to time and may represent mitral regurgitation, a common problem.

Clinical Manifestations

History

a. Usually seen in adolescents and young adults, with equal sex distribution.

b. Positive family history in 30% of the patients.

c. Easy fatigability, dyspnea, palpitation, or anginal pain may be present.

PE

a. A sharp upstroke of the arterial pulse is characteristic (in contrast to a slow upstroke seen with fixed aortic stenosis).

b. A left ventricular lift and a systolic thrill at the apex or along the LLSB.

c. The S2 is normal and an ejection click is generally absent. A late SEM of medium pitch, best audible at the middle and lower LSB or at the apex, is usually heard. A holosystolic murmur of mitral regurgitation is often present. The intensity and even the presence of the heart murmur vary from examination to examination.

ECG (Fig 18–2): Abnormal in the majority of the patients. The common ECG abnormalities are:

a. LVH by voltage criteria.

b. ST-T changes.

c. Abnormally deep Q waves (owing to septal hypertrophy) with diminished or absent R waves in the LPLs (Fig 18–2).

d. Arrhythmias.

X-Rays

Mild LV enlargement with globular-shaped heart may be present.

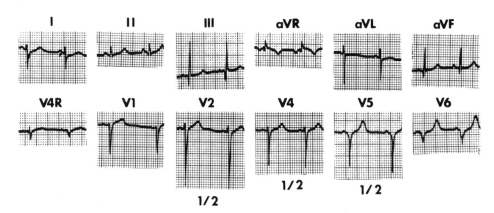

FIG 18–2.
Tracing from a 17-year-old girl with hypertrophic obstructive cardiomyopathy with marked septal hypertrophy. Note prominent Q waves with absent R waves in V5 and V6.

ECHO
ECHO is diagnostic. M-mode ECHO demonstrates:

  a. An asymmetric septal hypertrophy (ASH) of the interventricular septum. The septum is at least 1.3 times greater than the posterior LV wall.

  b. Systolic anterior motion (SAM) of the anterior mitral valve leaflet is also present in the obstructive subgroup.

2D ECHO can detect the wide morphological spectrum of the disease, including those that could be missed by M-mode ECHO.

Natural History and Complications

  a. The obstruction may be absent, stable, or slowly progressive.

  b. Sudden death may occur, particularly during exercise, even in patients with only mild obstruction, probably secondary to ventricular arrhythmias.

  c. Atrial fibrillation results in clinical deterioration, due to loss of the atrial "kick" needed for filling the thick LV.

  d. Heart failure with cardiac dilatation may develop later in life.

  e. Infective endocarditis rarely occurs on the mitral valve.

  f. Pregnancy is usually well tolerated.

Management

Medical

  a. Moderate restriction of physical activity is recommended.

  b. A β-adrenergic blocker (such as propranolol) is the drug of choice in the obstructive subgroup. This drug reduces the degree of outflow tract obstruction, decreases the incidence of anginal pain, and has antiarrhythmic effects.

    c. Calcium channel blockers such as verapamil and nifedipine may be equally effective. These agents reduce hypercontractile systolic function and improve diastolic filling.

    d. Digitalis is contraindicated as it increases the degree of obstruction. Avoid the cardiotonic drugs and vasodilators, since they tend to increase the pressure gradient.

    e. Prophylaxis against infective endocarditis is indicated.

Surgical

Indications: Symptomatic patients who are not responding to medical management and who have severe obstruction with resting pressure gradient of greater than 50 mm Hg.

Procedure: Transaortic left ventricular septal myotomy and myectomy (Morrow's myectomy) is the procedure of choice.

Mortality: 5%–10%.

Complications: (a) LBBB; (b) surgery does not entirely prevent death or abolish atrial fibrillation.

B. Dilated (or Congestive) Cardiomyopathy

Pathology and Pathophysiology

1. In this group, a weakening of systolic contraction is associated with dilatation of all four cardiac chambers and often with the development of CHF.

2. Histologic examination reveals extensive small areas of degeneration and necrosis. This may represent the end result of myocardial damage produced by a variety of infectious, toxic, or metabolic agents.

Clinical Manifestations

History

    a. Fatigue, weakness, and symptoms of left heart failure (dyspnea on exertion, orthopnea) may be elicited.

    b. History of prior viral infection is often obtained.

PE

    a. Findings of CHF (tachycardia, pulmonary rales, weak peripheral pulses, distended neck veins, hepatomegaly).

    b. Displaced apical impulse (cardiomegaly).

    c. The S2 may be normal or narrowly split with accentuated P2 if pulmonary hypertension develops. A soft systolic murmur (due to mitral or tricuspid regurgitation) with or without gallop rhythm may be audible.

ECG

    a. Sinus tachycardia, LVH, and ST-T changes are the most common findings.

    b. Atrial or ventricular arrhythmias and AV conduction disturbances may be seen.

X-Rays

a. Generalized cardiomegaly with predominant LV enlargement is usually present.

b. Signs of pulmonary venous hypertension or pulmonary edema are often seen.

ECHO

a. LV enlargement with increased end-diastolic and end-systolic dimensions.

b. Reduced fractional shortening and ejection fraction.

c. Pericardial effusion and intracavitary thrombus may be visualized.

Natural History

a. Progressive deterioration is the rule rather than the exception. About two-thirds of the patients die within 4 years after the onset of symptoms.

b. Arrhythmias develop with time.

c. Systemic and pulmonary embolism from dislodgement of intracavitary thrombi in the late stages of the illness.

d. Causes of death are CHF, sudden death from arrhythmias, massive embolization, and complications after cardiac transplantation.

Treatment

1. Treatment for CHF (with digoxin, diuretics, bed rest, restriction of activity, etc.).

2. Anticoagulants are recommended because of the frequency of embolization.

3. Vasodilator therapy (with hydralazine, nitrates, prazosin, or captopril) may prove to be salutary.

4. Cautious use of antiarrhythmic agents for arrhythmias.

5. Beneficial effects of β-adrenergic blocking agents (somewhat heretical given poor contractility) are under investigation.

6. Cardiac transplantation may be indicated.

C. Restrictive Cardiomyopathy

Pathology and Pathophysiology

1. The least common of the three types of cardiomyopathy in North America is characterized by abnormal diastolic ventricular filling owing to excessively stiff ventricular walls. Contractile function, on the other hand, is relatively unimpaired, thus functionally resembling constrictive pericarditis.

2. There is myocardial fibrosis, hypertrophy or infiltration of unknown cause. Secondary restrictive cardiomyopathy may be due to amyloidosis, hemochromatosis, glycogen deposit, neoplastic infiltration, etc.

Clinical Manifestations

1. History of exercise intolerance, weakness and dyspnea, or chest pain may be present.

2. Jugular venous distention, gallop rhythm, and a systolic murmur of AV valve regurgitation may be present.

3. Endomyocardial biopsy may be useful in identifying causes of restrictive cardiomyopathies.

Treatment

1. Diuretics are beneficial (but digoxin is not indicated, since systolic function is unimpaired).

2. Anticoagulants (warfarin) and antiplatelet drugs (aspirin and dipyridamole).

3. Corticosteroids and immunosuppressive agents have been suggested.

III. TUMORS OF THE HEART

Cardiac tumors are extremely rare in children. The most common primary tumor is intracavitary myxoma, especially left atrial myxoma. Rare benign mural tumors include fibromas and rhabdomyomas; the latter are commonly associated with tuberous sclerosis. The most common primary malignant tumor of the heart is sarcoma. Metastatic tumors of the heart, although extremely rare in children, are associated with leukemia or lymphosarcoma. They may involve the pericardium or myocardium.

Clinical manifestations vary, primarily in terms of the location of the tumor. Tumors involving the conduction tissues may manifest with arrhythmias. Intracavitary tumors, such as left atrial myxoma, may produce inflow obstruction. Fragmentation of intracavitary tumors may lead to embolism of the pulmonary or systemic circuits. Involvement of the myocardium (mural tumors) may result in myocardial failure. Pericardial tumors, which are usually malignant, may produce cardiac compression or features simulating infective pericarditis.

19 / Cardiovascular Infections

I. INFECTIVE ENDOCARDITIS

Infective endocarditis may be classified into two types according to the course: acute and subacute. Acute infective endocarditis is rare and develops during the course of septicemia. Preexisting heart disease is not a prerequisite, as it is in patients with subacute infective endocarditis. Acute endocarditis occurs mainly in infants and small children. The invading organism is more virulent than in the subacute type, and *Staphylococcus aureus* is the most commonly encountered organism. The mortality is very high (greater than 50%). Subacute infective endocarditis occurs in children usually older than 2 years of age with underlying cardiovascular abnormalities. *Only the subacute type will be discussed in depth.*

Incidence
0.5–1/1,000 hospital admissions, excluding postoperative endocarditis.

Pathogenesis
Two factors are important in the pathogenesis of subacute endocarditis:

1. The presence of structural abnormalities of the heart or great arteries with a significant pressure gradient or turbulence (with resulting endothelial damage and platelet-fibrin thrombus formation), and

2. Bacteremia, even transient.

Those with a prosthetic heart valve or prosthetic material in the heart are at particularly high risk to develop endocarditis. Drug addicts may develop endocarditis in the absence of known cardiac anomalies. Bacteremia results frequently following dental procedures in children who have had extraction of nondiseased teeth. The incidence of bacteremia following dental extraction is even higher in patients who had diseased teeth or disease of the gingiva. Bacteremia also occurs with such activities as chewing or brushing the teeth. Chewing with diseased teeth may be the most frequent cause of bacteremia. Therefore, good dental hygiene is more important in prevention of infective endocarditis than antibiotic coverage prior to dental procedures.

Pathology
All congenital heart defects, with the exception of secundum-type ASD, predispose to endocarditis. More frequently encountered defects are tetralogy of Fallot, ventricular septal defect, and aortic stenosis. Rheumatic valvular disease, particularly mitral insufficiency, is responsible in a small number of patients. Patients with other lesions, such as mitral valve prolapse syndrome (with mitral regurgitation) and hypertrophic obstructive cardiomyopathy (HOCM, or IHSS), have been reported to be vulnerable to infective endocarditis.

Vegetation of infective endocarditis is found usually in the low-pressure side of the defect, either around the defect or on the opposite surface of the defect where an endothelial damage is established by the jet effect of the defect. For example, vegetations are found in the pulmonary artery in PDA or systemic-pulmonary artery shunts, on the atrial surface of the mitral valve in mitral regurgitation, on the ventricular surface of the aortic valve and mitral chordae in aortic regurgitation, and on the superior surface of the aortic valve or at the site of a jet lesion in the aorta in patients with aortic stenosis.

Microbiology

a. *Streptococcus viridans, S. faecalis* (enterococcus), and *Staphylococcus aureus* are responsible for over 90% of the cases. Less commonly encountered organisms include pneumococcus, *Hemophilus influenzae, Pseudomonas, Escherichia coli, Proteus, Aerobacter,* and *Listeria.*

b. *Candida* endocarditis may occur in patients who are receiving long-term antibiotic or steroid therapy.

c. The organism most commonly found in postoperative endocarditis and in drug abusers is the *Staphylococcus.*

Clinical Manifestations

History

a. History of underlying heart defect is present in almost all patients.

b. History of recent dental procedures or tonsillectomy is occasionally present. History of toothache (from dental or gingival disease) is frequently found.

c. Insidious onset, with fever, fatigue, loss of appetite, and pallor, is common.

PE

a. Heart murmur (100%). Appearance of a new heart murmur and an increase in the intensity of the murmur are important.

b. Fever (80%–90%). Fluctuating fever between 101° and 103° F (38.3° and 39.4° C) is present.

c. Splenomegaly (70%).

d. Skin manifestations (50%), probably secondary to microemboli, are present in the following forms:

1) Petechiae on the skin, mucous membranes, or conjunctivas are the most frequent skin lesions.

2) Osler's nodes (tender red nodes at the ends of the fingers) are rare in children.

3) Janeway's lesions (small, painless, hemorrhagic areas on the palms or soles) are rare.

4) Splinter hemorrhage (linear hemorrhagic streaks beneath the nails) are also rare.

e. Embolic phenomena to other organs are present in 50% of the cases:

1) Pulmonary emboli in patients with VSD or TOF with a systemic-pulmonary artery shunt.

2) Seizures and hemiparesis are the result of embolization to the CNS (20%) and more common with left-sided defects such as aortic and mitral valve disease or with cyanotic heart disease.

3) Hematuria and renal failure.

f. Carious teeth or periodontal or gingival disease are frequently present.

g. Clubbing of fingers in the absence of cyanosis (rare).

Laboratory

a. Positive blood cultures.

b. Complete blood cell count shows anemia, with hemoglobin levels lower than 12 gm/100 ml (80%), and leukocytosis with shift to the left. Patients with polycythemia preceding the onset of subacute infective endocarditis may have normal hemoglobin.

c. Increased sedimentation rate (ESR).

d. Microscopic hematuria (30%).

ECHO

2D ECHO may actually demonstrate the vegetation. It is unlikely that vegetations less than 2 mm in maximum dimension will be seen by 2D ECHO. Negative ECHO does not rule out infective endocarditis; repeated ECHO studies are indicated when infective endocarditis is suspected. False positive diagnosis is also possible, especially with abnormal valves or improper gain of the ECHO machine. ECHO evidence of vegetations may persist for months or years after bacteriologic cure.

Diagnosis

A *presumptive* diagnosis of infective endocarditis is made when a patient with an underlying heart lesion has a fever of unknown origin of several days' duration, and any of the above-mentioned physical findings or laboratory changes is present. A *definitive* diagnosis is made by positive blood cultures. Demonstration of the vegetation by 2D ECHO provides a conclusive anatomical diagnosis.

Management

1. Draw 4–6 blood cultures in succession over 24–48 hours.

2. Start treatment with IV penicillin or oxacillin plus IV gentamicin or IM streptomycin while awaiting the results of blood cultures.
   Penicillin, 6–20 million units/day, IV bolus in 6 divided doses (every 4 hours).
   Oxacillin, 200–300 mg/kg/day, IV bolus in 6 divided doses (every 4 hours).
   Gentamicin, 7 mg/kg/day, IV in 3 divided doses.
   Streptomycin, 20 mg/kg/day, IM in 1–2 divided doses.

3. Final selection of antibiotics depends on the organism isolated and the result of antibiotic sensitivity test. In general, however, when *Str. viridans* is the causative agent, IV penicillin for a total of 4 weeks is recommended. Enterococcus-caused endocarditis usually requires a combination of IV penicillin for 4 weeks and IV gentamicin or IM streptomycin for 2 weeks. The drug of choice for *Staphylococcus* endocarditis is one of the semisynthetic penicillinase-resistant penicillins, such as oxacillin, methicillin, or cloxacillin, given for 4–6 weeks. Penicillin-allergic individuals may be treated with IV vancomycin (40 mg/kg/day in 4 divided doses) for the same duration as penicillin.

4. Patients with prosthetic valve endocarditis should be treated for 4–6 weeks based on organism isolated and the results of sensitivity test. Operative intervention may be necessary before completion of the antibiotic therapy if clinical situation warrants (such as progressive CHF, significant malfunction of prosthetic valves, persistently positive blood cultures after 2 weeks' therapy). Bacteriologic relapse after an appropriate course of therapy also calls for operative intervention.

Prognosis
Overall recovery rate is 80%–85%; 90% or better for *Str. viridans* and enterococcus; and 50% for *Staphylococcus*.

Prevention
More important than diagnosis and treatment of infective endocarditis is its prevention. Maintenance of good dental hygiene is more important than antibiotic prophylaxis (discussed below in detail). All patients with congenital or rheumatic heart disease, patients who have a prosthetic valve or conduit in the heart, and patients who have residual shunt, or obstructive or regurgitant lesions following cardiac surgery must receive antibiotic prophylaxis when they undergo certain dental or surgical procedures, or instrumentation of the upper respiratory tract, genitourinary, or GI tracts. Patients with prosthetic valve and surgically constructed systemic-pulmonary artery shunt or conduits are at higher risk of endocarditis than others. Patients with unoperated isolated secundum ASD and those who had secundum ASD repaired without a patch or PDA ligated six or more months earlier do not require prophylaxis.

Procedures for which endocarditis prophylaxis is indicated are as follows:

a) *All* dental procedures (including routine professional cleaning) which are likely to cause bleeding.

b) Tonsillectomy and/or adenoidectomy.

c) Surgical procedures or biopsy involving respiratory mucosa.

d) Bronchoscopy, especially with a rigid bronchoscope.

e) Incision and drainage of infected tissues.

f) Genitourinary and GI procedures (cystoscopy, GU tract surgery, gallbladder surgery, colonic surgery, esophageal dilatation, upper and lower GI endoscopy with biopsy.

Spontaneous shedding of deciduous teeth, simple adjustment of orthodontic appliances, endotracheal intubation, and insertion of tympanostomy tubes are not indications for antibiotic prophylaxis.

The following is an excerpt of the recommendation made by the Committee on Rheumatic Fever and Infective Endocarditis of the Council of Cardiovascular Disease of the Young of the American Heart Association, 1984 (used by permission). It is important to realize that the antibiotic prophylaxis should be initiated one hour before, *not several days before*, a procedure.

A. For dental and respiratory tract procedures:

   1. For most low-risk patients:
      Children <60 lb: Penicillin V, 1.0 gm one hour prior to procedure and then 0.5 gm 6 hours after the initial dose.
      Adults: Penicillin V, 2.0 gm one hour prior to procedure and then 1.0 gm 6 hours after the initial dose.

2. For high-risk patients (prosthetic heart valve, shunt procedures):
   Children*: Ampicillin, 50 mg/kg, plus gentamicin, 2.0 mg/kg, IM or IV, both given 30 minutes before procedure, then penicillin V, 0.5 gm, orally 6 hours after the initial dose.
   Adults: Ampicillin, 1.0–2.0 gm, plus gentamicin, 1.5 mg/kg, IM or IV, then penicillin V, 1.0 gm, orally 6 hours after the initial dose.

3. For those low-risk patients allergic to penicillin:
   Children*: Erythromycin, 20 mg/kg, orally one hour prior to procedure, and then, 10 mg/kg, 6 hours after the initial dose.
   Adults: Erythromycin, 1.0 gm, orally one hour prior to procedure, and then 0.5 gm 6 hours after the initial dose.

4. For high-risk patients allergic to penicillin:
   Children*: Vancomycin, 20 mg/kg, IV over 60 minutes, begun 60 minutes before procedure; no repeat dose is necessary.
   Adults: Vancomycin 1.0 gm IV over 60 minutes, begun 60 minutes before procedure; no repeat dose is necessary.

5. For those patients taking an oral penicillin for secondary prevention of rheumatic fever, one may choose either erythromycin as above or one of the parenteral regimens.

B. For genitourinary and GI tract surgery and instrumentation:

1. Standard regimen:
   Children*: Ampicillin, 50 mg/kg, plus gentamicin, 2.0 mg/kg, IM or IV, given 30 minutes before procedure. May repeat once 8 hours later.
   Adults: Ampicillin, 2.0 gm, plus gentamicin, 1.5 mg/kg, IM or IV. Same timing of medications as in children.

2. For patients allergic to penicillin:
   Children*: Vancomycin, 20 mg/kg, IV given over 60 minutes plus gentamicin, 2.0 mg/kg, IM or IV, each given 60 minutes before procedure. Doses may be repeated once 8–12 hours later.
   Adults: Vancomycin, 1.0 gm, IV plus gentamicin, 1.5 mg/kg, IM or IV. Timing as above.

3. For minor or repetitive procedures in low-risk patients:
   Children*: Amoxicillin, 50 mg/kg, orally one hour prior to procedure and 25 mg/kg 6 hours after the initial dose.
   Adults: Amoxicillin, 3.0 gm and 1.5 gm follow-up dose. Same timing of doses as above.

II. MYOCARDITIS

Incidence

Myocarditis severe enough to be recognized clinically is rare, but the incidence of mild and subclinical myocarditis is probably much higher.

Procedure

Macroscopically, inflamed myocardium is soft, flabby, and pale, with areas of scarring. Microscopic examination reveals patchy infiltrations by plasma cells,

---

*Children are those who weigh less than 60 lb. Children who weigh more than 60 lb may receive adult doses.

mononuclear leukocytes, and some eosinophils during the acute phase and giant cell infiltration in the later stages.

Etiology

1. Infections, most commonly by viruses, and rarely by bacteria, rickettsia, fungi, and parasites. More common viral agents include coxsackie viruses A and B (particularly in newborns and small infants), rubella, vaccinia, varicella, cytomegalovirus, herpesvirus, enterovirus, arbovirus, adenovirus, influenza, rubeola, hepatitis, mumps, and infectious mononucleosis.

2. Acute rheumatic fever.

3. Some "collagen diseases."

4. Toxic myocarditis (drug ingestion and other toxic and anoxic agents).

Clinical Manifestations

History

a. History of an upper respiratory infection may be present in older children.

b. Sudden onset of illness in newborns and small infants with anorexia, vomiting, lethargy, and occasional shock.

PE

a. Signs of CHF may be present: poor heart tone, tachycardia, gallop rhythm, tachypnea, and, rarely, cyanosis.

b. A soft, systolic heart murmur and hepatomegaly may be present.

c. Irregular rhythm caused by supraventricular or ventricular ectopic beats may be present.

ECG

Any one or combination of the following may be present: low QRS voltages, ST-T changes, prolongation of QT interval, or arrhythmias, especially premature contractions.

X-Rays

Cardiomegaly of varying degree is the most important clinical sign of myocarditis.

ECHO

ECHO reveals cardiac chamber enlargement and impaired LV function.

Natural History and Complications

a. The majority of the patients, especially those with mild inflammation, recover completely.

b. Some patients develop subacute or chronic myocarditis with persistent cardiomegaly with or without signs of CHF, and ECG evidence of LVH or CVH. Clinically, these patients are indistinguishable from those with dilated cardiomyopathy or endocardial fibroelastosis (see chap. 18).

Management

1. Virus identification by viral cultures from the blood, stool, or throat washing, and comparison of acute and convalescent sera for serologic titer rise.

2. Anticongestive measures include:

a. Rapid-acting diuretics (furosemide or ethacrynic acid, 1 mg/kg, each).

b. Oxygen.

c. "Cardiac chair" or "infant seat" to relieve respiratory distress.

d. Cautious digitalization (using half of the usual dose) is indicated as some patients with myocarditis may be exquisitely sensitive to the drug.

e. Other inotropic agents such as isoproterenol or dopamine may be useful.

3. The role of corticosteroids is unclear at this time except for severe rheumatic carditis (see also chap. 20).

III. PERICARDITIS

Etiology

1. Viral infection is probably the most common cause, particularly in infancy. Many viruses similar to those listed under myocarditis can cause pericarditis.

2. Acute rheumatic fever is a common cause of pericarditis, especially in certain parts of the world (see also chap. 20).

3. Bacterial infection (purulent pericarditis). Commonly encountered are *Sta. aureus, Streptococcus pneumoniae, H. influenzae, Neisseria meningitidis,* and streptococci.

4. Tuberculosis (an occasional cause of constrictive pericarditis).

5. Following heart surgery (postpericardiotomy syndrome, chap. 31).

6. Collagen disease such as rheumatoid arthritis (see chap. 22).

7. As a complication of oncologic disease or its therapy, including radiation.

8. Uremia (uremic pericarditis).

Pathology

There is an inflammation of the parietal and visceral surfaces of the pericardium. Serofibrinous, hemorrhagic, or purulent exudate may be completely absorbed or may result in pericardial thickening or chronic constriction (constrictive pericarditis).

Pathophysiology

Pathogenesis of symptoms and signs of pericardial effusion is determined by two factors: speed of fluid accumulation and competence of the myocardium. A rapid accumulation of a large amount of pericardial fluid produces more serious circulatory embarrassment. Even a slow accumulation of a relatively small amount of fluid may result in serious circulatory embarrassment if the extent of myocarditis is significant. Slow accumulation of a large amount of fluid may be well tolerated if the myocardium is intact.

With the development of pericardial tamponade, several compensatory mechanisms are called upon: (a) systemic and pulmonary venous constriction (to improve diastolic filling), (b) an increase in systemic vascular resistance (to raise falling blood pressure), and (c) tachycardia (to improve cardiac output).

Clinical Manifestations

History

a. History of upper respiratory tract infection may be present.

b. Precordial pain (dull, aching, or stabbing) with occasional radiation to the shoulder and neck.

c. Fever of varying degrees.

PE

a. Pericardial friction rub is the cardinal physical sign.

b. Quiet and hypodynamic heart in the presence of cardiomegaly.

c. Heart murmur is usually absent, although it may be present in acute rheumatic fever (see chap. 20).

d. In children with *purulent pericarditis*, septic fever (101°–105° F), tachycardia, chest pain, and dyspnea are almost always present.

e. Signs of *cardiac tamponade* may be present: distant heart sounds, tachycardia, pulsus paradoxus, hepatomegaly, venous distention, and occasional hypotension with peripheral vasoconstriction. Cardiac tamponade occurs more commonly in purulent pericarditis than other forms of pericarditis.

ECG

a. The low-voltage QRS complex due to pericardial effusion is not a constant finding.

b. The following time-dependent changes secondary to myocardial involvement may occur (see Fig 24–2):

1) Initial ST segment elevation,

2) Return of the ST segment to the baseline with an inversion of T waves, and

3) Inverted T waves with isoelectric ST segment.

X-Rays

a. Varying degree of cardiomegaly.

b. A "pear" or "water-bottle" shaped heart with large effusion.

c. Pulmonary venous markings may be increased in cardiac tamponade.

ECHO

a. ECHO is the most useful tool in establishing the diagnosis of pericardial effusion. Effusion is seen usually both anteriorly and posteriorly. 2D ECHO is more sensitive than M-mode ECHO, as it can detect loculated effusions as well.

b. ECHO is very helpful in detecting *cardiac tamponade*. Helpful 2D ECHO findings are as follows:

1) Collapse of the RA in (late) diastole (Fig 19–1).

2) Collapse or indentation of the RV free wall, especially the outflow tract.

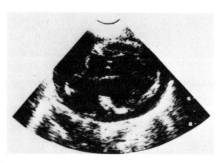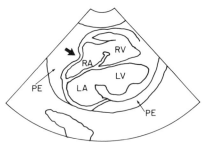

FIG 19–1.
Subcostal four-chamber view demonstrating pericardial effusion *(PE)* and collapse of the right atrial wall *(arrow)*, a sign of cardiac tamponade. LA = left atrium; LV = left ventricle; RA = right atrium; RV = right ventricle.

Management

1. Pericardiocentesis or surgical drainage to identify the etiology of the pericarditis is mandatory, especially when purulent pericarditis or tuberculous pericarditis is suspected.

2. No specific treatment for viral pericarditis.

3. Treatment of the basic disease itself (uremia, collagen disease, etc.).

4. Salicylates for precordial pain for nonbacterial pericarditis and rheumatic fever.

5. Corticosteroid therapy may be indicated in children with severe rheumatic carditis or postpericardiotomy syndrome.

6. For cardiac tamponade, urgent decompression by surgical drainage or pericardiocentesis is indicated. While preparing for pericardial drainage, fluid push with plasmanate to increase central venous pressure is indicated; this helps to improve cardiac filling.

7. Urgent surgical drainage of the pericardium is indicated when purulent pericarditis is suspected. This must be followed by IV antibiotic therapy for 4–6 weeks' duration.

8. Digitalis is contraindicated in cardiac tamponade (since it blocks tachycardia, the compensatory response to impaired venous return).

IV. CONSTRICTIVE PERICARDITIS

A fibrotic, thickened, and adherent pericardium restricts diastolic filling of the heart. Although rare in children, it may be associated with an earlier idiopathic or viral pericarditis, tuberculosis, incomplete drainage of purulent pericarditis, hemopericardium, mediastinal irradiation, neoplastic infiltration, or connective tissue disorders.

Diagnosis of constrictive pericarditis is suspected by the following clinical findings.

a. Signs of elevated jugular venous pressure.

b. Hepatomegaly with ascites and systemic edema.

c. Diastolic pericardial knock (which resembles the opening snap) is often heard along the left sternal border in the absence of heart murmur.

d. Calcification of the pericardium, enlargement of the SVC and the LA, and pleural effusion are common on chest x-rays.

e. The ECG may show low QRS voltages, T-wave inversion or flattening, and LAH.

f. ECHO may reveal two parallel lines representing the thickened visceral and parietal pericardia or multiple dense echoes (M-mode).

Cardiac catheterization may document the presence of constrictive physiology.

Treatment for constrictive pericarditis is complete resection of the pericardium; symptomatic improvement occurs in 75% of patients.

V. KAWASAKI'S DISEASE (MUCOCUTANEOUS LYMPH NODE SYNDROME)

Etiology

Etiology of this disease is not known. It affects children of all racial groups, although it is more common in orientals. It is a disease primarily of young children; 80% of the patients are younger than 4 years of age, 50% are younger than 2 years of age, and cases in children older than 8 years old are only rarely reported.

Pathology

This generalized febrile illness is accompanied by significant pathologies of the heart, which may be the cause of death. There is vasculitis of the coronary arteries with aneurysm formation, which may result in scar formation and calcification. Occasionally, massive myocardial infarction results. The elevated platelet count seen in this condition contributes to coronary thrombosis.

Clinical Manifestations

Clinical Course

Clinical course of the disease may be divided into three phases: acute, subacute, and convalescent. Each phase of the disease is characterized by unique symptoms and signs.

A. Acute Phase (first 10 days):

The following six signs which compose the diagnostic criteria for Kawasaki's disease (Table 19–1) are present: (a) fever, spiking up to 40° C, (b) conjunctival injection, (c) changes in the mouth and lips (strawberry tongue, diffuse reddening of the oral cavity, and fissuring of the lips), (d) reddening and

TABLE 19–1.

Diagnostic Criteria for Kawasaki's Disease

1. Fever, spiking up to 40° C, persisting for more than 5 days.
2. Conjunctival injection (without exudate).
3. Changes in the mouth and lips: strawberry tongue, reddening of oral cavity, and erythema and fissuring of the lips.
4. Changes in the hands and feet: reddening of the palms and soles and indurative edema of hands and feet.
5. Erythematous rash.
6. Cervical lymphadenopathy (greater than 1.5 cm in diameter)

edema of the hands and feet, (e) erythematous rash, and (f) cervical lymph-adenitis. In addition, there are other frequently associated findings, such as pyuria (70%), arthritis (40%), GI tract symptoms (25%), and aseptic meningitis (in almost all patients).

B. Subacute Phase (11–25 days after the onset):

a. Desquamation of the tips of fingers and toes is characteristic.

b. Rash, fever, and lymphadenopathy disappear.

c. Significant cardiovascular changes occur in this phase, including coronary aneurysm, pericardial effusion, CHF, or myocardial infarction.

d. Thrombocytosis also occurs during this phase.

e. Sedimentation rate (ESR) remains elevated.

C. Convalescent Phase (until elevated ESR and platelet count return to normal): Deep transverse grooves may appear across each fingernail and toenail.

Laboratory

a. Marked leukocytosis with shift to the left.

b. Increased sedimentation rate.

c. Thrombocytosis during the subacute phase, with platelet count of 600,000 to more than 1 million/cu mm.

d. ECG shows subtle changes (prolonged PR interval or nonspecific ST-T changes) in up to 60% of the patients. Abnormal Q waves are seen with myocardial damage.

Natural History and Complications
It is a self-limited disease for most patients. Cardiovascular involvement is the most serious complication of the disease.

a. Coronary artery aneurysm occurs in 25% of the patients and is responsible for myocardial infarction (less than 5%) and mortality (1%–2%).

b. Aneurysms have a tendency to regress within one year in about 50% of the patients, more likely in infants less than 1 year of age, and in females.

c. Mitral regurgitation (10%) and aortic regurgitation (less than 5%) occur during acute phase.

d. Pericardial effusion occurs during the subacute phase.

e. Involvement of other peripheral arteries (cervical, axillary, renal, iliac) has been reported.

Diagnosis

1. Diagnosis of Kawasaki's disease is based on clinical findings; there are no consistently reliable or pathognomonic laboratory tests for this disease. Five of six diagnostic criteria are required to make diagnosis (see Table 19–1). Over 90% of the patients have all of the five signs (1 through 5), and about 70% have the lymphadenopathy.

2. One must rule out diseases with similar manifestations by appropriate cultures and other laboratory investigations; scarlet fever, Stevens-Johnson syndrome, viral exanthems, sepsis, staphylococcal "scalded skin" syndrome, Rocky Mountain spotted fever, etc.

3. Diagnosis of coronary artery involvement can be made by 2D ECHO. It is nearly as reliable as coronary angiography in demonstrating aneurysm of the proximal coronary arteries. Distal coronary aneurysm without proximal coronary involvement can occur but is rare. Coronary angiography is not necessary, as surgical intervention is not advised.

4. Abnormal Q waves in the ECG almost always reflect myocardial damage from coronary artery involvement.

5. Higher plasma β-thromboglobulin levels (an indicator of increased platelet activation) have been reported in patients with coronary involvement.

Treatment

1. Aspirin at high anti-inflammatory dose (100 mg/kg/day) is the treatment of choice. Serum salicylate levels are monitored and are kept near 20 mg/100 ml. The dose is reduced to 10 mg/kg/day after fever subsides. Some authorities recommend the antiplatelet dose of aspirin from the outset, as the high dose may inhibit prostacyclin (a compound that may be a potent inhibitor of platelet aggregation). However, a significantly lower incidence of coronary aneurysm was found in patients who received the higher dose of aspirin. Low-dose aspirin therapy is continued for three months. Aspirin can be stopped if no aneurysm is identified, but if aneurysm is present, aspirin should be continued until the coronary artery appears normal by 2D ECHO.

2. Corticosteroids are considered to be contraindicated, since they may increase the incidence of coronary aneurysm.

3. High dose γ-globulin (400 mg/kg/day) given IV for four consecutive days during the acute phase has been shown to reduce incidence of coronary artery abnormalities.

4. Repeat 2D ECHO studies are recommended, at least during the acute phase and subacute phase, and at three months after the onset.

20 / Acute Rheumatic Fever

Incidence

Acute rheumatic fever is uncommon in the United States, but is a common cause of heart disease in underdeveloped countries.

Etiology

1. It is believed to be an immunologic lesion which occurs as a delayed sequela of group A hemolytic streptococcal infection of the pharynx (but not of the skin).

2. The attack rate of acute rheumatic fever following streptococcal infection varies with the severity of the infection, ranging from 0.3% to 3.0%.

3. Important predisposing factors are as follows:

    a. High family incidence of rheumatic fever.

    b. Low socioeconomic status (poverty, poor hygiene, medical deprivation, etc.).

    c. Age: common between 6 and 15 years, with peak incidence at 8 years of age.

Pathology

1. The inflammatory lesion is found in many parts of the body, notably in the heart, brain, joints, and skin.

2. Aschoff bodies in the atrial myocardium are believed to be characteristic of rheumatic fever.

3. Valvular damage most frequently involves the mitral, less commonly the aortic, and rarely the tricuspid and pulmonary valves.

Clinical Manifestations

History

a. Streptococcal pharyngitis, 1–5 weeks (average 3 weeks) prior to the onset of symptoms. The latent period may be as long as 2–6 months (average 4 months) in cases of isolated chorea.

b. Pallor, malaise, and easy fatigability.

c. Other nonspecific history may include epistaxis (5%–10%) and abdominal pain.

d. Family history of rheumatic fever is frequently positive.

Major Manifestations

a. Arthritis is the most common manifestation of acute rheumatic fever occurring in 60%–85% of the cases. It usually involves large joints (knees, an-

238

kles, elbows, wrists, etc.). Often more than one joint, either simultaneously or in succession, are involved with characteristic migratory nature. Heat, redness, swelling, pain, and tenderness are commonly present.

  b. Carditis occurs in 40%–50% of patients. Signs of carditis include some or all of the following:

    1) Tachycardia (out of proportion for the degree of fever).

    2) Significant heart murmurs (due to mitral and/or aortic regurgitation) are almost always present; without the significant heart murmurs, the diagnosis of carditis should not be made (see below for further discussion).

    3) Pericarditis (friction rub, pericardial effusion, chest pain, and ECG changes).

    4) Cardiomegaly on chest x-rays (due to pericarditis, pancarditis, or CHF).

    5) Signs of congestive heart failure (gallop rhythm, distant heart sounds, cardiomegaly).

  c. Erythema marginatum occurs in less than 10% of the patients with acute rheumatic fever. The characteristic nonpruritic serpiginous or annular erythematous rashes are most prominent on the trunk and the inner proximal portions of the extremities. The rashes are evanescent, disappearing on exposure to cold and reappearing after a hot shower or when the patient is covered with a warm blanket. They are seldom detected in air-conditioned hospital rooms.

  d. Subcutaneous nodules are found in 2%–10% of the cases, particularly in those with recurrences. They are hard, painless, nonpruritic, freely movable, swelling, 0.2–2.0 cm in diameter. They are usually found symmetrically, singly or in clusters, on the extensor surfaces of both large and small joints, over the scalp, or along the spine. They are not transient, lasting for weeks, and have a significant association with carditis.

  e. Sydenham's chorea (St. Vitus' dance) is found in 15% of the cases with acute rheumatic fever. It occurs more often in prepubertal girls (8–12 years) than boys. It starts with emotional lability and personality changes, which are soon replaced by loss of motor coordination. Characteristic spontaneous, purposeless movement then develops, followed by motor weakness. It is often an isolated manifestation; the patient may have no fever, and ESR and ASO titers may be normal (because of a long latent period of chorea).

Minor Manifestations

  a. Fever of 38° C (100.4° F) is usually present in the course of untreated rheumatic fever. Higher fever is unusual.

  b. Arthralgia refers to joint pain without the objective changes of arthritis.

  c. History of rheumatic fever or rheumatic heart disease. The history must be well documented, or the evidence of preexisting rheumatic heart disease clear-cut.

  d. Acute-phase reactants, e.g., ESR is elevated, and C-reactive protein (CRP) is positive. The ESR may be normal in the presence of CHF. Leukocytosis with shift to the left is usually present.

e. The ECG may show a prolongation of PR interval (first-degree AV block). It is not specific for acute rheumatic fever (and is also seen in other infectious diseases and in some normal persons) nor an indication of active carditis.

Evidence of Preceding Streptococcal Infection

a. History of recent scarlet fever is the best clinical evidence of antecedent streptococcal infection.

b. Positive throat culture for group A β-hemolytic streptococcus is less satisfactory than antibody tests.

c. Specific antibody tests are the most reliable laboratory evidence of antecedent streptococcal infection capable of producing acute rheumatic fever.

1) Antistreptolysin O (ASO) titer is well standardized and, therefore, is the most widely used test. It is elevated in 80% of the patients with acute rheumatic fever (and 20% of normal individuals). An ASO titer greater than 333 Todd units in children and that greater than 250 Todd units in adults is considered significant. A rise of two tubes or more, regardless of the initial level, is also evidence of recent streptococcal infection.

2) Other antibodies that can be tested include anti-DNase (antideoxyribonuclease), anti-NADase (anti-nicotinamide-adenine-dinucleotidase), anti-hyaluronidase, and anti-streptokinase, but these tests are less well standardized.

3) Streptozyme test: This simple agglutination test determines antibodies to a number of streptococcal extracellular antigens. Its sensitivity is reported to be good, but its specificity is questionable.

Diagnosis

Diagnosis of acute rheumatic fever is made by the use of revised Jones's criteria (Table 20–1) which consist of three groups of important clinical and laboratory findings: (a) five major criteria, (b) five minor criteria, (c) supporting evidence of preceding streptococcal infection. Diagnosis of acute rheumatic fever is probable when (a) two major criteria or one major plus two minor criteria are present, and (b) the positive evidence of preceding streptococcal infection is present.

TABLE 20–1.
Jones Criteria (Revised)

Major Manifestations	Minor Manifestations
Polyarthritis	Clinical:
Carditis	Fever
Chorea	Arthralgia
Erythema marginatum	Hx of RF or RHD
Subcutaneous nodules	Laboratory:
	Acute phase reactants
	(↑ ESR, +CRP)
	Prolonged PR interval

Plus

Supporting Evidence of Streptococcal Infection
Increased ASO titer
Positive throat culture for Grp A strep
Recent scarlet fever

The following are helpful tips in applying the Jones criteria:

a. Two major criteria are always stronger than one major plus two minor criteria.

b. Arthralgia or prolonged PR interval cannot be used as minor criteria in the presence of their corresponding major criteria; i.e., arthritis and carditis, respectively.

c. Polyarthritis + fever + acute-phase reactants are particularly weak criteria, as many other febrile illnesses may satisfy the criteria.

d. The absence of evidence of preceding streptococcal infection is a warning sign against acute rheumatic fever (with the exception of chorea).

e. Chorea is often an isolated manifestation without positive acute-phase reactants or elevated ASO titers.

Misdiagnosis of rheumatic fever is still common. A common cause of the misdiagnosis is misinterpretation of physical and laboratory findings by physicians, for which the following comments apply:

a. A *significant* heart murmur must be present before the diagnosis of carditis can be made. The significant heart murmurs are due to regurgitation of the mitral and/or aortic valve. An apical regurgitant systolic murmur is almost always present, and apical diastolic (Carey-Coombs) and aortic diastolic murmurs are rarely present. The vibratory systolic murmur, one of the most common innocent murmurs in school-aged children, is best audible near or at the apex and is frequently misinterpreted as a significant murmur of mitral regurgitation. The mitral regurgitation murmur of acute rheumatic fever is a regurgitant systolic murmur that starts with the S1 and is usually soft (grade 2/6 or less).

b. A prolonged PR interval is not a sign of active carditis in many patients and should not be taken as a major criterion.

e. The possibility of early suppression of full clinical manifestations should be sought during the history taking. Subtherapeutic doses of aspirin or aspirin-containing analgesics (Bufferin, Anacin, etc.) may suppress full manifestations.

d. Although increased ASO titer is an essential part of diagnosis of acute rheumatic fever, it is not specific for rheumatic fever.

Clinical Course

1. Only carditis can cause permanent cardiac damage. A mild carditis disappears rapidly in weeks, while severe carditis may last for 2–6 months.

2. Arthritis subsides in a few days to weeks even without treatment and does not cause permanent damage.

3. Chorea gradually subsides in 2–3 months and usually does not cause neurologic sequelae.

Management

1. When acute rheumatic fever is suspected by history and physical examination findings, obtain the following laboratory studies:

   a. Complete blood cell count (CBC).

   b. Acute phase reactants (ESR, CRP).

   c. Throat culture.

   d. ASO titer (and a second antibody titer, particularly with chorea).

   e. Chest x-ray.

   f. ECG.

   g. Echocardiogram if pericardial effusion is suspected.

2. Give benzathine penicillin G, 0.6–1.2 million units IM, for eradication of
   Streptococcus. This serves as the first dose of penicillin prophylaxis as well
   (see below for prophylaxis).

3. *DO NOT* start anti-inflammatory or suppressive therapy with salicylates or
   steroids until definite diagnosis is made. Early suppressive therapy may interfere with the definite diagnosis of acute rheumatic fever, since it suppresses
   full development of joint manifestations, suppresses acute phase reactants, and
   might even suppress antibody response to streptococcal infection.

4. Bed rest is recommended for the duration of the inflammatory process. The
   ESR is a helpful guide to the rheumatic activity, at least in the early stages.
   The duration of bed rest depends on the kind and severity of manifestations
   and may range from one week to a few months (Table 20–2).

5. Therapy with anti-inflammatory agents should be started as soon as the diagnosis of acute rheumatic fever is made. Prednisone is indicated only in cases
   of moderate to severe carditis. For minimal carditis or isolated arthritis, aspirin alone is recommended. Table 20–3 shows suggested dosage and duration
   of anti-inflammatory drug therapy. An adequate blood level of salicylates is
   20–25 mg/100 ml.

TABLE 20–2.

General Guide for Bed Rest and Ambulation*

	Arthritis Alone	Minimal Carditis	Moderate Carditis	Severe Carditis
Bed rest	1–2 wk	3 wk	6 wk	3–6 mo
Indoor ambulation	2 wk	3 wk	6 wk	3 mo
Outdoor activity (school)	3 wk	4 wk	3 mo	> 3 mo
Full activity	After 6–8 wk	After 10 wk	After 6 mo	Variable

*Minimal carditis = questionable cardiomegaly; moderate carditis = definite but mild cardiomegaly;
severe carditis = marked cardiomegaly or CHF.

TABLE 20–3.

Recommended Anti-Inflammatory Agents

	Arthritis Alone	Minimal Carditis	Moderate Carditis	Severe Carditis
Prednisone	0	0	2–4 wk*	2–6 wk*
Aspirin	1–2 wk	2–4 wk†	6–8 wk	2–4 mo

   Dosages: Prednisone = 2 mg/kg/day, in 4 divided doses.
            Aspirin   = 100 mg/kg/day, in 4–6 divided doses.

*The dose of prednisone should be tapered and aspirin started during the
final week.
†Apirin may be reduced by 60/mg/kg/day after two weeks of therapy.

6. Treatment for congestive heart failure includes (see also chap. 27):

   a. Complete bed rest with orthopneic position.

   b. Moist, cool oxygen.

   c. Morphine sulfate, 0.2 mg/kg, at 4-hour intervals for severe CHF with respiratory distress.

   d. Restriction of sodium and fluid intake.

   e. Prednisone for carditis of recent onset (see Table 20–3).

   f. Digoxin should be used with caution, as certain patients with rheumatic carditis are supersensitive to digitalis. Start with half of the usual recommended dose (see chap. 27).

   g. Furosemide, 1 mg/kg every 6–12 hours, if indicated.

7. Management of Sydenham's chorea:

   a. Protective measures.

   b. Reduce physical and mental stress.

   c. Benzathine penicillin G, 1.2 million units, is given initially for eradication of *Streptococcus* and also every 28 days for prevention of recurrence, just as in patients with other rheumatic manifestations. Without the prophylaxis, about 25% of patients with isolated chorea (without carditis) develop rheumatic valvular heart disease in 20-year follow-up.

   d. Any of the following drugs may be used: phenobarbital, chlorpromazine (Thorazine), diazepam (Valium), haloperidol, or steroids.

Prognosis

The presence or absence of permanent cardiac damage determines the prognosis. The presence of residual heart disease is determined by the following three factors:

1. Cardiac status at the start of treatment: the more severe the cardiac involvement at the time the patient is first seen, the greater the incidence of residual heart disease.

2. Recurrence of rheumatic fever: there is increasing severity of valvular involvement with each recurrence.

3. Regression of heart disease: evidence of cardiac involvement at the first attack may disappear in 10%–25% of patients 10 years after the initial attack.

Prevention

1. Who needs prophylaxis? Any patients with documented history of rheumatic fever, including those with isolated chorea and those without evidence of rheumatic heart disease, must receive the prophylaxis.

2. How long? Ideally, the patients should receive prophylaxis indefinitely. However, many cardiologists recommend discontinuing the prophylaxis at the age of 21–25 provided that:

   a. The patient does not have evidence of valvular involvement.

   b. The patient is not in a high-risk occupation (e.g., school teachers, physicians, nurses, career military personnel).

If the patient has rheumatic valvular disease, the prophylaxis is recommended for a longer (possibly indefinite) period of time. The chance of recurrence is highest in the first five years.

3. Methods: The method of choice for secondary prevention is benzathine penicillin G, 1.2 million units given IM every 28 days (not once a month). Alternative methods, although not as effective as above, are:

   a. Oral penicillin, 200,000–250,000 units twice daily.

   b. Oral sulfadiazine, 0.5 gm once a day for children less than 60 lb, and 1.0 gm once a day for children over 60 lb. Note that the sulfonamides are not effective for the prevention of infective endocarditis.

   c. If the patient is allergic to penicillin, 250 mg of erythromycin twice daily is recommended.

4. Primary prevention of rheumatic fever is possible with a 10-day course of penicillin therapy for streptococcal pharyngitis. However, the primary prevention will not be able to cover those who develop subclinical pharyngitis and therefore do not seek medical treatment. Thirty percent of patients who develop acute rheumatic fever have no symptoms suggestive of streptococcal pharyngitis.

21 / Valvular Heart Disease

Acquired valvular heart diseases are usually of rheumatic origin. Mitral valve involvement occurs in about three-fourths and aortic valve involvement in about one-fourth of all cases with rheumatic heart disease. Stenosis and regurgitation of the same valve usually occur together. Isolated aortic stenosis of rheumatic origin is extremely rare. Involvement of the tricuspid valve is very rare and that of the pulmonary valve almost never occurs. Therefore, only mitral stenosis, mitral regurgitation, and aortic regurgitation of rheumatic origin will be discussed. Although etiology of mitral valve prolapse syndrome is not entirely clear, it will be discussed in this chapter, since it involves a cardiac valve.

I. MITRAL STENOSIS

Incidence

Although rare in children (as it requires 5–10 years from the initial attack), it is the most common valvular involvement in adult rheumatic patients. In certain parts of the world where rheumatic fever is prevalent, severe mitral stenosis occurs in children under the age of 15 years.

Pathology

Thickening of the leaflets and fusion of the commissures dominate pathologic findings. Calcification with immobility of the valve results in time.

Clinical Manifestations

History

    a. Asymptomatic in mild cases.

    b. Dyspnea with or without exertion, orthopnea, nocturnal dyspnea, or palpitations in more severe cases.

PE (Figure 21–1 shows cardiac findings.)

    a. Increased RV impulse.

    b. Peripheral pulses may be weak with narrow pulse pressure.

    c. A loud S1 at the apex, and a narrowly split S2, with accentuated P2 if pulmonary hypertension is present. An opening snap (a short snapping sound accompanying the opening of the mitral valve) is present at the apex or LLSB (see Fig 21–1).

    d. A low-frequency middiastolic rumble following the opening snap is audible at the apex (see Fig 21–1). A crescendo presystolic murmur may be audible at the apex. Occasionally, a high-frequency diastolic murmur of pulmonary regurgitation (Graham Steell's murmur) is present at the ULSB (see Fig 21–1).

245

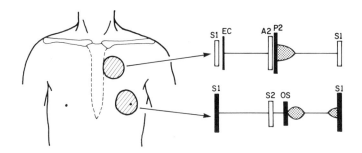

FIG 21–1.
Cardiac findings of mitral stenosis. Abnormal sounds are shown in *black* and include a loud S1, an ejection click (EC), a loud S2, and an opening snap (OS). Also note the middiastolic rumble and presystolic murmur. The murmur of pulmonary insufficiency indicates long-standing pulmonary hypertension.

ECG

   a. RAD, RVH, and LAH or CAH are commonly present.

   b. Atrial fibrillation is rare in children.

X-Rays

   a. Enlargement of the LA and RV and prominence of the MPA segment are usually present.

   b. Lung fields may show the following:

   1) Pulmonary venous congestion.

   2) Interstitial edema shown as Kerley's B lines. These are dense, short, horizontal lines most commonly seen in the costophrenic angles.

   3) Redistribution of PBF (increased pulmonary vascularity) to the upper lobes.

ECHO

   a. M-mode ECHO may show (1) diminished EF slope (diastolic closure of the anterior mitral leaflet), (2) anterior movement of the posterior leaflet during diastole, (3) multiple echoes from thickened mitral leaflets, and (4) large LA dimension.

   b. 2D ECHO shows (1) doming of thick mitral leaflets, and (2) small mitral valve orifice inscribed by the thickened valve.

   c. Doppler studies can estimate the valve area.

Natural History and Complications

   a. Most children with mitral stenosis are asymptomatic but become symptomatic with recurrence of rheumatic fever.

   b. Thromboembolism is rare in children (related to chronic atrial fibrillation).

   c. Infective endocarditis.

   d. Atrial flutter/fibrillation, rare in children, may be seen during active carditis.

e. Hemoptysis (pulmonary edema).

f. Hoarseness with recurrent laryngeal nerve palsy.

Management

Medical

a. Maintenance of good dental hygiene and antibiotic prophylaxis against infective endocarditis.

b. Prevention of recurrence of rheumatic fever with penicillin or sulfonamide (see chap. 20).

c. Varying degrees of restriction of activity may be indicated.

d. Limited experience with balloon valvuloplasty suggests it may delay surgical intervention or result in satisfactory relief of the stenosis.

Surgical

a. Indications

1) Symptomatic patients (dyspnea on exertion, pulmonary edema, paroxysmal dyspnea).

2) Atrial fibrillation.

3) Intractable CHF or progressive cardiomegaly.

b. Procedures and Mortality

1) Closed commissurotomy, approaching blindly via the LA or via a left ventriculotomy for those with noncalcified valves. The mortality is less than 5%; it may be higher in patients with CHF.

2) Open heart procedures

a) Reconstruction of the valve (valvuloplasty). The hospital mortality for the procedure is less than 1% in the adult (slightly higher in children).

b) Artificial valve replacement (for older children with calcified valves and those with combined lesions). The hospital mortality is 5%–10%. The valve of choice varies widely. Prosthetic valves (Starr-Edwards, Bjork-Shiley, St. Jude) have the advantage of longer durability but require long-term anticoagulation therapy with its attendant risks. The bioprostheses (porcine valve, heterograft valve) do not require anticoagulation but tend to deteriorate, more rapidly in the young.

3) Complications

a) Postoperative CHF, the most common cause of early postoperative death.

b) Arterial embolization.

c) Postperfusion syndrome (see chap. 32).

d) Bleeding diathesis, if anticoagulated for prosthetic valve replacement.

II. MITRAL REGURGITATION

Incidence

The most common valvular involvement in children with RHD. Males are more commonly affected than females.

Pathology

1. Mitral valve leaflets are shortened and adherent to the ventricular wall.

2. The mitral valve ring may be dilated.

3. Dilatation of the LA and LV is present.

Clinical Manifestations

History

a. Usually asymptomatic during childhood.

b. Rarely, fatigue and palpitation.

PE (Figure 21–2 shows cardiac findings.)

a. The S1 is normal or diminished. The S2 may split widely (as a result of shortening of LV ejection and early aortic closure). The S3 is commonly present and loud.

b. A regurgitant systolic murmur (starting with the S1), grade 2–4/6, is present at the apex and often transmits to the left axilla (best demonstrated on left decubitus position) (see Fig 21–2).

c. A short, low-frequency diastolic flow rumble may be present at the apex (see Fig 21–2).

ECG

a. Normal in mild mitral regurgitation.

b. LVH or LV dominance is usually present.

c. Occasional LAH.

X-Rays (Fig 21–3)

a. Enlargement of the LA and LV.

b. Pulmonary vascularity is usually within normal limits.

c. Pulmonary venous congestion if CHF develops.

ECHO

a. 2D ECHO may show dilated LA and LV.

b. Doppler studies detect high-velocity turbulent flows within the LA.

Natural History and Complications

a. Relatively stable for a long time, but mitral stenosis eventually supervenes in some patients.

b. Infective endocarditis.

c. Left ventricular failure and consequent pulmonary hypertension may occur in adult life.

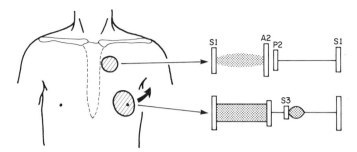

FIG 21–2.
Cardiac findings of mitral regurgitation. *Arrow* near the apex indicates the direction of radiation of the murmur toward the axilla.

Management

Medical

    a. Preventive measures against infective endocarditis.

    b. Prophylaxis against recurrence of rheumatic fever (see chap. 20).

    c. Restriction of activity is not indicated in most mild cases.

    d. Anticongestive measures if CHF develops.

Surgical

    a. Indications: Intractable CHF, progressive cardiomegaly with symptoms, and pulmonary hypertension.

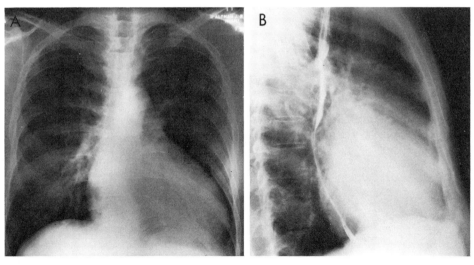

FIG 21–3.
PA **(A)** and lateral **(B)** views of chest roentgenogram in a patient with moderately severe mitral regurgitation of rheumatic origin. The lateral view was obtained with barium swallow. The CT ratio is increased (0.64), and the apex is displaced downward and laterally in the PA view. The lateral view shows an indentation of the barium-filled esophagus by an enlarged LA, and the LV is displaced posteriorly.

b. Procedures and Mortality: Mitral valvuloplasty or valve replacement during cardiopulmonary bypass. Valvuloplasty is preferred over valve replacement in children; it carries lower mortality (less than 10%) and complication rate than does valve replacement.

c. Complications: Similar to those listed for mitral stenosis.

III. AORTIC REGURGITATION

Incidence

Most patients have associated mitral valve disease. More common in males than females.

Pathology

Semilunar cusps are deformed and shortened and the valve ring is dilated, so that the cusps fail to appose tightly.

Clinical Manifestations

History

a. Asymptomatic with mild regurgitation.

b. Decreased exercise tolerance with more severe regurgitation or CHF.

PE (Figure 21–4 shows cardiac findings.)

a. Increased LV impulse, and occasional diastolic thrill at 3LICS (see Fig 21–4).

b. Wide pulse pressure and bounding water-hammer pulse.

c. The S1 is decreased in intensity. The S2 may be normal or single.

d. A high-pitched diastolic decrescendo murmur, best audible at the 3LICS or 4LICS. This murmur is more easily audible with the patient sitting up and leaning forward. The longer the murmur, the more severe the regurgitation (see Fig 21–4).

e. A systolic ejection murmur of varying intensity may be present at 2RICS, owing to relative AS, with increased stroke volume. The combination of the diastolic and systolic murmurs gives rise to the to-and-fro murmur.

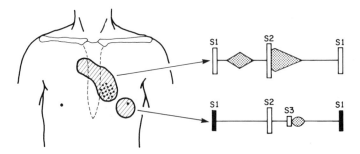

FIG 21–4.
Cardiac findings of aortic regurgitation. The S1 is abnormally soft *(black bar)*. The predominant murmur is a high-pitched, diastolic decrescendo murmur at 3LICS.

f. A middiastolic mitral rumble (Austin-Flint murmur) is occasionally present (see Fig 21–4 and chap. 10 for pathophysiology of this murmur).

ECG

a. Normal or LVH.

b. LAH in long-standing cases.

X-Rays

a. Cardiomegaly involving the LV.

b. Dilated ascending aorta or prominent aortic knob may be present.

Natural History and Complications

a. Asymptomatic for a long time, but if symptoms begin, many patients deteriorate rapidly.

b. Anginal pain, CHF, or multiple PVCs are unfavorable signs.

c. Infective endocarditis.

Management

Medical

a. Maintenance of good dental hygiene and antibiotic prophylaxis against infective endocarditis.

b. Prophylaxis against recurrence of rheumatic fever with penicillin or sulfonamides (see chap. 20).

c. No restriction of activity for mild cases, but varying degrees of restriction may be indicated in more severe cases.

d. Anticongestive measures if CHF develops.

Surgical

a. Indications

   1) Symptoms such as anginal pain, dyspnea on exertion.

   2) Even in asymptomatic patients, significant cardiomegaly (CT ratio greater than 55% on chest x-rays), ejection fraction less than 40%, or stress test-induced symptoms may be an indication.

b. Procedure: Aortic valve replacement under cardiopulmonary bypass. The antibiotic sterilized aortic homograft appears to be the device of choice. The porcine heterograft has the risk of accelerated degeneration. The Bjork-Shiley and the St. Jude prostheses are less suited for young patients.

c. Mortality: 2%–5%. Postoperative acute cardiac failure is the most common cause of death.

d. Complications

   1) Thromboembolism, chronic hemolysis and anticoagulant-induced hemorrhage may occur with prosthetic valve.

   2) Early calcification of porcine valve in children.

   3) Prosthetic valve endocarditis.

IV. MITRAL VALVE PROLAPSE SYNDROME (MVPS)

Incidence

A reported incidence of 5% in pediatric population is probably an overestimation. Usually in older children and adolescents (more common in adults), with female preponderance (M:F = 1:2).

Pathology

1. Thick and redundant mitral valve leaflets (due to myxomatous degeneration) bulge into the mitral anulus.

2. The posterior leaflet is more commonly and more severely affected than the anterior leaflet.

Etiology

1. Idiopathic in more than 50% of the cases.

2. Congenital heart disease in one-third of the patients with MVPS.

   a. Secundum-type ASD is the most commonly found defect.

   b. Other CHDs include VSD and Ebstein's anomaly.

3. Marfan's syndrome: 4% of the patients with MVPS have Marfan's syndrome, and nearly all patients with Marfan's syndrome have MVPS.

4. Other connective tissue disorders.

5. Familial in the primary form (with autosomal dominant mode of inheritance).

Clinical Manifestations

History

   a. Usually asymptomatic.

   b. Nonexertional chest pain, palpitation, and, rarely, syncope may be elicited.

PE

   a. Asthenic build with high incidence of thoracic skeletal anomalies (80%), including pectus excavatum (50%), straight back (20%), and scoliosis (10%). (Straight-back syndrome refers to a condition in which there is a loss of the normal dorsal curvature of the spine, resulting in a shortening of the anteroposterior diameter of the chest.)

   b. The midsystolic click and late systolic murmur are the hallmarks of this syndrome and are best audible at the apex (Fig 21–5).

   c. The presence or absence of the click and murmur, as well as their timing, are variable from one examination to the next.

      1) They may be brought out by held expiration, left decubitus position, sitting, standing, or leaning forward. They may disappear on inspiration.

      2) Various maneuvers can alter the timing of the click and the murmur (see Fig 21–5).

         a) The click moves toward the S1 and the murmur lengthens by maneuvers that decrease the LV volume—such as standing, sitting, Valsalva's (strain phase), tachycardia, administration of amyl nitrite, etc.

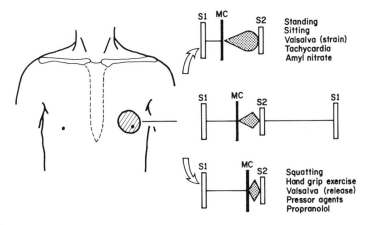

FIG 21–5.
Diagram of auscultatory findings in MVPS and the effect of various maneuvers on the timing of the midsystolic click *(MC)* and the murmur. The maneuvers that reduce ventricular volume enhance leaflet redundancy and move the click and murmur earlier in systole. An increase in LV dimension has the opposite effect.

> **b)** The click moves toward the S2 and the murmur shortens by maneuvers that increase the LV volume—such as squatting, hand grip exercise, Valsalva's (release), bradycardia, administration of pressor agents or propranolol, etc.

ECG

> **a.** Superiorly directed T vector (flat or inverted T waves in II, III, and aVF) is the most common and a more specific ECG finding occurring in 20%–60% of the patients (Fig 21–6).
>
> **b.** Arrhythmias are relatively uncommon and include PAT, PACs, and PVCs.
>
> **c.** Conduction disturbances (first-degree AV block, WPW syndrome or its variants, prolonged QT interval, or RBBB) are occasionally reported.
>
> **d.** LVH or LAH is rarely present.

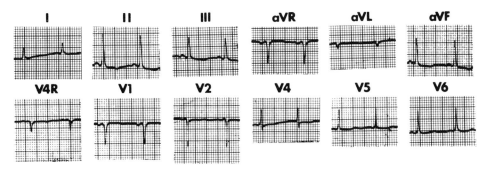

FIG 21–6.
Tracing from a 14-year-old girl with mitral valve prolapse syndrome. The T wave in aVF is inverted.

X-Rays

Unremarkable except for LA enlargement in patients with severe mitral regurgitation.

ECHO

Although there are false positives and false negatives, ECHO is usually diagnostic of the condition.

    a. M-mode ECHO shows posterior motion of the posterior and/or anterior leaflets of the mitral valve.

    b. 2D ECHO is more reliable and shows prolapsing of the mitral valve leaflet(s) superior to the plane of the AV junction, best seen in the parasternal long axis and apical four-chamber views.

    c. Doppler demonstration of mitral regurgitation confirms the diagnosis.

Natural History and Complications

    a. The majority of patients are asymptomatic, particularly during childhood.

    b. Complications that are rare in childhood include sudden death (from ventricular arrhythmias), infective endocarditis, spontaneous rupture of chordae tendineae, progressive mitral regurgitation, CHF, and arrhythmias and conduction disturbances (see ECG findings above).

Management

    1. Asymptomatic patients require no treatment or restriction of activity.

    2. Preventive measures against infective endocarditis (see chap. 19).

    3. Patients who are symptomatic (palpitation, lightheadedness, dizziness, or syncope) or who have arrhythmias should undergo ambulatory ECG monitoring and/or treadmill exercise testing. Propranolol is the drug of choice for ventricular arrhythmias. Other drugs, such as calcium blockers, quinidine, or Pronestyl, may prove to be effective in some patients.

    4. Chest pain may be treated with propranolol (it is not relieved by nitroglycerin, but may worsen).

    5. Reconstructive surgery or mitral valve replacement may be indicated in rare patients with severe mitral regurgitation.

22 / Cardiac Involvement in Systemic Diseases

Many collagen, neuromuscular, and endocrine diseases as well as other systemic diseases may manifest with cardiac involvement. Involvement of the cardiovascular system usually becomes evident when the diagnosis of the primary disease is well established, but occasionally cardiac manifestations may precede evidence of the basic disease. Brief listing of cardiac manifestations will be presented for selected systemic diseases.

Periarteritis Nodosa

a. Coronary arteritis is common and may lead to myocardial infarction. (There may be an overlap between periarteritis nodosa and Kawasaki's disease). Systemic hypertension, probably secondary to renal involvement, may contribute to the cardiac involvement. Signs of pericarditis (friction rub, chest pain, etc.) are occasionally present. CHF may be a terminal event.

b. The ECG abnormalities occur in 85% of the cases and consist most commonly of ST segment shift and T wave changes. LVH and myocardial infarction pattern have also been reported.

Disseminated Lupus Erythematosus

a. Approximately 40% of the patients demonstrate signs and symptoms of cardiac involvement.

b. Pericarditis and pericardial effusion are most commonly encountered (up to 75% of patients with cardiac manifestations). Pericardial tamponade or constrictive pericarditis is less frequent.

c. Heart valve involvement in the form of Libman-Sacks verrucous valvular lesions may occur in 40% of adult patients with mild regurgitation of AV valves. Cardiac enlargement with CHF occurs in 25% of the patients. Raynaud's phenomenon occurs in 25% of the patients.

d. The ECG often shows flat or inverted T waves.

Rheumatoid Arthritis

a. Pericarditis is the most common finding, occurring in 30% of the clinical population and 45% of autopsy cases. Occasionally, constrictive pericarditis may result. Chest pain and friction rub signify pericarditis.

b. Endocardium is rarely involved, with thickening of mitral and aortic valve edges (20%), but myocardium is usually spared. Signs of mitral regurgitation are occasionally present and are more likely in females. (If a male patient has valvular involvement, it is more likely to be aortic regurgitation.)

255

   c. Occasionally, coronary arteritis, focal or diffuse myocarditis, and involvement of the conduction system with heart block can occur.

   d. Tachycardia and nonspecific systolic murmurs are commonly present.

   e. ECG abnormalities occur in 20% of the cases. The most common changes are ST segment shift and T wave changes. Pericarditis may be associated with normal ECG.

Friedreich's Ataxia

   a. Diffuse interstitial fibrosis, fatty degeneration of the myocardium, and hypertrophy of ventricles, especially the left ventricle, are frequently found. CHF is the terminal event, occurring in 70% of the patients.

   b. ECG abnormalities are very common. The most common findings are T vector changes in the limb leads and/or left precordial leads. LVH, RVH, or abnormal Q waves are occasionally present.

   c. Chest x-rays are usually normal, but rarely moderate cardiomegaly is present.

   d. ECHO reveals concentric hypertrophy of the LV, asymmetric septal hypertrophy, or globally decreased LV function, approximately 10% each.

Muscular Dystrophy

   a. Significant cardiac involvement is seen only in Duchenne's type and is manifest clinically during adolescence.

   b. Cardiac enlargement, with endocardial thickening of the LV and LA, is present on gross examination. Fatty degeneration and lymphocytic infiltration are present on microscopic examination.

   c. Exertional dyspnea and tachypnea are common symptoms. A loud P2 secondary to pulmonary hypertension or mitral regurgitation murmur may develop. CHF is an ominous, terminal sign.

   d. ECG abnormalities occur in 90% of teenagers with Duchenne's type. RVH or RBBB is the most common abnormality. Deep Q waves in LPLs are frequently present. T vector changes may be present in the limb leads or LPLs.

Marfan's Syndrome

   a. Clinically evident cardiovascular involvement occurs in over 50% of the patients by the age of 21. Microscopic changes may be present in almost all patients, even during infancy and childhood.

   b. The common cardiovascular abnormalities include aneurysmal dilatation of the ascending aorta with/without dissection or rupture, aortic valve regurgitation, aneurysm of the sinus of Valsalva, aneurysmal dilatation of the main pulmonary artery with/without pulmonary insufficiency, mitral valve prolapse and regurgitation, and, rarely, myocardial fibrosis and infarction.

   c. The ECG findings may include LVH, first-degree AV block, and T vector changes in leads that represent the LV.

   d. Chest x-rays may show cardiomegaly, generalized or involving the LV and LA, or prominence of the aorta or main pulmonary artery.

Acute Glomerulonephritis

   a. Significant myocardial damage is present in 10% of patients on postmortem examination.

   b. Clinically the evidence of cardiac involvement is found in 30%–40%, manifested by pulmonary edema, systemic venous congestion, and cardiomegaly. It is usually accompanied by hypertension; signs of CHF may be related to, but not wholly dependent on, the hypertension.

   c. Systemic hypertension is commonly present, sometimes with hypertensive encephalopathy, and may be responsible for signs of CHF. Although hypertension probably reflects fluid expansion (secondary to impaired salt and water excretion), peripheral resistance has been found to be elevated. Increased renin activity may be responsible for the latter (normal renin levels found in these patients may be inappropriately elevated in the presence of fluid overload and hypertension).

Hyperthyroidism

   a. Persistent tachycardia and systolic hypertension with a wide pulse pressure are frequent findings.

   b. A nonspecific systolic murmur is commonly audible at the ULSB. High-output cardiac failure may occur.

   c. The ECG does not show specific abnormalities. Atrial fibrillation, which is common in adults (20%), is rare in children.

   d. Chest x-ray may reveal cardiomegaly when CHF is present.

Cretinism (Congenital Hypothyroidism)

   a. PDA and PS are frequently associated cardiac defects.

   b. Relatively slow heart rate. Hepatomegaly and peripheral edema may be present.

   c. ECG abnormalities are quite common (over 90%) and consist of some or all of the following:

   1) Low QRS voltages, especially in the limb leads.

   2) Low T wave amplitude, not affecting the T axis.

   3) Prolongation of PR and QT intervals.

   4) Dome-shaped T wave with an absent ST segment ("mosque" sign).

   d. Chest x-rays are usually normal.

Mucopolysaccharidosis

   a. Accumulation of mucopolysaccharides in the myocardium and coronary artery pathology are commonly found.

   b. Over half of the cases show evidence of heart involvement; regurgitation of the mitral, tricuspid, and aortic valves is common. Occasionally systemic hypertension is present.

   c. Chest x-rays may show cardiomegaly.

   d. The ECG may show prolonged QT interval, RVH, LVH, or LAH.

PART VI

Electrocardiography II

Steps in routine interpretation of an ECG and two common ECG abnormalities in children, hypertrophy and ventricular conduction disturbances, were discussed in chapter 3, Electrocardiography I. In this section, arrhythmias, AV conduction disturbances, pacemaker ECGs, and ECG abnormalities involving ST segments and T waves will be discussed.

23 / Arrhythmias and Disturbances of Atrioventricular Conduction

The frequency and clinical significance of arrhythmias differ between children and adults. Although arrhythmias are relatively infrequent in infants and children, the widely practiced monitoring of cardiac rhythm in children makes it important for average pediatricians to be able to recognize and to manage common arrhythmias. Only basic arrhythmias with clearly defined mechanisms will be presented in terms of their characteristics, cause, clinical significance, and therapy.

Normal heart rate varies with age: the younger the child, the faster the heart rate. Therefore, the definitions used for adults of bradycardia (fewer than 60/min) and tachycardia (in excess of 100/min) have little significance for children. Tachycardia is present when the heart rate is beyond the upper limit of normal for the patient's age, and bradycardia is present when the heart rate is slower than the lower limit of normal. Normal resting heart rates according to age are presented in Table 23–1.

I. BASIC ARRHYTHMIAS

Common basic arrhythmias will be presented according to their origin of the impulse.

I. RHYTHMS ORIGINATING IN THE SINUS NODE

All rhythms that originate in the sinoatrial (SA) node (sinus rhythm) have two important characteristics (Fig 23–1):

   a. P waves preceding each QRS complex with a regular PR interval. (The PR interval may be prolonged as in first-degree AV block.)

   b. The P axis between 0° and +90°, an often neglected criterion. This produces upright P waves in lead II and inverted P waves in aVR. (Refer to chap. 3 for detailed discussion of sinus rhythm.)

A. Regular Sinus Rhythm

Description.—The rhythm is regular and the rate is normal for age. The two characteristics of sinus rhythm described above must be present (see Fig 23–1).

Significance.—Normal rhythm at any age.

Treatment.—None.

B. Sinus Tachycardia

Description.—Characteristics of sinus rhythm are present (see above). The rate is faster than the upper limit of normal for age (see Table 23–1). A rate in excess

TABLE 23–1.
Normal Ranges of Resting
Heart Rate

Age	Beats/Min
Newborn	110–150
2 yr	85–125
4 yr	75–115
Over 6 yr	60–100

of 140/min in children and in excess of 160/min in infants may be significant. The heart rate is usually lower than 200/min in sinus tachycardia (see Fig 23–1).

Causes.—Anxiety, fever, hypovolemia or circulatory shock, anemia, CHF, catecholamines, thyrotoxicosis, myocardial disease.

Significance.—Increased cardiac work is well tolerated by healthy myocardium.

Treatment.—Treat underlying cause.

C. Sinus Bradycardia

Description.—Characteristics of sinus rhythm are present (see above), but the heart rate is slower than the lower range of normal for age (see Table 22–1). A rate slower than 80/min in newborn infants and slower than 60/min in older children may be significant (see Fig 23–1).

Causes.—Normal athletes, vagal stimulation, increased intracranial pressure, hypothyroidism, hypothermia, hypoxia, hyperkalemia, and drugs such as digitalis and β-adrenergic blockers.

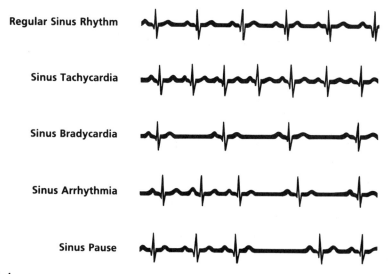

FIG 23–1.
Normal and abnormal rhythms originating in the SA node. (From Park MK, Guntheroth WG: *How to Read Pediatric ECGs,* ed 2. Chicago, Year Book Medical Publishers, 1987. Used by permission.)

Significance.—In some patients, marked bradycardias may not maintain normal cardiac output.

Treatment.—Treat underlying cause.

D. Sinus Arrhythmia

Description.—Sinus arrhythmia is a phasic variation in the heart rate, increasing during inspiration and decreasing during expiration. Arrhythmia is present while characteristics of sinus rhythm are maintained (see Fig 23–1).

Causes.—This is a normal phenomenon and is due to phasic variation in the firing rate of cardiac autonomic nerves with the phase of respiration.

Significance.—No significance, as it is a normal finding in children and sign of good cardiac reserve.

Treatment.—No treatment is indicated.

E. Sinus Pause

Description.—In *sinus pause*, there is a momentary cessation of sinus node pacemaker activity, resulting in the absence of P wave and QRS complex for a relatively short duration (see Fig 23–1). *Sinus arrest* is of longer duration and usually results in an escape beat (see below) by other pacemakers such as the nodal tissue (nodal escape).

Causes.—Increased vagal tone, hypoxia, digitalis toxicity, and sick sinus syndrome.

Significance.—It usually has no hemodynamic significance, but may result in decreased cardiac output.

Treatment.—Treatment is rarely indicated except in the sick sinus syndrome (see below) and digitalis toxicity (see chap. 27).

F. Sick Sinus Syndrome

Description.—The sinus node fails to function as the dominant pacemaker of the heart or at least performs abnormally slowly, resulting in a variety of arrhythmias. The arrhythmias include profound sinus bradycardia, sinoatrial exit block, sinus arrest with junctional escape, paroxysmal atrial tachycardia (PAT), ectopic atrial or nodal rhythm, and bradytachyarrhythmia.

Causes.

1) Extensive cardiac surgery, particularly involving the atria, such as the Mustard or Senning procedure.

2) Rarely, arteritis or focal myocarditis.

3) Occasionally idiopathic, involving an otherwise normal heart without structural defect.

Significance.—Bradytachyarrhythmia is the most worrisome. Profound bradycardia following a period of tachycardia (overdrive suppression) can cause syncope and even death.

Treatment.

1) Antiarrhythmic drugs, such as propranolol or quinidine, to suppress tachycardia (see Appendix for dosage) are indicated.

2) Demand ventricular pacemaker may be required for symptomatic patients with episodes of extreme bradycardia.

II. RHYTHMS ORIGINATING IN THE ATRIUM (ECTOPIC ATRIAL RHYTHM)

Atrial arrhythmias are characterized by (Fig 23–2):

1) P waves of unusual contour (abnormal P axis), and/or

2) Abnormal number of P waves per QRS complex.

QRS complexes are usually of normal configuration, but may occasionally exhibit *aberrancy* with wide, bizarre QRS complexes (see below).

A. Premature Atrial Contraction (PAC)

Description.—The QRS complex occurs prematurely. The P waves may be upright in lead II when the ectopic beat is high in the atrium. It is inverted when the ectopic focus is low in the atrium ("coronary sinus rhythm"). There is an

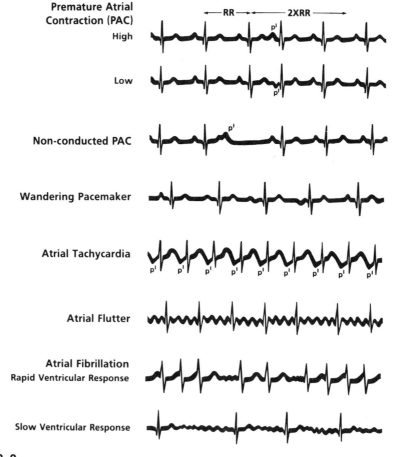

FIG 23–2.
Arrhythmias originating in the atrium. (From Park MK, Guntheroth WG: *How to Read Pediatric ECGs,* ed 2. Chicago, Year Book Medical Publishers, 1987. Used by permission.)

incomplete compensatory pause; i.e., the length of two cycles, including one premature beat, is less than the length of two normal cycles (see Fig 23–2). Occasional PACs are not followed by QRS complexes (nonconducted PAC) (see Fig 23–2).

Causes.—Healthy children, including the newborn, following cardiac surgery, and digitalis toxicity.

Significance.—No hemodynamic significance.

Treatment.—Usually no treatment is indicated, except in digitalis toxicity.

B. Wandering Atrial Pacemaker

Description.—It is characterized by gradual changes in the shape of P waves and PR intervals (see Fig 23–2). The QRS complex is normal.

Causes.—It is seen in otherwise healthy children. It is the result of a gradual shift of the site of impulse formation in the atria through several cardiac cycles.

Significance.—It is a benign arrhythmia and has no clinical significance.

Treatment.—No treatment is indicated.

C. Atrial Tachycardia

Description.

1) The heart rate is extremely rapid and regular (usually 240 ± 40 beats/min). The P wave is buried in the T wave and invisible, but when visible, usually has an abnormal P axis (see Fig 23–2). The QRS duration is usually normal. Occasionally, aberrancy will cause prolongation of QRS duration making differentiation of this arrhythmia from ventricular tachycardia difficult (see below).

2) Atrial tachycardia is difficult to separate from the rarer nodal tachycardia. This has led to the use of the term *supraventricular tachycardia* (SVT) to include both atrial and nodal tachycardia.

3) There are three different mechanisms for SVT: two distinct forms of atrial tachycardia and nodal tachycardia.

   a) *AV reentry or reciprocating tachycardia* is not only the most common mechanism of SVT but also the most common tachyarrhythmia seen in the pediatric age group. This was formerly called *paroxysmal atrial tachycardia* (PAT) because the onset and termination of this arrhythmia were characteristically abrupt. The retrograde conduction of a PVC through the bundle of Kent is responsible for the initiation and maintenance of the tachycardia. A PAC can also initiate and maintain the tachycardia if the bypass tract does not allow an antegrade conduction of the PAC but allows a subsequent retrograde conduction of an impulse from the ventricle. When the heart rate is normal, WPW syndrome may be present because of an antegrade conduction and a premature depolarization of a portion of the ventricle (see preexcitation in chap. 3), but with the initiation of the tachycardia (with a retrograde conduction), the QRS complex becomes normal.

   b) *Ectopic or nonreciprocating atrial tachycardia* is a rare mechanism of SVT, in which rapid firing of a single focus in the atrium is responsible for the tachycardia. Unlike reciprocating atrial tachycardia, in ectopic atrial tachycardia, the heart rate may vary substantially during a course of a day, and second-degree AV block may develop.

c) *Nodal tachycardia* may superficially resemble atrial tachycardia because the P wave is buried in the T wave of the preceding beat and becomes invisible in the latter, but the rate of nodal tachycardia is relatively slower (120–200 beats/min) than atrial tachycardia.

Causes.

1) No demonstrable heart disease (idiopathic) is present in about half of the patients. The idiopathic type occurs more commonly in young infants than in older children.

2) WPW syndrome is present in 10%–20% of the cases (evident only after conversion to sinus rhythm).

3) Some congenital heart defects (Ebstein's anomaly, single ventricle, L-TGA) are more prone to this arrhythmia.

Significance.

1) It may decrease cardiac output and result in CHF.

2) Many infants tolerate PAT well for 24 hours, but within 48 hours about 50% of the patients develop heart failure.

3) Clinical manifestation of CHF includes irritability, tachypnea, poor feeding, and pallor. When CHF develops, the infant's condition can deteriorate rapidly.

Treatment.

1) Vagal stimulatory maneuvers (carotid sinus massage, gagging, pressure on an eyeball) may be effective in older children, but are rarely effective in infants.

2) Placing an icebag on the face (up to 10 seconds) is often successful in infants.

3) Initial cardioversion may be performed in infants with CHF and those with wide QRS complexes in which differentiation between ventricular tachycardia and atrial tachycardia with an aberrancy is difficult. The initial dose of 0.5 w-sec/kg may be increased step-by-step up to 2 w-sec/kg. This is followed by digitalization.

4) Digitalization is the method of choice in infants without CHF and those with mild CHF (see chap. 27 for details of digitalization). Cardioversion carries a risk of inducing ventricular tachycardia in digitalized patients. This is why an initial cardioversion is preferred in patients with CHF.

5) If the patient is not in CHF and digitalis is not effective, but a rapid conversion to sinus rhythm is desirable, IV infusion of phenylephrine may be tried. It raises blood pressure abruptly and converts the tachycardia by reflex increase in vagal tone. This method is not recommended in infants with CHF, since increasing afterload may be detrimental to a failing heart. Add 10 mg (one ampule) to 200 ml IV solution and drip it rapidly while monitoring blood pressure frequently, not to exceed systolic pressure of 160–170 mm Hg.

6) Intravenous administration of propranolol or verapamil may be tried, but they are certainly not the treatment of choice. These drugs may produce extreme bradycardia and hypotension in infants less than 1 year of age and should be avoided when possible. When the decision is made to administer

these drugs, they should be given step-by-step in small doses with careful monitoring of vital signs and with readiness to respond to adverse effects.

7) Overdrive suppression by atrial pacing in the cardiac catheterization laboratory may be indicated in children who are already digitalized.

8) Prevention of recurrence of PAT with maintenance dose of digoxin (see Table 27–3) for 3–6 months is recommended. In patients with WPW syndrome, propranolol may be effective in preventing further attacks. In occasional patients with WPW syndrome, surgical interruption of accessory pathways should be considered, if medical management fails.

D. Atrial Flutter

Description.—The pacemaker lies in an ectopic focus, and "circus movement" in the atrium is the mechanism of this arrhythmia. It is characterized by the atrial rate ("F" wave with "saw-tooth" configuration) of about 300/min, the ventricle responding with varying degrees of block (2:1, 3:1, 4:1, etc.), and normal QRS complexes (see Fig 23–2).

Causes.—Structural heart disease with dilated atria, myocarditis, previous surgery involving atria (Mustard's procedure or ASD repair), or digitalis toxicity.

Significance.—The ventricular rate determines eventual cardiac output; rapid ventricular rate may decrease cardiac output. Atrial flutter usually indicates the presence of a significant cardiac pathology.

Treatment.

1) Digitalization, if the arrhythmia is not the result of digitalis toxicity (digitalis increases the AV block and slows the ventricular rate).

2) Propranolol may be added (1.0–4.0 mg/kg/day orally in 3–4 divided doses).

3) Electric cardioversion may be required. Digitalis should be discontinued for at least 48 hours prior to cardioversion.

4) Quinidine may prevent recurrence (see Appendix for dosage).

E. Atrial Fibrillation

Description.—The mechanism of this arrhythmia is "circus movement" as in atrial flutter. It is characterized by an extremely fast atrial rate ("f" wave at a rate of 350–600/min), and an irregularly irregular ventricular response with normal QRS complexes (see Fig 23–2).

Causes.—Usually associated with structural heart disease with dilated atria, myocarditis, digitalis toxicity, or previous intra-atrial surgery.

Significance.

1) As in atrial tachycardia, rapid ventricular rate, in addition to the loss of co-ordinated contraction of the atria and ventricles, decreases the cardiac output.

2) Usually indicates the presence of a significant cardiac pathology.

Treatment.

1) Digoxin to slow the ventricular rate (see Table 27–3).

2) Propranolol may be added if necessary (1.0–4.0 mg/kg/day orally in 3–4 divided doses).

3) Cardioversion may be indicated, but recurrence is common.

4) Quinidine to prevent recurrence (see Appendix for dosage).

III. RHYTHMS ORIGINATING IN THE AV NODE

Rhythms originating in the AV node are characterized by the following (Fig 23–3):

1) The P wave may be absent, or inverted P waves may follow the QRS complex, and

2) The QRS complex is usually normal in duration and configuration

Only the lower part (NH region) of the AV node has pacemaking ability. The upper (AN region) and middle (N region) parts do not function as a pacemaker, but provide delay in the conduction of an impulse, either antegrade or retrograde.

A. Nodal Premature Beats

Description.—A normal QRS complex occurs prematurely. P waves are usually absent, but inverted P waves may follow QRS complexes (see Fig 23–3). The compensatory pause may be complete or incomplete.

Causes.—Usually idiopathic in an otherwise normal heart, folowing cardiac surgery, and digitalis toxicity.

Significance.—Usually no hemodynamic significance.

Treatment.—Treatment is not indicated unless the cause is digitalis toxicity.

B. Nodal Escape Beat

Description.—When there is failure of the SA node impulse to reach the AV node, the NH region of the AV node will initiate an impulse (nodal or junctional escape beat). The QRS complex occurs later than the anticipated normal beat. The P wave may be absent or an inverted P wave follows the QRS complex (see Fig 23–3). The duration and configuration of QRS complexes are normal.

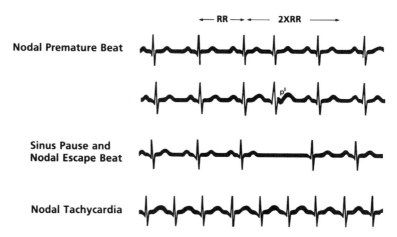

FIG 23–3.
Arrhythmias originating in the AV node. (From Park MK, Guntheroth WG: *How to Read Pediatric ECGs,* ed 2. Chicago, Year Book Medical Publishers, 1987. Used by permission.)

Causes.—Cardiac surgery involving the atria (the Mustard or Senning procedure) or otherwise healthy children.

Significance.—Little hemodynamic significance.

Treatment.—Generally no specific treatment is required.

C. Nodal or Junctional Rhythm

Description.—If there is a persistent failure of the SA node, the AV node may function as the main pacemaker of the heart with a relatively slow rate (40–60/min). Nodal rhythm is characterized by no P waves or inverted P waves following QRS complexes, and normal QRS complexes with a rate of 40–60/min.

Causes.—Otherwise normal heart, following cardiac surgery, and increased vagal tone (increased intracranial pressure, pharyngeal stimulation), and digitalis toxicity.

Significance.—The slow heart rate may significantly decrease cardiac output and produce symptoms.

Treatment.

1) Treat known causes such as digitalis toxicity.

2) No treatment is indicated if asymptomatic.

3) Atropine or electric pacing if symptomatic.

D. Accelerated Nodal Rhythm

Description.—In the presence of normal sinus rate and AV conduction, if the AV node (NH region) with enhanced automaticity captures the pacemaker function at a faster rate (60–120/min), the rhythm is called accelerated nodal (or AV junctional) rhythm. P waves are either absent, or inverted P waves follow QRS complexes. The QRS complex is normal, and the heart rate is between 60 and 120/min.

Causes.—Idiopathic, digitalis toxicity, myocarditis, following cardiac surgery.

Significance.—Little hemodynamic significance.

Treatment.—No treatment is necessary unless caused by digitalis toxicity.

E. Nodal Tachycardia

Description.—The ventricular rate varies from 120 to 200/min. The P waves are either absent, or inverted P waves follow QRS complexes (see Fig 23–3). The QRS complex is usually normal but rarely *aberration* may occur as in atrial tachycardia. Nodal tachycardia is difficult to separate from atrial tachycardia. Therefore, both arrhythmias are grouped as supraventricular tachycardia (SVT).

Causes.—Similar to those of atrial tachycardia.

Significance.—Similar to atrial tachycardia.

Treatment.—Treatment is not indicated if the rate is slower than 130/min. Although digoxin is the drug of choice for most cases of supraventricular tachycardia (of atrial origin), it may be contraindicated in *true* form of nodal tachycardia. In that instance, quinidine is probably the drug of choice.

IV. RHYTHMS ORIGINATING IN THE VENTRICLE

Ventricular arrhythmias are characterized by (Fig 23–4):

1) Bizarre and wide QRS complexes,

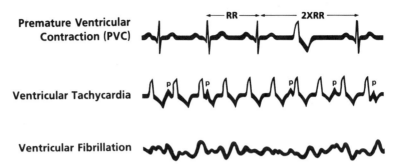

FIG 23–4.
Ventricular arrhythmias. (From Park MK, Guntheroth WG: *How to Read Pediatric ECGs,* ed 2. Chicago, Year Book Medical Publishers, 1987. Used by permission.)

2) T waves pointing in directions opposite to QRS complexes, and

3) QRS complexes randomly related to P waves, if visible.

A. Premature Ventricular Contraction (PVC)

Description.

1) A bizarre, wide QRS complex comes earlier than anticipated, with T wave pointing in the opposite direction (see Fig 23–4). There is a full compensatory pause (the length of two cycles, including the premature beat, is the same as that of two normal cycles) (see Fig 23–4).

2) Ventricular *"fusion" complex* may be seen. This is a QRS complex that is produced in part by a normally conducted supraventricular impulse and in part by an ectopic ventricular impulse. The resulting QRS complex is intermediate in appearance between the patient's normal conducted beat and the pure ectopic ventricular beat. The presence of a "fusion" complex is a reliable sign of PVC and helps to differentiate it from a supraventricular rhythm with aberrant ventricular conduction.

3) Depending on the configuration, number, and regularity of the bizarre QRS complex, PVC may be classified into several types:

a) Uniform PVCs: QRS complexes have the same configuration in a single lead.

b) Multifocal PVCs: QRS complexes have different configuration in a single lead.

c) Ventricular bigeminy or coupling: Each abnormal QRS complex alternates with normal QRS complex regularly.

d) Ventricular trigeminy: Each abnormal QRS complex follows two normal QRS complexes regularly.

Causes.—Otherwise healthy children, myocarditis, long QT syndrome, congenital heart disease, following heart surgery, digitalis toxicity, or drugs such as catecholamines, theophylline, caffeine, and amphetamines.

Significance.—Occasional PVCs are benign in children, particularly if they are unifocal and disappear or decrease in frequency with exercise. PVCs are more likely significant if:

1) They are multifocal, particularly couplets.

2) They are precipitated by, or increase in frequency with, activity.

3) They are associated with underlying cardiac conditions.

4) There are runs of PVCs with symptoms.

Treatment.

1) Frequent PVCs may require treatment with IV bolus injection of lidocaine (1 mg/kg/dose), followed by IV drip of lidocaine (1–3 mg/kg/hour).

2) Antiarrhythmic drugs such as propranolol, quinidine, diphenylhydantoin (Dilantin), or procainamide (Pronestyl) may be indicated (see Appendix for dosage).

3) PVCs that are more likely to be significant warrant electrophysiologic studies.

B. Ventricular Tachycardia (VT)

Description.—Ventricular tachycardia is a series of PVCs with a heart rate of 120–200/min. QRS complexes are abnormally wide and bizarre, with T waves pointing in the opposite direction (see Fig 23–4). It is sometimes difficult to differentiate VT from supraventricular tachycardia (SVT) with aberrant conduction (see below).

Causes.—Similar to those listed for PVCs, except for normal children.

Significance.—Usually signifies a serious myocardial pathology or dysfunction. Cardiac output may decrease notably and may deteriorate to ventricular fibrillation.

Treatment.

1) It must be treated promptly with synchronized cardioversion, if the patient is unconscious.

2) If the patient is conscious, an IV bolus of lidocaine (1 mg/kg/dose over 1–2 minutes) followed by IV drip of lidocaine (1–3 mg/kg/hour) may be effective.

3) Recurrence may be prevented with administration of propranolol, quinidine, or diphenylhydantoin (see Appendix for dosage).

ABERRATION

When a supraventricular impulse prematurely reaches the AV node or bundle of His, it may find one bundle branch excitable and the other still refractory. Therefore, the resulting QRS complex resembles a bundle branch block pattern. The right bundle branch usually has a longer refractory period than the left bundle branch, producing QRS complexes similar to those of RBBB.

The following features are helpful in differentiating aberrant ventricular conduction from ectopic ventricular impulses:

1) An rsR' pattern in V1 and a qRs pattern in V6, resembling QRS complexes of RBBB, suggest aberration. In a ventricular ectopic beat, the QRS morphology is bizarre and does not resemble the classic form of RBBB or LBBB.

2) Occasional wide QRS complexes following P waves with regular PR intervals suggest an aberration.

3) The presence of ventricular "fusion" complex (see above) is a reliable sign of ventricular ectopic rhythm.

C. Ventricular Fibrillation

Description.—Ventricular fibrillation is characterized by bizarre QRS complexes of varying sizes and configurations. The rate is rapid and irregular (see Fig 23–4).

Causes.—Postoperative, severe hypoxia, hyperkalemia, digitalis or quinidine toxicity, myocarditis, myocardial infarction, and drugs (catecholamines, anesthetics, etc.).

Significance.—It is usually the terminal arrhythmia, since it results in ineffective circulation.

Treatment.—Immediate cardiopulmonary resuscitative procedures, including electric defibrillation at the dose of 2 w-sec/kg.

II. DISTURBANCES OF ATRIOVENTRICULAR CONDUCTION

Atrioventricular block (AV block) is a disturbance in conduction between the normal sinus impulse and the eventual ventricular response. It is assigned to one of three classes depending on the severity of the conduction disturbance. First-degree AV block is a simple prolongation of the PR interval. In second-degree AV block, some atrial impulses are not conducted into the ventricle. None of the atrial impulses is conducted into the ventricle in third-degree AV block (complete heart block) (Fig 23–5).

A. First-degree AV Block

Description.—There is a prolongation of the PR interval beyond the upper limits of normal for the patient's age and heart rate (see Table 3–2 and Fig 23–5). This is produced by an abnormal delay in conduction through the AV node.

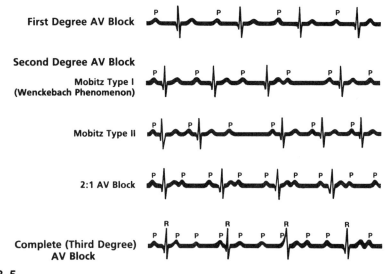

FIG 23–5.
Atrioventricular block. (From Park MK, Guntheroth WG: *How to Read Pediatric ECGs,* ed 2. Chicago, Year Book Medical Publishers, 1987. Used by permission.)

Causes.—Some healthy children, acute rheumatic fever, cardiomyopathies, congenital heart defect (ASD, Ebstein's anomaly, ECD, etc.), following cardiac surgery, and digitalis toxicity.

Significance.—It does not produce symptoms of hemodynamic disturbance. Sometimes it may progress to a more advanced AV block.

Treatment.—No treatment is indicated, with the exception of digitalis toxicity (see chap. 27).

B. Second-degree AV Block

Some, but not all, P waves are followed by QRS complexes (dropped beats). There are several types:

1. Mobitz Type I (Wenckebach Phenomenon):

Description.—The PR interval becomes progressively prolonged until one QRS complex is dropped completely (see Fig 23–5).

Causes.—Otherwise healthy children, myocarditis, cardiomyopathy, myocardial infarction, congenital heart disease, following surgery, and digitalis toxicity.

Significance.—The block is at the level of the AV node. It usually does not progress to complete heart block.

Treatment.—Treat underlying causes.

2. Mobitz Type II:

Description.—The AV conduction is "all or none": there is either normal AV condution or the conduction is completely blocked (see Fig 23–5).

Causes.—Same as for Mobitz Type I.

Significance.—The block is at the level of His bundle. It is more serious than type I block, since it may progress to complete heart block.

Treatment.—(a) Treat underlying causes. (b) Prophylactic pacemaker therapy may be indicated.

3. Two-to-One (or higher) AV Block:

Description.—A QRS complex follows every seond (third or fourth) P wave resulting in 2:1 (3:1 or 4:1) AV block (see Fig 23–5).

Causes.—Similar to other second-degree AV blocks.

Significance.—The block is usually at the AV nodal level and occasionally at the level of His bundle. It may occasionally progress to complete heart block.

Treatment.—(a) Treat underlying causes. (b) Electrophysiologic studies may be necessary to determine the level of the block. (c) Occasional pacemaker therapy.

C. Third-degree AV Block (Complete Heart Block)

Description.—In third-degree AV block, the atrial and ventricular activities are entirely independent of each other (see Fig 23–5):

1) The P waves are regular (regular PP interval) with a rate comparable to the heart rate of the patient's age.

2) The QRS complexes are also quite regular (regular RR interval) with a rate much slower than the P rate.

3) In *congenital* complete heart block, the duration of the QRS complex is normal (since the pacemaker for the ventricular complex is at a level higher than the bifurcation of the His bundle). The ventricular rate is faster (50–80/min) than that in the acquired type.

4) In *surgically induced* or *acquired* (postmyocardial infarction) complete heart block, the QRS duration is prolonged and the ventricular rate is in the range of 40–50/min (idioventricular rhythm). The pacemaker for the ventricular complex is at a level below the bifurcation of the His bundle.

Causes.

1) Congenital type: An isolated anomaly (without associated structural heart defect), maternal lupus erythematosus or mixed connective tissue disease, or structural heart disease such as L-TGA.

2) Acquired type: Cardiac surgery is the most common cause of acquired complete heart block in children. Other rare causes include severe myocarditis, acute rheumatic fever, mumps, diphtheria, cardiomyopathies, tumors in the conduction system, overdose of certain drugs, and following myocardial infarction. Some of these causes produce temporary heart block.

Significance.

1) CHF may develop in infancy, particularly when there is associated CHD.

2) Patients with isolated congenital heart block who survive infancy are usually asymptomatic, with normal growth and development and normal physical working capacity.

3) Syncopal attacks (Stokes-Adams attack) may occur with the heart rate below 40–45/min.

4) Sudden onset of acquired heart block may result in death, unless the heart rate is maintained in the acceptable range by treatment.

5) Chest x-rays show cardiomegaly.

Treatment.

1) No treatment is required for asymptomatic children with congenital complete heart block.

2) Atropine or isoproterenol in symptomatic children and adults until temporary ventricular pacing is secured.

3) A temporary transvenous ventricular pacemaker is indicated in patients with heart block or prophylactically in those patients who might develop heart block.

4) Permanent artificial ventricular pacemaker is indicated in patients with surgically induced heart block and in patients with congenital heart block who are symptomatic or have CHF. Dizziness or light-headedness may be an early warning sign for the need of a pacemaker.

5) A variety of problems may arise after pacemaker placement in children. Stress placed on the lead system by the linear growth of the child, fracture of the lead system in a physically active child, electrode malfunction (scarring of the

myocardium around the electrode, especially in infants), and the limited life span of the pulse generator require regular follow-up of children with artificial pacemakers.

III. ECGs OF ARTIFICIAL CARDIAC PACEMAKERS

Increasing numbers of children receive pacemaker therapy, most frequently for symptomatic bradycardia resulting from congenital or acquired causes of AV block or sinus node dysfunction (sick sinus syndrome). More recently, the electrical device has been used for the termination of supraventricular tachycardia and less frequently of ventricular tachycardia. Discussion will be limited to the pacemakers installed for treatment of bradycardia.

Temporary pacing is indicated for advanced second-degree or complete heart block secondary to overdose, myocarditis, or myocardial infarction; for patients with a malfunctioning permanent pacemaker prior to replacement of a new permanent pacemaker; and for certain patients immediately after cardiac surgery. The most common indication for a permanent pacemaker is symptomatic bradycardia with syncope, dizziness, exercise intolerance, or CHF. Symptomatic bradycardia may be intermittent or permanent and may be the result of complete heart block (either congenital or acquired including surgically induced) or sick sinus syndrome.

Three letters are used as a shorthand notation to identify the different types of pacemakers; the first letter indicates the chamber paced, the second letter the chamber sensed, and the third letter the mode of response, but the discussion of the letter code is beyond the scope of this book. Emphasis will be placed on the recognition of different ECG patterns produced by different types of pacemakers, accomplished by the position and number of the pacemaker spikes. Thus, the pacemaker may be classified into (a) ventricular pacemaker, (b) atrial pacemaker, and (c) P-wave triggered ventricular pacemaker. When the pacemaker stimulates the ventricle, the ventricle stimulated (or the ventricle on which the pacemaker electrode is placed) can be determined by the morphology of QRS complexes. With an RV pacemaker, the QRS complex resembles LBBB pattern and vice versa.

A. Ventricular Pacemaker (ventricular sensing and pacing)

This mode of pacing is recognized by vertical pacemaker spikes that initiate ventricular depolarization with wide QRS complexes (Fig 23–6,A). The electrical spike has no fixed relationship to atrial activity (P wave). The pacemaker rate may be fixed (as in Fig 23–6,A) or it may be on a demand (or standby) mode in which the pacemaker fires only after a long pause between the patient's own ventricular beats.

B. Atrial Pacemaker (atrial sensing and pacing)

The atrial pacemaker is recognized by a pacemaker spike followed by an atrial complex; when there is normal AV conduction, a QRS complex of normal duration will follow (Fig 23–6,B). This type of pacemaker is indicated in patients with sinus node dysfunction with bradycardia. When there is high-degree or complete AV block in addition to sinus node dysfunction with sinus bradycardia, a ventricular pacemaker may also be required (AV sequential pacemaker, not illustrated). The AV sequential pacemaker is recognized by two sets of electronic spikes, one before the P wave and another before the wide QRS complex.

C. P Wave-Triggered Ventricular Pacemaker (atrial sensing, ventricular pacing)

This pacemaker may be recognized by pacemaker spikes that follow the patient's own P waves, at regular PR intervals, and with wide QRS complexes (Fig 23–

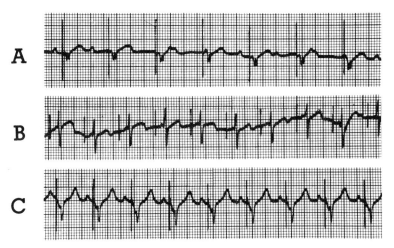

FIG 23–6.
Examples of some artificial pacemakers. **A,** fixed-rate ventricular pacemaker. Note the regular rate of the electronic spikes with no relationship to the P waves. **B,** atrial pacemaker. This tracing is from a 2-year-old child in whom extreme, symptomatic bradycardia developed following the Mustard operation. **C,** P-wave triggered pacemaker. This tracing is from a child in whom surgically induced complete heart block developed following repair of tetralogy of Fallot. (From Park MK, Guntheroth WG: *How to Read Pediatric ECGs,* ed 2. Chicago, Year Book Medical Publishers, 1987. Used by permission.)

6,C). The patient's own P waves are sensed, which trigger a ventricular pacemaker after an electronically preset PR interval. This type of pacemaker is most physiologic and indicated when there is an AV block but the sinus mechanism is normal. Advantages of this type of pacemaker are that (1) the heart rate varies with physiologic needs, and (2) the atrial contraction contributes to ventricular filling and improves cardiac output.

24 / ST Segment and T Wave Changes

ECG changes involving the ST segment and the T wave are quite common in adults but they are relatively rare in children. This is because of a high incidence of ischemic heart disease, bundle branch blocks, myocardial infarction, and other myocardial disorders in adults.

I. NONPATHOLOGIC ST SEGMENT SHIFT

Not all ST segment shifts are abnormal. Slight shift of the ST segment is common in normal children. Elevation or depression up to 1 mm in the limb leads and up to 2 mm in the precordial leads is within normal limits.

Two common types of nonpathologic ST segment shift are J depression and early repolarization. The T vector remains normal in these conditions. J depression is a shift of the J point (the junction between the QRS complex and the ST segment) without sustained shift of the ST segment (Fig 24–1,A). In early repolarization, all leads with an upright T wave have elevated ST segments and leads with inverted T waves have depressed ST segments. The T vector remains normal. This condition, seen in healthy adolescents and young adults, resembles the ST segment shift seen in acute pericarditis, but in the former, the ST segment is stable, while the ST segment returns to the isoelectric line in the latter.

II. PATHOLOGIC ST SEGMENT SHIFT

Abnormal shifts of the ST segment are often accompanied by T wave inversion. A pathologic ST segment shift assumes one of the following two forms:

a. Downward slanting followed by diphasic or inverted T wave (Fig 24–1,B).

b. Horizontal elevation or depression sustained for over 0.08 second (Fig 24–1,C).

Pathologic ST segment shifts are seen in (1) LVH or RVH with "strain" (see chap. 3), (2) digitalis effect (see chap. 27), (3) pericarditis, including postoperative state, (4) myocarditis, (5) myocardial infarction, and (6) some electrolyte disturbances (hypokalemia and hyperkalemia).

T wave changes are usually associated with the above conditions. Other conditions associated with T wave changes with or without ST segment shift, discussed in previous chapters, include bundle branch block, preexcitation (WPW syndrome), and ventricular arrhythmias. Only those conditions not covered previously will be briefly discussed in this chapter.

277

J-Depression   Abnormal ST-Segments

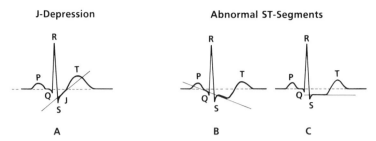

A   B   C

FIG 24–1.
Nonpathologic (nonischemic) and pathologic (ischemic) ST and T changes. **A,** characteristic nonischemic ST segment change called J depression; note that the ST slope is upward. **B** and **C** are examples of pathologic ST segment changes; note that the downward
slope of the ST segment **(B)** or the horizontal segment is sustained **(C).** (From Park MK,
Guntheroth WG: *How to Read Pediatric ECGs,* ed 2. Chicago, Year Book Medical Publishers, 1987. Used by permission.)

I. Pericarditis

The ECG changes seen in pericarditis are the results of subepicardial myocardial damage and/or pericardial effusion, and consist of the following:

a. Pericardial effusion may produce low QRS voltages (QRS voltages less than
5 mm in every one of the limb leads).

b. Subepicardial myocardial damage produces the following time-dependent
changes in the ST segment and T wave (Fig 24–2):

1) ST segment elevation in the leads representing the LV.

2) The ST segment shift returns to normal within 2–3 days.

3) T wave inversion (with isoelectric ST segment), 2–4 weeks after the onset
of pericarditis.

II. Myocarditis

ECG findings of myocarditis (rheumatic or viral) are relatively nonspecific and
may include changes in all phases of the cardiac cycle. Various arrhythmias

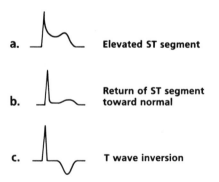

a.   Elevated ST segment

b.   Return of ST segment
toward normal

c.   T wave inversion

FIG 24–2.
Time-dependent changes of ST segment and T wave in pericarditis. (From Park MK,
Guntheroth WG: *How to Read Pediatric ECGs,* ed 2. Chicago, Year Book Medical Pub-
lishers, 1987. Used by permission.)

have also been associated with myocarditis. One or more of the following changes are seen in myocarditis:

a. Disturbances in AV conduction (first- or second-degree AV block).

b. Low QRS voltages (5 mm or less in all six limb leads).

c. Decreased amplitude of the T wave.

d. Prolongation of QT interval.

e. Arrhythmias or ectopic beats.

III. Myocardial Infarction

Although myocardial infarction is rare in infants and children, a brief discussion will be included for the sake of completeness. ECG findings of myocardial infarction in pediatric patients may be caused by anomalous origin of the left coronary artery from the pulmonary artery, coronary artery embolization from infective endocarditis or from diagnostic procedures performed in the left side of the heart, inadvertent surgical interruption of the coronary artery, endocardial fibroelastosis, coronary arteritis seen in Kawasaki's disease, and some cardiac tumors. All other conditions that have been associated with myocardial infarction in adults have been described to cause myocardial infarction in children. These conditions include atherosclerosis, inflammatory disease of the myocardium, lupus erythematosus, syphilis, polyarteritis nodosa, hypertension, and diabetes mellitus.

The ECG findings of myocardial infarction are time-dependent and are illustrated in Figure 24–3. Changes seen during the hyperacute phase are short-lived. The more commonly encountered ECG findings of myocardial infarction are those seen during the early evolving phase. These consist of pathologic Q waves (abnormally deep and abnormally wide, at least 0.03 second), ST segment elevation, and T wave inversion. During the next few weeks, there is a gradual return of the elevated ST segment toward the baseline with persistence of inverted T waves (late evolving phase). The pathologic Q waves persist for years after myocardial infarction (see Fig 24–3). Leads that show these abnor-

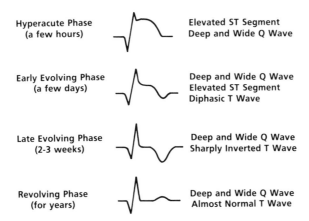

FIG 24–3.
Sequential changes of ST segment and T wave in myocardial infarction. (From Park MK, Guntheroth WG: *How to Read Pediatric ECGs*, ed 2. Chicago, Year Book Medical Publishers, 1987. Used by permission.)

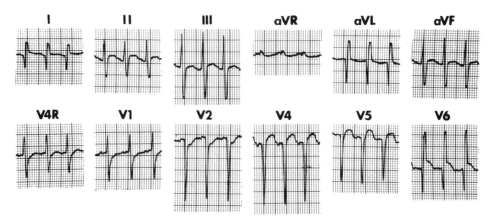

FIG 24–4.
Tracing from a 2-month-old infant who has anomalous origin of the left coronary artery from the pulmonary artery.

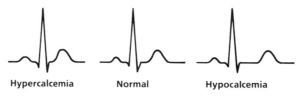

Hypercalcemia   Normal   Hypocalcemia

FIG 24–5.
ECG findings of hypercalcemia and hypocalcemia. Hypercalcemia shortens and hypocalcemia lengthens the ST segment. (From Park MK, Guntheroth WG: *How to Read Pediatric ECGs,* ed 2. Chicago, Year Book Medical Publishers, 1987. Used by permission.)

SERUM K

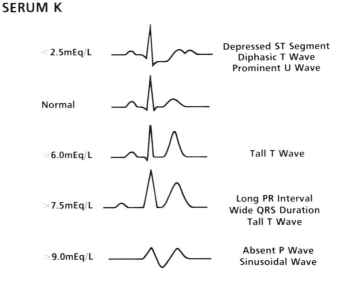

FIG 24–6.
ECG findings of hypokalemia and hyperkalemia. (From Park MK, Guntheroth WG: *How to Read Pediatric ECGs,* ed 2. Chicago, Year Book Medical Publishers, 1987. Used by permission.)

TABLE 24–1.

Leads Showing Abnormal ECG Findings in Myocardial Infarction

	Limb Leads	Precordial Leads
Lateral	I, aVL	V5, V6
Anterior		V1, V2, V3
Anterolateral	I, aVL	V2–V6
Diaphragmatic	II, III, aVF	
Posterior		V1–V3*

*None of the leads is oriented toward the posterior surface of the heart. Therefore, in posterior infarction, changes that would have been present in the posterior surface leads will be seen in the anterior leads as a mirror image, e.g., tall and slightly wide R waves in V1 and V2, and tall and wide symmetric T waves in V1 and V2.

malities vary with the location of the infarction and are summarized in Table 24–1.

Figure 24–4 is an example of myocardial infarction pattern seen in an infant with anomalous origin of the left coronary artery from the PA. The most important abnormality is the presence of deep and wide Q wave (0.04 second) in leads I, aVL, and V6. A QS pattern is present in leads V2 through V5, indicating anterolateral myocardial infarction (see Table 24–1).

III. ELECTROLYTE DISTURBANCES

Two important serum electrolytes that produce ECG changes are calcium and potassium. Although T wave changes are not seen with hypocalcemia and hypercalcemia, these conditions will be discussed here, since they change the relative position of the T wave.

I. Calcium

Calcium ion affects only the duration of the ST segment without changing the ST segment or the T vector. Hypocalcemia produces prolongation of the ST segment with resulting prolongation of QTc (Fig 24–5). The T wave duration remains normal. Hypercalcemia shortens the ST segment without affecting the T wave, with resultant shortening of QTc (see Fig 24–5).

II. Potassium

Hypokalemia produces one of the least specific ECG changes. When the serum potassium (K) level is below 2.5 mEq/L, ECG changes consist of a prominent U wave (with apparent prolongation of QTc), flat or diphasic T waves, and ST segment depression (Fig 24–6). With further lowering of serum K, the PR interval becomes prolonged, and sinoatrial block may occur.

A progressive increase in serum K level (hyperkalemia) produces the following ECG changes (see Fig 24–6):

a. Tall "tented" T waves, best seen in the precordial leads.

b. Prolongation of QRS duration (intraventricular block).

c. Prolongation of PR interval (first-degree AV block).

d. Disappearance of P wave.

e. Wide, bizarre diphasic QRS complex ("sine wave").

f. Eventual asystole.

PART VII

Neonates With Cardiac Problems

In the following two chapters are discussed the physical findings, ECG, and chest x-ray findings that are unique to the neonatal period as well as problems frequently encountered in this period.

25 / Special Features in Cardiac Evaluation of the Newborn

Because of progressive postnatal changes in the cardiovascular system, the physical findings, chest x-rays, and ECGs of not only normal newborns but also neonates with CHD are different from those of older children and adults. Furthermore, these findings change rapidly with age, making cardiac evaluation of a newborn infant a real challenge.

Newborn infants at the time of birth have RV dominance, with a thick RV wall and elevated pulmonary vascular resistance (PVR) secondary to a thick medial layer of pulmonary arterioles. The thick pulmonary artery smooth muscle gradually becomes thinner and by 6–8 weeks of age resembles that of the adult. Most perinatal changes in hemodynamics are related to the normal evolution (thinning) of pulmonary vascular smooth muscle, resulting in a gradual fall in PVR and loss of RV dominance of the newborn (see chap. 8).

Without repeating what has been described in earlier chapters, some important aspects of normal and abnormal findings in physical examination, ECG, and chest x-rays will be briefly reviewed in this chapter.

I. PHYSICAL EXAMINATION

A. Normal Physical Findings

1. The following is a list of some physical findings that are unique in normal full-term newborn infants:

    a. Heart rate is in general faster than in older children and adults (it is usually over 100/min with ranges from 70 to 180/min).

    b. A varying degree of acrocyanosis is a rule rather than an exception.

    c. Mild arterial desaturation with arterial Po_2 as low as 60 mm Hg is not unusual in an otherwise normal neonate. This may be caused by an intrapulmonary shunt through an as yet unexpanded portion of the lungs or by a right-to-left atrial shunt through the patent foramen ovale.

    d. There is a relative overactivity of the RV, with the PMI at the LLSB rather than at the apex.

    e. The S2 may be single on the first days of life.

    f. An ejection click is occasionally present in the first hours of life (representing pulmonary hypertension).

    g. An innocent heart murmur may be present (see chap. 26).

    h. Peripheral pulses are easily palpable in all extremities, including the feet, in *every* normal infant.

i. Blood pressure. Although blood pressure is not routinely measured in the normal newborn, its measurement becomes essential when one suspects COA. The conventional auscultatory method is difficult to apply in the newborn. A Doppler method or an oscillometric method (Dinamap) appears to be more suitable. No matter which method is used, the selection of an appropriate cuff should be about 50% of the circumference of the extremity on which blood pressure is being measured. The same size cuff may be used for the arm and the calf. The normal BP values for the arm by a Doppler method and by Dinamap method are presented in Tables 2–2, and 2–3, respectively. The mean BP values by the Dinamap method are almost identical in the arm and the calf in a quiet newborn.

2. Premature infants have additional features that need to be kept in mind when examining them:

   a. The incidence and the loudness of the pulmonary flow murmur of the newborn are greater in premature than in full-term infants because of their thin chest walls.

   b. The incidence of PDA murmur is greater in premature infants.

   c. The peripheral pulses normally appear bounding because of the lack of normal amount of subcutaneous tissue. One needs to become familiar with the normal volume of peripheral pulses in prematures.

B. Abnormal Physical Findings

The following abnormal physical findings suggest the presence of cardiac malformation (see chap. 26 for further discussion). Repeated examination is important, since physical findings change rapidly in normal infants as well as in infants with cardiac problems.

   a. Cyanosis, particularly when it does not improve with oxygen administration.

   b. Peripheral pulses: decreased or absent peripheral pulses in the lower extremities suggest coarctation of the aorta. Generalized weak peripheral pulses suggest hypoplastic left heart syndrome or circulatory shock. Bounding peripheral pulses suggest aortic run-off lesions such as PDA or persistent truncus arteriosus.

   c. Tachypnea of greater than 60/min with or without retraction.

   d. Hepatomegaly may suggest a heart defect. A midline liver suggests asplenia or polysplenia syndrome.

   e. A heart murmur may be a presenting sign of congenital heart disease (see chap. 26).

   f. Irregular rhythm and abnormal heart rate (see chaps. 23 and 26).

II. ELECTROCARDIOGRAPHY

A. Normal ECG

The normal ECG of a newborn is different from that of an adult and may show the following (see chap. 3):

   1) Sinus tachycardia with a rate as high as 180/min.

   2) Rightward deviation of the QRS axis with the mean of $+125°$ and the maximum of $+180°$.

3) Relatively small QRS voltages.

4) Low voltage of T waves.

5) RV dominance with tall R waves in the right precordial leads (V4R, V1, and V2).

6) Occasional q waves in V1.

7) Benign arrhythmias (see chap. 26).

In interpreting neonatal ECGs, one must use normal standards for the particular age rather than those for older children or adults (see chap. 3 for normal standards).

B. Abnormal ECG

An abnormal ECG may be in the form of abnormal P axis, abnormal QRS axis, hypertrophy of ventricles or atria, or ventricular conduction disturbance. Because of the wide ranges of normal values, many infants with significant CHD may have a normal ECG for their age.

1. P axis:

a. A P axis in the right lower quadrant suggests atrial situs inversus, asplenia syndrome or incorrectly placed electrodes.

b. A superior P axis suggests ectopic atrial rhythm or polysplenia syndrome.

2. QRS axis:

a. A superiorly oriented QRS axis between $0°$ and $-150°$ (left anterior hemiblock) suggests ECD or tricuspid atresia.

b. A QRS axis less than $+30°$ is abnormal and indicates LAD for the patient's age. The axis between $+30°$ and $+60°$ is unusual and indicates relative LAD. LAD may be seen with LVH.

c. A QRS axis greater than $+180$ degrees (in the range of $-150°$ to $-180°$) may indicate RAD. It may occur with RVH or RBBB.

3. LVH is suggested when the following are present (see chap. 3):

a. LAD or relative LAD (less than $+60°$) for the newborn.

b. R/S progression in precordial leads that resembles adult R/S progression.

c. QRS voltages demonstrating abnormal leftward and posterior forces or abnormal inferior forces for age (see chap. 3 for normal data).

4. RVH is difficult to diagnose because of the normal dominance of the RV at this age. However, the following are helpful clues to RVH in the newborn.

a. Pure R wave (with no S wave) in V1 greater than 10 mm.

b. R in V1 greater than 25 mm or R in aVR greater than 8 mm.

c. A qR pattern in V1 (also present in 10% of normal newborns).

d. Upright T in V1 after 3 days of age.

e. RAD greater than $+180°$.

5. Atrial hypertrophy:

a. Right atrial hypertrophy (RAH) is present when P wave amplitude is greater than 3 mm in any lead.

    b. Left atrial hypertrophy (LAH) is present when P wave duration is 0.08 second or greater (usually with notched P waves in the limb leads and biphasic P waves in V1).

6. Ventricular conduction disturbance (such as RBBB, LBBB, WPW syndrome, etc.) is present when the QRS duration is greater than the upper limit of normal for age; 0.07 second or greater in the newborn (not 0.1 second or greater as in the adult). The QRS duration increases with age in normal persons (see Table 3–2).

    a. RBBB may be associated with Ebstein's anomaly, COA in infants, ASD, or PAPVR. It may be seen in otherwise normal neonates. RBBB is frequently misinterpreted as RVH.

    b. LBBB is extremely rare in the newborn.

    c. Intraventricular block with a widening of the QRS complex throughout the QRS duration is more significant than RBBB. It is often associated with significant metabolic abnormalities, such as hypoxia, acidosis, hyperkalemia, or diffuse myocardial disease. It may be seen with CHD or as a terminal ECG in a dying patient.

    d. WPW syndrome may be an isolated finding or may be associated with CHD such as Ebstein's anomaly or L-TGA. It is a frequent cause of supraventricular tachycardia. Voltage criteria for hypertrophy do not apply in the presence of WPW syndrome.

III. CHEST ROENTGENOGRAPHY

A. Normal Chest X-Rays

The cardiothoracic (CT) ratio of normal newborn infants is greater than 0.5, the normal value in older children and adults. No single figure can be given as a normal CT ratio in neonates because multiple variables contribute to an abnormal CT ratio. Inadequate inspiratory expansion of the lungs and the large thymic shadow are important contributors to this difficulty. Therefore, evaluation of heart size should take into consideration the degree of inspiration, judged from the level of the diaphragm.

Thymic shadow may have many different shapes. It may show a classic "sail" sign (see Fig 4–9) or may have undulant or smooth borders on upper mediastinum. The thymic shadow may be unilateral or bilateral. The thymus occupies anterosuperior mediastinal space and is best appreciated on the lateral view of the chest x-rays.

Cardiac silhouette is not always as well defined in neonates as in older children. The main pulmonary artery often does not form a prominence in the left middle cardiac border. The lateral chest x-ray is quite sensitive to enlargement of the LV. Evaluation of pulmonary vascular markings in the neonate poses difficulties similar to those of cardiac size and silhouette for the same reasons.

Pulmonary vascular markings pose special problems in the neonate. Increased vascularity is not always apparent in the chest x-ray when the pulmonary blood flow is large. Distinction beween inreased PBF and pulmonary venous congestion is often difficult. Reduced PBF is usually easier to detect and indicates serious cyanotic CHD.

B. Abnormal Chest X-Rays

A cardiac problem is suggested by an abnormal size, position, or silhouette of the heart, by an abnormal shape or position of the liver, or by increased or decreased pulmonary vascularity on chest x-ray film.

1. Heart Size

Unfortunately, there are no reliable criteria with which to assess cardiomegaly in newborn infants. The CT ratio, which is quite useful in evaluating cardiomegaly in older children and adults (see Fig 4–1), is of limited value, since the CT ratio of normal neonates is usually greater than 0.5. This difficulty arises from many factors; the more important ones are: (A) lack of deep inspiration in newborns; (B) the presence of a large thymic shadow; and (C) the presence of an atelectatic area which may give the spurious impression of cardiomegaly.

Unequivocal cardiomegaly may be due to:

a. Congenital heart defects, with or without CHF (VSD, PDA, TGA, Ebstein's anomaly, etc.).

b. Myocarditis or cardiomyopathy.

c. Pericardial effusion.

d. Metabolic disturbances: hypoglycemia, severe hypoxemia, and acidosis.

e. Overhydration or overtransfusion.

It is important to remember that many serious CHDs that eventually will result in cardiomegaly may show normal heart size in the newborn period.

2. Abnormal Cardiac Silhouette

An abnormal shape of the heart may be of considerable help in suspecting correct diagnosis. For example:

a. "Boot-shaped" heart (coeur en sabot) is seen in TOF or tricuspid atresia (see Fig 14–12).

b. "Egg-shaped" heart with narrow waist may be seen in TGA (see Fig 14–2).

c. A large globular heart is seen with Ebstein's anomaly.

d. The "snowman" sign of TAPVR is usually not evident in the neonatal period.

3. Dextrocardia or Mesocardia

When the heart is located predominantly in the right side of the chest (dextrocardia) or in the midline of the thorax (mesocardia), the segmental approach of van Praagh should be used to deduce the nature of the segmental relationship of the atria and ventricles (refer to Chamber Localization in chap. 14).

Four common situations in which the heart is located in the right side of the chest or in the midline are (see Fig 16–5):

a. Situs inversus totalis with normal heart.

b. Hypoplasia of the right lung with displacement of a normally formed heart to the right (dextroversion).

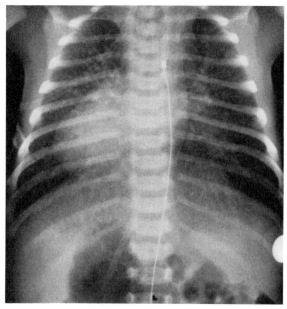

FIG 25–1.
An x-ray film of chest and upper abdomen of a newborn infant with polysplenia syndrome. Note a symmetric liver ("midline liver"), a stomach bubble in the midline, dextrocardia, and increased pulmonary vascularity.

    c. Complex cyanotic heart defect including atrial or ventricular inversion.

    d. Asplenia or polysplenia syndrome with midline liver.

4. The Situs of Abdominal Viscera
The location of the liver or the stomach bubble, and the shape of the liver provide important clues to the nature of the cardiac defect.

    a. A midline liver indicates asplenia or polysplenia syndrome with complex cyanotic CHD (Fig 25–1).

    b. A left-sided liver (or right-sided stomach bubble) with the heart in the right side of the chest indicates situs inversus totalis with a mirror-image dextrocardia (normal).

    c. The liver and the cardiac apex on the same side usually suggest complex cardiac defects.

5. Pulmonary Vascular Markings
Evaluation of pulmonary vascular markings is an integral part of the interpretation of cardiac x-rays.

    a. Increased pulmonary vascularity in a cyanotic infant suggests TGA, persistent truncus arteriosus, or single ventricle. In an acyanotic newborn infant, increased pulmonary vascularity suggests VSD, PDA, or ECD.

    b. Decreased pulmonary vascularity with "black" lung fields suggests critical cyanotic heart defects with decreased PBF, such as pulmonary atresia, tricuspid atresia, or TOF with pulmonary atresia. The heart size is usually normal in these conditions. Decreased pulmonary vascular markings with marked cardiomegaly are seen in Ebstein's anomaly.

c. "Ground-glass" appearance or a reticulated pattern of lung fields is characteristic of pulmonary venous obstruction and suggests hypoplastic left heart syndrome (HLHS) (see Fig 26–2) or TAPVR with obstruction.

26 / Cardiac Problems of the Newborn

The majority of cardiology consultations are requested during the newborn period for one or more of the following reasons: (a) a heart murmur, (b) cyanosis, (c) suspected congestive heart failure (CHF), (d) arrhythmias, (e) abnormal chest x-ray findings, or (f) abnormal ECG findings. The first four topics will be discussed in this chapter; abnormal ECG and chest x-ray findings are discussed in chapter 25.

I. HEART MURMURS

A. Innocent Heart Murmurs

As in older infants and children, not all heart murmurs in the neonatal period are pathologic. It has been reported that more than 50% of full-term newborn infants who were examined frequently were found to have an innocent systolic murmur at some time during the first week of life. The incidence of heart murmur in premature infants is even higher than in full-term infants. The four most common innocent murmurs in the newborn period are: (a) pulmonary flow murmur of the newborn; (b) transient systolic murmur of PDA; (c) transient systolic murmur of tricuspid regurgitation; and (d) vibratory systolic murmur.

1. Pulmonary flow murmur of the newborn

This innocent heart murmur is probably the most common heart murmur in the newborn infant. It is more common in premature and small-for-gestational-age infants than in full-term infants. It is heard best at the ULSB and transmits well to both sides of the chest, axillae, and the back. The murmur is soft, usually not greater than grade 2/6 in intensity. It is not transient, lasting for weeks or months, but usually disappearing by 6 months of age (see also chap. 2 for the mechanism of the murmur).

2. Transient systolic murmur of PDA

This murmur is best audible at the ULSB and in the left infraclavicular area on the first day, and it usually disappears shortly thereafter. It is believed to originate from a closing ductus arteriosus. It is grade 2/6 or less in intensity. It is usually only systolic and crescendic up to the S2.

3. Transient systolic murmur of tricuspid regurgitation

This murmur is indistinguishable from that of VSD in that it is regurgitant (starting with the S1) and is maximally audible at the LLSB. It disappears in a day or two. It is believed that a minimal tricuspid valve abnormality produces regurgitation in the presence of high PVR, but the regurgitation disappears as the PVR falls. Therefore, this murmur is more common in infants who had fetal distress or neonatal asphyxia, since they tend to maintain high PVR for a longer period.

4. **Vibratory innocent murmur**

This murmur is a counterpart of Still's murmur in older children (see also Innocent Heart Murmur in chap. 2). It is best audible at the LLSB or near the apex and has a low-frequency, vibratory quality. Therefore, differentiation of this murmur from that of VSD may pose some difficulties. It is best audible with the bell of the stethoscope in light contact with the chest wall, but it disappears when the bell is pressed against the chest wall.

B. **Pathologic Heart Murmurs**

Most pathologic murmurs should be audible during the first month of life, with the exception of an atrial septal defect. However, there are differences in the time of appearance of a heart murmur depending on the nature of the defect.

1. Heart murmurs of stenotic lesions (AS, PS, COA, etc.) are audible immediately after birth and persist.

2. Heart murmurs of left-to-right shunt lesions that depend on the reduction of PVR (dependent shunt) may appear later. For example, a heart murmur of a small VSD in which the reduction of the PVR is normal becomes audible shortly after birth, whereas the heart murmur of a large VSD does not become audible for some time, until the PVR falls significantly. The appearance of a murmur of large VSD may be delayed until 2–3 weeks of age.

3. The continuous murmur of a large PDA may not appear for 2–3 weeks. Instead, it is a crescendo systolic murmur with slight or no diastolic component; it is best audible at the ULSB and left infraclavicular area.

4. The murmur of ASD appears late in infancy with insidious onset. It becomes loud after a year or two, when the distensibility of the RV becomes maximal.

It is important to understand that even careful, repeated examinations may not detect a heart murmur in a newborn infant who eventually receives a diagnosis of a serious heart disease such as a large VSD. Even in the absence of a heart murmur, a newborn infant may have a serious heart defect that requires immediate attention; e.g., severe cyanotic heart disease, such as transposition of the great arteries or pulmonary atresia with a closing PDA. Infants who are in severe CHF may not have a loud murmur until the myocardial function is improved with anticongestive measures.

II. CYANOSIS IN THE NEWBORN

A. **Detection**

Most patients with cyanotic heart disease, particularly those with a more severe form, have cyanosis at birth. Early detection of cyanosis in a newborn is crucial, but is not always easy. One must look for cyanosis not only on the lips but also on the tip of the tongue, fingernails and toenails, oral mucous membrane, conjunctivas, and the tip of the nose. When in doubt, blood gases should be obtained for arterial Po_2 to confirm or rule out central cyanosis. Normal Po_2 of a 1-day-old infant may be as low as 60 mm Hg.

B. **Etiology**

Central cyanosis (with low arterial Po_2) may be due to: (a) CNS depression, (b) lung disease, or (c) cyanotic congenital heart disease. Table 26–1 lists some of the characteristic physical and routine laboratory findings of each type of cyanosis.

TABLE 26–1.

Causes and Clinical Characteristics of Central Cyanosis

A. CNS depression
  Causes
    Perinatal asphyxia
    Heavy maternal sedation
    Intrauterine fetal distress
  Findings
    Shallow irregular respiration
    Poor muscle tone
    Cyanosis disappears when stimulated or given oxygen
B. Pulmonary disease
  Causes
    Parenchymal lung disease (hyaline membrane disease, atelectasis, etc.)
    Pneumothorax or pleural effusion
    Diaphragmatic hernia
    Persistent pulmonary hypertension of newborn (or PFC syndrome)
  Findings
    Tachypnea and respiratory distress with retraction and expiratory grunting
    Rales and/or decreased breath sounds on auscultation
    Chest x-ray may reveal causes (as listed above)
    Oxygen administration improves or abolishes cyanosis
C. Cardiac disease
  Causes
    Cyanotic CHD with right-to-left shunt
  Findings
    Tachypnea but usually without retraction
    No rales or abnormal breath sounds unless CHF supervenes
    Heart murmur may be absent in serious forms of cyanotic CHD
    A continuous murmur (of PDA) may be present and indicates restricted pulmonary
      blood flow through the ductus
    Chest x-rays may show cardiomegaly, abnormal cardiac silhouette, increased or
      decreased pulmonary vascular markings
    Little or no increase in Po_2 with oxygen administration

C. Suggested Approach to Patients With Central Cyanosis

Determination of arterial blood gases clarifies the type of cyanosis (central or peripheral). Once central cyanosis has been confirmed by direct measurement of arterial Po_2, one tests the response of arterial blood gases to 100% oxygen inhalation (hyperoxitest). This test helps to differentiate cyanosis due to cardiac disease from that due to pulmonary disease. Oxygen should be administered through a plastic hood (such as Oxyhood) for at least 10 minutes to replace the alveolar air completely with oxygen (Table 26–2). With pulmonary disease, arterial Po_2 usually rises to more than 100 mm Hg. When there is a significant intracardiac right-to-left shunt, the arterial Po_2 does not exceed 100 mm Hg, and the rise is not more than 10–30 mm Hg. It should be pointed out, however, that some infants with cyanotic CHD with increased PBF, such as total anomalous pulmonary venous return, may have a rise in the arterial Po_2 to 100 mm Hg or higher. On the other hand, infants with massive intrapulmonary shunt (but with a normal heart) may not have a rise in arterial Po_2 to 100 mm Hg.

Whenever possible, arterial blood samples should be obtained from the right upper body (right radial, brachial or temporal artery) to avoid falsely low values

TABLE 26–2.

Suggested Steps in Management of Cyanotic Newborns

1. Chest x-ray films

   Chest x-rays may reveal pulmonary causes of cyanosis and urgency of the problem. It will also hint the presence or absence and the type of cardiac defects

2. Arterial blood gases in room air

   Arterial blood gases in room air will confirm or reject central cyanosis. Elevated PCO_2 suggests pulmonary or CNS problems. Low pH may be seen in sepsis, circulatory shock, or severe hypoxemia.

3. Hyperoxitest

   Repeating arterial blood gases while breathing 100% oxygen helps to separate cardiac causes of cyanosis from pulmonary or CNS causes.

4. ECG if cardiac origin of cyanosis is suspected

5. An umbilical artery line

   A PO_2 value in a preductal artery (such as right radial artery) higher than that in a postductal artery (an umbilical artery line) by 10–15 mm Hg suggests a right-to-left ductal shunt. (The umbilical line placed high in the descending aorta can be used for aortogram during cardiac catheterization, reducing the time spent in the lab and eliminating the risk of arterial complications.)

6. Prostaglandin E_1

   If a cyanotic CHD is suspected based on the above laboratory tests, Prostin VR Pediatric (PGE_1) should be started or made available.

due to right-to-left ductal shunt. If a low arterial PO_2 is obtained from an umbilical artery line or from the lower extremity, another sample from the right upper body should be obtained and compared with a simultaneously obtained sample from the lower part of the body to clarify the presence or absence of a right-to-left ductal shunt. An arterial PO_2 from the right radial artery higher than that from an umbilical artery catheter by 10–15 mm Hg is significant. In severe cases of right-to-left ductal shunt, differential cyanosis may be noticeable; a pink upper and cyanotic lower parts of the body. Such a differential cyanosis or differential arterial PO_2 suggests persistent pulmonary hypertension of the newborn (PPHN, or PFC syndrome), or obstructive lesions of the left heart (severe AS, interrupted aortic arch, preductal COA, etc.) with a right-to-left ductal shunt (see Table 26–2).

If cyanotic CHD is suspected, especially a defect which appears to be ductus dependent (pulmonary atresia with or without VSD, tricuspid atresia, HLHS, interrupted aortic arch, preductal COA, etc.), one should have prostaglandin E_1 (Prostin VR Pediatric) available for IV infusion as soon as an indication is established. The starting dose of Prostin is 0.1 μg/kg/min, administered in a continuous IV drip. When the desired effects (increased PO_2, increased systemic blood pressure, and improved pH) are achieved, the dose should be reduced step-by-step to 0.01 μg/kg/min. When there is no effect with the initial starting dose, it may be increased up to 0.4 μg/kg/min. Three common side effects of Prostin IV infusion are apnea (12%), fever (14%), and flushing (10%). Less common side effects include tachycardia or bradycardia, hypotension, and cardiac arrest.

Discussion of individual cyanotic heart defect is found in chapter 14. Only persistent pulmonary hypertension of the newborn will be discussed in this section.

PERSISTENT PULMONARY HYPERTENSION OF THE NEWBORN (PPHN) (Persistence of the fetal circulation, PFC syndrome)

This neonatal condition is characterized by persistence of pulmonary hypertension, which in turn causes a right-to-left shunt through the PDA or the PFO in the absence of intracardiac defects.

Etiology

Pulmonary hypertension seen in the newborn may be caused by a powerful pulmonary vasoconstriction from various etiologies in the presence of a normally developed pulmonary vascular bed, or by structural abnormalities (hypertrophy, decreased cross-sectional area) of the pulmonary vascular bed (Table 26–3). In general, pulmonary hypertension secondary to the latter conditions is more difficult to reverse.

Clinical Manifestations

1. The idiopathic form usually affects full-term or postterm neonates. There is usually history of meconium staining or birth asphyxia. Maternal ingestion of nonsteroidal anti-inflammatory drugs may be present.

2. Marked cyanosis and tachypnea (with grunting and retraction) are always present.

3. Single and loud S2 and increased RV impulse.

4. Varying degrees of ventricular dysfunction ranging from a faint systolic murmur of tricuspid regurgitation to CHF with systemic hypotension may be present.

5. Arterial PO_2 is lower in the descending aorta or legs than in the right arm (because of right-to-left ductal shunt), and differential cyanosis may be evident.

6. ECG is usually normal for age, but occasional RVH or T wave changes suggestive of myocardial dysfunction may be present.

7. Chest x-rays reveal hyperinflated lungs and varying degrees of cardiomegaly.

TABLE 26–3.
Etiology of Persistent Pulmonary Hypertension of the Newborn

---

1. Pulmonary vasoconstriction in the presence of a normally developed pulmonary vascular bed may be caused by or seen in:
   a. Alveolar hypoxia (meconium aspiration syndrome, hyaline membrane disease, hypoventilation due to CNS anomalies)
   b. Birth asphyxia
   c. LV dysfunction or circulatory shock
   d. Infections (such as group B hemolytic streptococcal infection)
   e. Hyperviscosity syndrome (polycythemia)
   f. Hypoglycemia and hypocalcemia
2. Increased pulmonary vascular smooth muscle development (hypertrophy) may be caused by:
   a. Chronic intrauterine asphyxia
   b. Maternal use of prostaglandin synthesis inhibitors (aspirin, indomethacin) results in early ductal closure
3. Decreased cross-sectional area of pulmonary vascular bed may be seen in association with:
   a. Congenital diaphragmatic hernia
   b. Primary pulmonary hypoplasia

Differential Diagnosis

This condition must be differentiated from cyanotic CHD early in the course of the disease.

1) Hyperoxitest with or without hyperventilation: A good response to 100% oxygen breathing with arterial PO_2 greater than 100 mm Hg fairly well excludes cyanotic CHD.

2) Preductal vs. postductal arterial PO_2: A significantly higher arterial PO_2 (greater than 10–15 mm Hg) obtained from the right arm than from an umbilical artery catheter indicates a right-to-left ductal shunt. It may result from PPHN or CHD such as preductal COA or interrupted aortic arch. No difference in PO_2 between the two sites in the presence of a low arterial PO_2 suggests a large right-to-left atrial or ventricular shunt; this may result from PPHN (with closed ductus and atrial right-to-left shunt) or cyanotic CHD.

3) A thorough 2D ECHO study should be performed to rule out cyanotic CHD and to identify patients with myocardial dysfunction. ECHO may confirm the right-to-left shunt at the atrial (Fig 26–1) or ventricular level.

Treatment

The goal of therapy is to lower pulmonary vascular resistance by administration of oxygen, induction of respiratory alkalosis, and the use of pulmonary vasodilators.

1) Hyperventilation (to produce respiratory alkalosis) and administration of oxygen (to improve arterial PO_2), by the use of FIO_2 up to 1.0, respiratory rates 40–60/min, peak inspiratory pressure (PIP) up to 40 cm H_2O, and inspiratory:expiratory (I:E) ratio of 1 or less. The patient may be paralyzed with pancuronium (Pavulon) 0.1 mg/kg IV.

2) Tolazoline (Priscoline) infusion through a vein on the scalp or upper extremity or via a catheter placed in the pulmonary artery. A loading dose of 1–2 mg/kg by slow IV, followed by IV infusion of 1–2 mg/kg/min, may be used. During the vasodilator therapy, blood pressure should be monitored carefully, since there may be a greater lowering of the SVR than of the PVR, resulting in lowering of systemic blood pressure. Adequate circulating blood volume should be maintained.

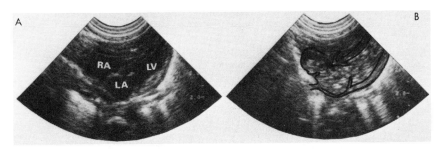

FIG 26–1.
Contrast echocardiography. **A,** the subcostal four-chamber view shows clearly defined, echo-free RA, LA, and LV cavities. **B,** following injection of a small amount of saline in the peripheral IV line, heavy echoes are seen in the LA and LV and higher echoes in the RA, demonstrating the presence of a large right-to-left atrial shunt in a newborn with PPHN.

3) Dopamine is often used concomitantly since tolazoline frequently causes systemic hypotension. The usual dose is 10 μg/kg/min.

4) Dobutamine (a β-adrenergic agent) may be used if signs of CHF are present.

5) Correction of hypocalcemia and hypoglycemia and treatment of acid-base imbalance help to improve myocardial function.

6) Extracorporeal membrane oxygenation (ECMO) has been shown to be effective in selected patients with severe PPHN.

7) Several experimental agents (PGD$_2$, PGI$_2$, leukotriene antagonists) have been tried with favorable results.

III. HEART FAILURE IN THE NEWBORN

A neonate with CHF usually suffers from a congenital heart defect, but may have nonstructural heart disease such as myocardial dysfunction (ischemia, myocarditis) or serious disturbances of heart rate. Metabolic and hematologic abnormalities as well as overtransfusion or overhydration may also be responsible for CHF. (Table 26–4 shows causes of CHF in the newborn).

The clinical picture of CHF in the newborn period may simulate other disorders, such as meningitis, sepsis, pneumonia, or bronchiolitis. Tachypnea, tachycardia, pulmonary rales or rhonchi, hepatomegaly, and weak peripheral pulses are common presenting signs. In premature infants with large PDA, apnea may be an early symptom of CHF. Heart murmur is frequently absent. Cardiomegaly, with or with-

TABLE 26–4.

Causes of Heart Failure in the Newborn

A. Structural heart defects
  At birth
    Hypoplastic left heart syndrome (HLHS)
    Severe tricuspid or pulmonary regurgitation
    Large systemic AV fistula
  First wk
    TGA
    Premature infant with large PDA
    TAPVR below diaphragm
  1–4 wk
    Critical AS or PS
    Preductal COA
B. Noncardiac causes
  1) Birth asphyxia (resulting in transient myocardial ischemia)
  2) Metabolic: hypoglycemia, hypocalcemia
  3) Severe anemia (as seen in hydrops fetalis)
  4) Neonatal sepsis
C. Primary myocardial disease
  1) Myocarditis
  2) Tansient myocardial ischemia (w/wo birth asphyxia)
  3) Cardiomyopathy (seen in infant of diabetic mother)
D. Disturbances in heart rate
  1) Supraventricular tachycardia (SVT, or PAT)
  2) Atrial flutter/fibrillation
  3) Congenital heart block (when associated with CHD)

out increased pulmonary vascularity, or pulmonary edema on chest x-rays confirms the diagnosis. Detailed discussion of treatment of CHF is presented in chapter 27.

Two important structural abnormalities of the cardiovascular system which present with CHF in the newborn period are hypoplastic left heart syndrome (HLHS) and premature infants with large PDA. Two nonstructural heart conditions which can present with CHF are transient myocardial ischemia and infants of diabetic mothers. These four conditions will be presented in this chapter. Other structural heart defects have been presented under specific conditions in earlier chapters. Arrhythmias that can cause CHF are presented in this chapter under Arrhythmias of the Newborn.

A. HYPOPLASTIC LEFT HEART SYNDROME (HLHS)

Incidence
One to two percent of all congenital heart disease. The most common cause of death from cardiac defect during the first month of life.

Pathology
This syndrome includes a group of closely related anomalies characterized by hypoplasia of the LV and encompasses atresia or severe stenosis of the aortic and/ or mitral valves and hypoplasia of the aortic arch (Fig 26–2,B).

Pathophysiology
During fetal life, the PVR is higher than the SVR because of alveolar hypoxia and the low-resistance placental circulation. The dominant RV maintains normal perfusing pressure in the descending aorta through the ductal right-to-left shunt, even in the presence of the nonfunctioning hypoplastic LV. However, difficulties arise after birth, primarily from two factors: (a) reversal of the vascular resistance in the two circuits, with higher vascular resistance in the systemic circulation as the result of expansion of the lungs and elimination of the placenta, and (b) closure of the ductus arteriosus. The end result is a marked decrease in systemic cardiac output and aortic pressure, producing circulatory shock and metabolic

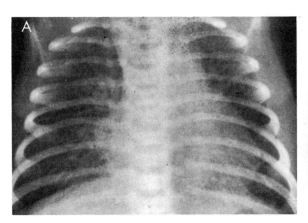 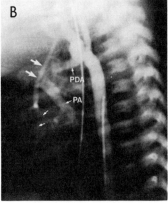

FIG 26–2.
An AP view of chest film **(A)** and a lateral view of an aortogram **(B)** in a 1-day-old newborn with hypoplastic left heart syndrome. The heart is enlarged and the pulmonary vascularity is increased, with marked pulmonary venous congestion and pulmonary edema **(A)**. The aortogram, obtained with injection of a radiopaque dye through an umbilical artery catheter, shows a hypoplastic ascending aorta *(thick arrows)* with small coronary arteries *(thin arrows)* filling retrogradely, a large PDA, and pulmonary arteries.

acidosis. An increase in PBF in the presence of the nonfunctioning LV results in an elevated LA pressure and pulmonary edema.

Clinical Manifestations

History
Critically ill in the first few hours to days of life.

PE
a) Mild cyanosis, pallor, and mottling.

b) Tachycardia, tachypnea, dyspnea, and pulmonary rales are always present.

c) Poor peripheral pulses and vasoconstricted extremities are also characteristic.

d) The S2 is loud and single.

e) Heart murmur is usually absent. Occasionally, a grade 1–3/6 nonspecific systolic murmur may be present over the precordium.

ECG: RVH is almost always present.

X-Rays
Pulmonary venous congestion or pulmonary edema (Fig 26–2,A) is a characteristic finding. The heart is only mildly to moderately enlarged.

Laboratory
Arterial blood gas determination reveals slightly decreased Po_2. Severe metabolic acidosis out of proportion to the Po_2 (because of markedly decreased cardiac output) is characteristic of this condition.

ECHO
ECHO findings are diagnostic and usually obviate cardiac catheterization. Severe hypoplasia of the aorta and aortic anulus and absent or distorted mitral valve are usually present. The LV cavity is diminutive, but the RV cavity is markedly dilated and the tricuspid valve is large.

Natural History and Complications
a) CHF in the first week of life.

b) Progressive hypoxemia and acidosis, resulting in death, usually in the first month of life.

Management

1. **Medical**

   a) Intubation, administration of oxygen, and correction of metabolic acidosis.

   b) IV infusion of prostaglandin E_1 (Prostin VR Pediatric) may produce temporary improvement by reopening the ductus arteriosus.

   c) Balloon atrial septostomy may help decompress the LA.

2. Surgical procedures carry either high mortality or are still in experimental stages.

   a) The first stage Norwood operation is followed by a Fontan-type operation later.

      1. A Norwood operation is performed in the neonatal period and involves the following three procedures (Fig 26–3):

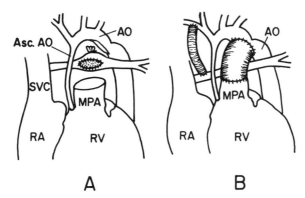

FIG 26–3.
The Norwood operation. **A,** the main pulmonary artery *(MPA)* is divided, and the distal PA is closed. **B,** the proximal MPA is connected to the descending aorta with the use of conduit. A right-sided Gore-Tex shunt is performed.

(a) The MPA is divided and the proximal stump is connected to the descending aorta with or without the use of conduit. The distal MPA is closed.

(b) A right-sided Gore-Tex shunt is performed to maintain PBF.

(c) The excision of the atrial septum for adequate interatrial mixing.

2. The second-stage Fontan-type operation is performed at 6–24 months of age, and involves

(a) Closure of the Gore-Tex shunt.

(b) A direct anastomosis between the RA and PA (see Fig 14–23,A).

(c) Closure of the surgically created ASD.

3. Mortality: Even in the experienced hands, the mortality of the initial Norwood procedure is very high (as high as 75%). The second stage mortality is also high (up to 50%).

b) Cardiac transplantation is in the experimental stage.

B. HEART FAILURE IN PREMATURE INFANTS WITH PDA

This represents a special problem in premature infants who have been recovering from hyaline membrane disease. With improvement in oxygenation, the PVR drops rapidly, but the ductus remains patent, and its responsiveness to oxygen is lower in premature newborns than in full-term newborns. The resulting large left-to-right ductal shunt makes the lungs stiff, and it becomes impossible to wean the infant from the respirator. Early recognition and appropriate management are keys to improving the prognosis of these infants. Infants who remain on the respirator and oxygen therapy for an extended period develop bronchopulmonary dysplasia, with resulting pulmonary hypertension (cor pulmonale) and right heart failure.

Incidence
CHF occurs in 15% of prematures whose birth weight is less than 1,750 gm and in 40%–50% of those whose birth weight is less than 1,500 gm.

Clinical Manifestations

History

History usually reveals that a premature infant with hyaline membrane disease has made some improvement during the first few days after birth, but this is followed by inability to wean the infant from the respirator or a need to increase respirator settings or oxygen requirement in 4–7-day-old premature infants. These are strong clues of the ductal contribution to the respiratory problem of the premature infant. Apneic spells or episodes of bradycardia may be initial signs in infants who are not on a respirator.

PE

a) Bounding peripheral pulses with hyperactive precordium.

b) Tachycardia with or without gallop rhythm.

c) Pulmonary rales may be present owing to left heart failure or to the pulmonary disease.

d) A systolic murmur is best audible at the middle and upper LSB. The classic continuous murmur at the ULSB is diagnostic, but the murmur is sometimes only systolic.

ECG: Usually not helpful but shows normal ECG or occasional LVH.

X-Rays

a) Increasing cardiomegaly (involving the LA and LV).

b) Evidence of pulmonary edema or increased pulmonary venous markings.

ECHO

2D ECHO and Doppler study confirm the diagnosis. 2D ECHO actually visualizes the patency and the diameter and length of the ductus from either the parasternal or suprasternal notch approach (Fig 26–4). Indirect estimate of the magnitude of the shunt can be made by measuring LA and LV dimensions by M-mode or 2D ECHO. The Doppler study with sample volume positioned in the ductus or pulmonary artery shows a continuous flow throughout systole and diastole.

Management

For symptomatic infants, either pharmcologic or surgical closure of the ductus is indicated. A small PDA that is not causing CHF should be followed up medically

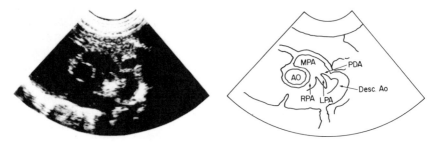

FIG 26–4.
Parasternal short-axis view demonstrating patent ductus arteriosus *(PDA)* which connects the main pulmonary artery *(MPA)* and the descending aorta *(Desc Ao)*. AO = aorta; LPA = left pulmonary artery; RPA = right pulmonary artery.

for 6 months without surgical ligation because of the possibility of spontaneous closure of PDA.

1. **Medical**

   a) Fluid restriction to 120 ml/kg/day, and a diuretic, such as furosemide, 1 mg/kg, 2–3 times a day for 24–48 hours may be tried initially.

   b) Many pediatric cardiologists do not recommend using digitalis in premature infants with PDA. It has not always been helpful and has been associated with a high incidence of digitalis toxicity. If digoxin is used, a smaller dose should be used (see Table 27–3).

   c) Pharmacologic manipulation of the PDA with a prostaglandin synthetase inhibitor (indomethacin, 0.2 mg/kg, PO or IV every 12 hours, up to 3 doses) may be used on selected cases. Contraindications to the use of indomethacin include a high BUN (>25 mg/dl) or creatinine levels (>1.8 mg/dl), low platelet count (<80,000/cu mm), bleeding tendency (including intracranial hemorrhage), necrotizing enterocolitis, and hyperbilirubinemia.

2. **Surgical:** If the above medical treatment is unsuccessful, or if the use of indomethacin is contraindicated, a surgical ligation of the ductus is indicated. In some institutions, an initial surgical ligation is preferred to medical management with indomethacin.

C. TRANSIENT MYOCARDIAL DYSFUNCTION

Severe perinatal stress can produce myocardial dysfunction of varying degrees in the newborn infant. Perinatal asphyxia is the most important cause of this condition. Hypoglycemia, hypocalcemia, and polycythemia may also contribute to it.

A wide spectrum of clinical manifestations is recognized, depending on the severity of myocardial dysfunction.

1. Transient tachypnea of the newborn is the mildest form of the condition. Mild LV dysfunction leads to fluid retention, elevated pulmonary capillary pressure and reduced lung compliance. In certain "hyperreactors," resulting alveolar hypoxia causes pulmonary vasoconstriction and pulmonary hypertension. Pulmonary hypertension may lead to bidirectional shunting at the atrial or ductal level.

2. Tricuspid (or mitral) valve insufficiency results from papillary muscle infarction.

3. Severe CHF with cardiogenic shock is the most severe form of myocardial dysfunction.

Physical examination reveals an early onset of respiratory difficulty with tachypnea, usually in a full-term newborn. The S2 is loud but usually split. A systolic murmur of tricuspid or mitral regurgitation is common. Signs of CHF with gallop rhythm develop in severe cases. Some infants progress to vascular collapse with hypotension. Chest x-rays reveal cardiomegaly of varying degrees. Pulmonary venous congestion ("wet lung") is present in severe cases. Common ECG abnormalities are generalized flat T waves and ST segment depression. ECHO reveals enlarged LA and LV dimensions and decreased contractility of the LV.

Most patients recover with proper management. Clinical improvement usually occurs within a week, and abnormalities in ECG and LV function studies return to normal in a few months. All or some of the measures described under Management of CHF are indicated (see chap. 27).

D. INFANTS OF DIABETIC MOTHERS

Although severe symptomatic CHF is rare, mild cardiomegaly is quite common in these infants of diabetic mothers. Hypoglycemia and hypocalcemia are at least in part responsible for this manifestation.

The heart shows increased size and weight owing to increased myocardial fiber size and number, rather than to excess glycogen. Incidence of CHD is higher in these infants (2%–4% of live births) than in general population; TGA, VSD and COA are frequently encountered defects. Hypertrophic cardiomyopathy with or without obstruction is seen in 10%–20% of the patients. Profound hypoglycemia and concomitant hypocalcemia may cause myocardial failure and cyanosis from a right-to-left atrial shunt.

This large-for-gestational-age infant may have diverse signs of hypoglycemia and hypocalcemia. Tachypnea is common during the first 5 days of life. A systolic ejection murmur is common along the LSB, and signs of CHF may develop in 5%–10% of the infants. Chest x-rays may show cardiomegaly with or without increased pulmonary vascularity. ECG findings are variable and nonspecific. ECHO may reveal an asymmetric septal hypertrophy, usually with a supernormal contractility of the LV. (The degree of septal thickening is not related to the severity of the maternal diabetes.) In infants with dilated cardiomyopathy, LV function is diminished. The septal hypertrophy usually resolves by 2–12 months of age.

General supportive therapy and correction of hypoglycemia and hypocalcemia are indicated. CHF from hypertrophic obstructive cardiomyopathy may be treated with β-adrenergic blockers. Anticongestive measures may be indicated in infants with dilated cardiomyopathy.

IV. ARRHYTHMIAS OF THE NEWBORN

Although once thought to be rare, arrhythmias are not uncommon in healthy premature and full-term newborn infants. In a way, the newborn is at more of a disadvantage. Continued postnatal development of the conduction system (the SA node, AV node, and His bundle) and of the sympathetic nervous system of the heart may predispose the newborn to arrhythmias. In addition, unfavorable environmental factors may also contribute to the occurrence of arrhythmias. These factors include maternal disease state (diabetes mellitus, toxemia), pharmacologic agents given to the mother or neonate, and postnatal difficulties of the newborn (hypoxia, acidosis, hypothermia, metabolic disorders, electrolyte imbalance, etc.).

The normal resting heart rate of the newborn is 110–115/min. Depending on the state of sleep or activity, the rate may range from 80 to 190/min. Rates above and below this range require investigation with ECG documentation. A detailed discussion of arrhythmias is presented in chapter 23.

1. Sinus Arrhythmia

Phasic variation in the heart rate is quite common in healthy full-term and premature infants. Unlike a similar variation in older children, this may or may not be related to respiration. It has no clinical significance. In fact, the lack of sinus arrhythmia (or the presence of "fixed rate") may be more serious, since it may be observed in asphyxiated newborns. No treatment is needed.

2. Sinus Tachycardia

Transient tachycardia of rates up to 180–190/min is commonly seen in normal newborns and does not require treatment. Persistent tachycardia may be caused by hypovolemia, hyperthermia, catecholamines, or hyperthyroidism. Detection and correction of the underlying etiology is indicated.

3. Sinus Bradycardia

Transient bradycardia (less than 70 beats/min) may be seen in normal neonates and requires no treatment. It may be associated with defecation, yawning, deep sleep, or nasopharyngeal stimulation. Prolonged bradycardia may be related to apnea (either preceded or followed by), maternal medications (such as reserpine), or neonatal asphyxia. Treatment should be directed to correct or improve underlying causes.

4. Sinus Pause or Arrest

It may occasionally occur in normal full-term and premature neonates, but digitalis toxicity or hyperkalemia should be considered as possibilities.

5. Wandering Atrial Pacemaker

It may occur in healthy newborn infants and does not require therapy.

6. Premature Contractions

Premature contractions are quite common, occurring in up to 30% of healthy premature and full-term neonates. Supraventricular (atrial or nodal) premature contractions are encountered more frequently than premature ventricular contractions (PVCs). These premature contractions are occasionally associated with CHDs, severe respiratory distress syndrome, sepsis, digitalis toxicity, or hypoxemia.

Treatment is not indicated for premature contractions per se, unless they are frequent PVCs. Treatment should be directed toward correcting the underlying causes, such as digitalis toxicity, sepsis, or hypoxemia. Frequent PVCs may be treated with IV lidocaine or oral phenytoin (Dilantin).

7. Supraventricular Tachycardia

Supraventricular tachycardia (SVT) is the most frequently encountered arrhythmia of significance in the newborn period. The heart rate is usually 240 ± 40 beats/min with a normal appearing QRS complex (Fig 26–5). The Wolff-Parkinson-White syndrome is responsible in about 50% of neonatal cases. Structural heart diseases (such as Ebstein's anomaly, tricuspid atresia, and cardiac tumors), viral myocarditis, and thyrotoxicosis are less frequent causes of SVT in neonates.

The great majority of SVT are due to atrioventricular (AV) reentry or reciprocating AV tachycardia, which is associated with a bypass tract such as the bundle of Kent (see chap. 23). Newborns with SVT usually develop signs of CHF within 24–48 hours after the onset. They are restless and tachypneic or "wheezy," and eventually develop signs of CHF (pallor, apathy, circulatory shock).

Cardioversion is the treatment of choice when CHF is present in a neonate, followed by digitalization and diuretics. In SVT of short duration without signs of CHF, digoxin alone is used. Application of an icebag on the face has been employed successfully in the neonate. Verapamil or propranolol is not the drug of choice and is indicated only when other measures fail. They should be given step-by-step in a small dose with careful monitoring and readiness to resuscitate

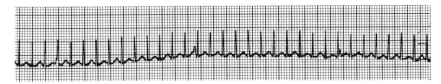

FIG 26–5.
A rhythm strip showing supraventricular tachycardia, with the heart rate 300 beats per minute.

the infant. In refractory cases, atrial overdrive with an electrode catheter may be effective.

8. **Atrial Flutter/Fibrillation**

This arrhythmia is relatively rare. The diagnosis is made occasionally in utero. It is often associated with congenital heart disease (such as Ebstein's anomaly, mitral stenosis, tricuspid atresia), viral myocarditis, and systemic infections. Severe CHF may develop. Cardioversion is the treatment of choice in infants who are in CHF, followed by digoxin. In the infant without CHF, the use of digoxin is indicated to prevent CHF by controlling ventricular rate within an acceptable range.

9. **Ventricular Tachycardia**

Ventricular tachycardia is rare but more serious than any other arrhythmia. It may be associated with congenital heart disease, myocarditis, cardiomyopathy, or cardiac tumors as well as hyperkalemia or asphyxia. Rarely, long QT syndrome (Jervell and Lange-Nielsen syndrome and Romano-Ward syndrome) may be responsible for the arrhythmia (see Table 1–2). Treatment consists of termination of the arrhythmia with lidocaine infusion or cardioversion, correction of the underlying cause when possible, and prevention of recurrence with antiarrhythmic agents (phenytoin, propranolol).

10. **Atrioventricular Block**

First-degree AV block (prolongation of PR interval) may be benign, although it may be a sign of digitalis toxicity, congenital heart defect (ECD, ASD, and Ebstein's anomaly), or metabolic abnormalities.

Second-degree AV block is a sign of digitalis toxicity until proved otherwise.

Third-degree AV block (complete heart block) is due to a structural defect in the conduction system, usually above the bifurcation of the His bundle. Therefore, the QRS duration is not prolonged. About one-third of the cases are associated with CHD and may result in CHF, requiring pacemaker therapy. When not associated with CHD, treatment is usually not indicated, and prognosis is good. There is frequent association of maternal lupus erythematosus or mixed connective tissue disease with congenital complete heart block in the offspring.

PART VIII

Special Problems

In this section some common pediatric cardiac problems not discussed in previous chapters are examined. The topics include congestive heart failure, systemic hypertension, pulmonary hypertension, hyperlipidemia, child with chest pain or syncope, and postoperative syndromes.

27 / Congestive Heart Failure

Definition

Congestive heart failure (CHF) is a clinical syndrome in which the heart is unable either to pump enough blood to the body to meet its needs or to dispose of venous return adequately or a combination of the two.

Etiology

CHF may result from congenital or acquired heart diseases with volume and/or pressure overload or from myocardial insufficiency.

1. *Congenital heart disease* (CHD) with volume or pressure overload is the most common cause of CHF in the pediatric age group. Volume overload lesions such as VSD, PDA, and ECD are the most common cause of CHF in the first 6 months of life. The time of onset of CHF varies rather predictably with the type of the defect. Table 27–1 lists common CHDs according to the age at which CHF develops. A few important comments need to be made in relation to Table 27–1.

   a. Children with tetralogy of Fallot do not develop CHF unless they have received a large aorta–pulmonary artery shunt procedure (such as Waterston's or Potts' operation).

   b. ASD rarely causes CHF in the pediatric age group, although it causes CHF in adulthood.

   c. Large left-to-right shunt lesions, such as VSD and PDA, do not cause CHF before 6–8 weeks of age. This is due to the fact that the PVR does not fall low enough to cause a large left-to-right shunt until this age. The onset of CHF from left-to-right shunt lesions may be earlier in premature infants (within the first month) because of an earlier fall in the PVR in these infants.

2. *Acquired heart disease*, notably acute rheumatic carditis and rheumatic heart disease, can cause CHF. Rheumatic myocarditis associated with acute rheumatic fever occurs primarily in school-aged children. Rheumatic heart diseases, usually volume overload lesions such as mitral or aortic regurgitation, cause CHF in older children and adults.

3. *Myocardial dysfunction* of various etiologies can cause CHF at any age. The age at onset of CHF secondary to myocardial dysfunction is not as predictable as that of CHD, but the following generalizations can be made:

   a. Endocardial fibroelastosis (EFE), a rare primary myocardial disease, causes CHF in infancy (90% of the cases occur in the first 8 months of life).

   b. Viral myocarditis tends to be more common in small children, older than 1 year of age. It occurs occasionally in the newborn period, with a fulminating clinical course.

309

TABLE 27–1.

Causes of Congestive Heart Failure Due to Congenital Heart Disease According to Age

At birth	a. Hypoplastic left heart syndrome (HLHS)
	b. Volume overload lesions:
	Severe tricuspid or pulmonary insufficiency
	Large systemic AV fistula
First week	a. Transposition of the great arteries (TGA)
	b. PDA in small premature infants
	c. HLHS (with more favorable anatomy)
	d. TAPVR, particularly those with pulmonary venous obstruction
	e. Others:
	Systemic AV fistula
	Critical AS or PS
1–4 wk	a. Coarctation of the aorta (preductal, with associated anomalies)
	b. Critical aortic stenosis
	c. Large left-to-right shunt lesions (VSD, PDA) in premature infants
	d. All other lesions listed above
4–6 wk	Some left-to-right shunt lesions such as endocardial cushion defect
6 wk–4 mo	a. Large VSD
	b. Large PDA
	c. Others such as anomalous left coronary artery from the pulmonary artery

    c. Anomalous origin of the left coronary artery from the pulmonary artery (resulting in myocardial infarction) causes CHF around 2–3 months of age.

    d. Metabolic abnormalities (severe hypoxia and acidosis as well as hypoglycemia and hypocalcemia) may cause CHF in newborn infants.

    e. Congestive cardiomyopathies and other cardiomyopathies associated with muscular dystrophy and Friedreich's ataxia may cause CHF in older children and adolescents.

4. *Miscellaneous causes:*

    a. Paroxysmal atrial tachycardia (PAT) causes CHF usually in early infancy.

    b. Complete heart block associated with other structural heart defects causes CHF in the newborn period or early infancy.

    c. Severe anemia may be a cause of CHF at any age; hydrops fetalis in the newborn period, and severe sicklemia at a later age.

    d. Acute hypertension as seen in acute glomerulonephritis causes CHF in school-aged children. Fluid overload is more critical with poor renal function.

    e. Bronchopulmonary dysplasia seen in prematurely born infants causes predominantly right heart failure in the first few months of life.

    f. Acute cor pulmonale may cause CHF at any age, but more commonly during early childhood.

Clinical Manifestations

The diagnosis of CHF relies on several sources of clinical findings, including history, physical examination, and chest x-rays. In addition to physical findings to be discussed below, cardiomegaly on a chest film is almost necessary for the diagnosis of CHF; an ECG is perhaps the least important. It should be emphasized that no single test is specific for CHF; it is a clinical diagnosis based on clinical judgment.

History

The following histories are suggestive of CHF: (1) poor feeding of recent onset, (2) tachypnea which worsens during feeding, (3) poor weight gain, and (4) cold sweat on the forehead.

PE

Physical findings of CHF may be classified as follows depending on their pathophysiologic mechanisms. The more common findings are in italic.

   a. Compensatory response to impaired cardiac function:

     1) *Tachycardia, gallop rhythm,* weak and thready pulse.

     2) *Cardiomegaly* is almost always present. Chest x-rays are more reliable than physical examination in demonstrating cardiomegaly.

     3) Increased sympathetic discharges (*growth failure, perspiration,* cold wet skin, etc.).

   b. Pulmonary venous congestion (left-sided failure):

     1) *Tachypnea.*

     2) Dyspnea on exertion (*poor feeding* in small infants).

     3) Orthopnea in older children.

     4) Wheezing and pulmonary *rales.*

   c. Systemic venous congestion (right-sided failure):

     1) *Hepatomegaly.* It is not always indicative of CHF; a large liver may be palpable in the absence of CHF, such as in conditions with hyperinflated lungs (asthma, bronchiolitis, hypoxic spell) and infiltrative liver disease. On the other hand, the absence of hepatomegaly does not rule out CHF; hepatomegaly may be absent in (early) left-sided failure.

     2) *Puffy eyelids.*

     3) Distended neck veins and ankle edema, which are common in adults, are not seen in infants.

     4) Splenomegaly is not indicative of chronic CHF, but usually indicates infection.

X-Ray

It is important to demonstrate the presence of cardiomegaly by chest x-rays. The absence of cardiomegaly almost rules out the diagnosis of CHF. However, the presence of cardiomegaly per se does not mean CHF is present, as many infants with large left-to-right shunt lesions have cardiomegaly without heart failure.

ECG

ECGs are helpful in determining the type of the defects, but are not very helpful in deciding whether CHF is present.

ECHO

ECHO may confirm the presence of chamber enlargement or impaired LV function (decreased fractional shortening or ejection fraction, increased LPEP/

LVET). A more important role of ECHO may be its capability to determine the cause of CHF. ECHO is also useful in serial evaluation of the efficacy of therapy.

Management

1. General Measures

a. "Cardiac chair" or "infant seat" to relieve respiratory distress.

b. Oxygen (40%–50%) with humidity in infants with respiratory distress.

c. Sedation with morphine sulfate (0.1–0.2 mg/kg/dose SC every 4 hours prn) or phenobarbital (2–3 mg/kg/dose PO or IM every 8 hours prn) for 1–2 days is occasionally indicated.

d. Salt restriction in the form of a low-salt formula and severe fluid restriction are not indicated in infants. Use of a diuretic has replaced these measures. In older children, salt restriction (less than 0.5 gm/day) and avoidance of salty snacks (chips, pretzels) and table salt are recommended.

e. Daily weight measurement is essential in hospitalized patients.

f. Elimination of predisposing factors, such as fever (reduction of fever), anemia (packed cell transfusion to raise hematocrit to 35% or higher), and infection.

g. Treatment of underlying causes such as hypertension (see chap. 28), arrhythmias (see chap. 23), or thyrotoxicosis.

2. Drug Therapy

Every child with CHF should be given digitalis unless its use is contraindicated (HOCM [or IHSS], complete heart block, or cardiac tamponade). Diuretics are almost always used in conjunction with digitalis.

a. Diuretics
Patients with CHF may improve rapidly after a dose of a fast-acting diuretic, such as ethacrynic acid or furosemide, even before digitalization. Table 27–2 shows dosages of commonly available diuretic preparations.

1) Types of diuretics and their dosages (see Table 27–2): Three major classes of diuretics are commercially available.

a) Thiazide diuretics (chlorothiazide, hydrochlorothiazide) which act at the proximal and distal tubules are less popular.

b) Furosemide and ethacrynic acid ("loop diuretics") which act primarily at the loop of Henle are probably the drug of choice.

c) Aldosterone antagonists (such as spironolactone) are indicated in the treatment of the hyperaldosteronism component of CHF. In addition, these drugs have value in preventing hypokalemia produced by other diuretics.

2) Side effects of diuretic therapy:
Diuretic therapy may produce alterations in the serum electrolyte balance and acid-base equilibrium.

a) Hypokalemia is a common problem with diuretic therapy (except Aldactone). It is more profound with potent loop diuretics. Hypokalemia may increase the likelihood of digitalis toxicity.

TABLE 27–2.

Diuretic Agents and Dosages

Preparation	Route	Dosage
Thiazide diuretics		
Chlorothiazide (Diuril)	Oral	20–40 mg/kg/day in 2–3 divided doses
Hydrochlorothiazide (HydroDiuril)	Oral	2–4 mg/kg/day in 2–3 divided doses
Loop diuretics		
Furosemide	IV	1 mg/kg/dose
(Lasix)	Oral	2–3 mg/kg/day in 2–3 divided doses
Ethacrynic acid	IV	1 mg/kg/dose
(Edecrin)	Oral	2–3 mg/kg/day in 2–3 divided doses
Aldosterone antagonist		
Spironolactone (Aldactone)	Oral	2–3 mg/kg/day in 2–3 divided doses

   b) Hypochloremic alkalosis: There is a greater loss of chloride than sodium ion through the kidneys, with resultant increase in bicarbonate. Alkalosis also predisposes to digitalis toxicity.

b. Digitalis Glycosides

   1) Digitalis dosage:
   Digoxin is the most commonly used digitalis preparation in pediatric patients. The total digitalizing dose (TDD) and maintenance doses of digoxin by oral (and IV) routes are shown in Table 27–3. (Dosage of digitoxin appears in the Appendix).

   2) How to digitalize:
   Loading doses of the TDD are given in 12 to 18 hours. This results in a pharmacokinetic steady state in 3–5 days. An IV route is preferred over the oral route, particularly when dealing with infants in severe heart failure. An IM route is not recommended, as absorption of the drug from the injection site is unreliable. When an infant is in mild heart failure, the maintenance dose may be administered orally, without loading doses; this results in a steady state in 5–8 days.

TABLE 27–3.

Digoxin Dosage (Oral)

	TDD*† (μg/kg)	Maintenance†‡ (μg/kg/day)
Prematures	20	5
Newborns	30	8
Under 2 yr	40–50	10–12
Over 2 yr	30–40	8–10

*TDD = total digitalizing dose.
†IV dose is 75% of the oral dose.
‡Maintenance dose is 25% of the TDD in 2 divided doses.

3) The following is a suggested step-by-step method of digitalization:

   a) Obtain a baseline ECG (rhythm and PR interval) and baseline levels of serum electrolytes. Changes in ECG rhythm and PR interval are important signs of digitalis toxicity (see below). Hypokalemia and hypercalcemia predispose to digitoxicity.

   b) Calculate the TDD (see Table 27–3). Two persons should calculate the TDD independently and compare findings, since a common mistake is in the magnitude of a decimal point.

   c) Give ½ TDD stat, followed by ¼ and the final ¼ of the TDD at 6–8-hour intervals.

   d) Obtain an ECG strip before the final ¼ TDD, and give the final ¼ TDD if no ECG signs of toxicity are present.

   e) Start the maintenance dose 12 hours after the final TDD. Obtain another ECG strip before starting the maintenance dose.

4) Monitoring for digitalis toxicity
   Detection of digitalis toxicity is best accomplished by ECG monitoring. Table 27–4 lists ECG signs of digitalis effect and toxicity. In general, digitalis effect is confined to *ventricular repolarization,* whereas toxicity involves disturbances in the *formation and conduction of the impulse.* A sound rule is to assume that any arrhythmia or conduction disturbance occurring *with* digitalis is *caused* by digitalis until proved otherwise. Whether the patient is "fully" digitalized is a clinical decision and cannot be answered by ECG tracings or by serum digoxin level determinations. Routine determination of serum digoxin levels and use of those levels for therapeutic goals are not wise and not recommended.

5) Digitalis toxicity
   With the relatively low dosage recommended in Table 27–3 and with careful monitoring of the ECG, digitalis toxicity is unlikely. However, the possibility of digitalis toxicity should be kept in mind for every child receiving digitalis preparations. An accidental ingestion of digoxin is not uncommon among toddlers.

TABLE 27–4.
ECG Changes Associated With Digitalis

Effects
Shortening of QTc, the earliest sign of digitalis effect
Sagging ST segment and diminished amplitude of T wave (the T vector does not change)
Slowing of heart rate
Toxicity
Prolongation of PR interval
Some normal children have prolonged PR interval making it mandatory to obtain a baseline ECG. The prolongation may progress to second-degree AV block.
Profound sinus bradycardia or sinoatrial block
Supraventricular arrhythmias, such as atrial or nodal ectopic beats and tachycardias (particularly if accompanied by AV block) are more common than ventricular arrhythmias in children.
Ventricular arrhythmias such as ventricular bigeminy or trigeminy are extremely rare in children, although they are common in adults with digitalis toxicity. Ventricular premature beats are not uncommon in children as a sign of toxicity.

Diagnosis of digitalis toxicity, again, is a clinical decision and is usually based on the following clinical and laboratory findings:

a) History of accidental ingestion.

b) Noncardiac symptoms in digitalized children: anorexia, nausea, vomiting, or diarrhea, restlessness, drowsiness, fatigue, and visual disturbances in older children.

c) Worsening of heart failure.

d) ECG signs are probably more reliable and appear early (see Table 27–4).

e) Serum digoxin levels: Determination of serum digoxin level is helpful in evaluation of possible toxicity, and it is definitely indicated in case of accidental overdose. An elevated serum level, greater than 2 ng/ml, is likely to be associated with toxicity in a child if the clinical findings are suggestive of digitalis toxicity. However, a lower serum level does not rule out the toxicity, and a higher level does not necessarily indicate digitalis toxicity.

Patients with any of the conditions listed in Table 27–5 are more likely to develop toxicity. It is important to understand these factors in the prevention and management of the toxicity.

When the diagnosis of digitalis toxicity is established, take the following measures:

a) General therapy include discontinuation of digitalis, discontinuation of diuretics, unless absolutely indicated, and continuous ECG monitoring. Do not give glucose without K^+. Evaluate predisposing factors (see Table 27–5) and eliminate or treat these factors.

b) Specific therapy:

(1) For frequent premature beats or supraventricular arrhythmias, administer KCl. It counteracts arrhythmia-producing effects of digi-

TABLE 27–5.

Factors That May Predispose to Digitalis Toxicity

High serum digoxin level
  High-dose requirement as in treatment of certain arrhythmias
  Decreased renal excretion
    Premature infants
    Renal disease
  Hypothyroidism
  Drug interaction (e.g., quinidine, verapamil, amiodarone)
Increased sensitivity of myocardium (without high serum digoxin level)
  Status of myocardium
    Myocardial ischemia
    Myocarditis (rheumatic, viral)
  Systemic changes
    Electrolyte imbalance (hypokalemia, hypercalcemia)
    Hypoxia
    Alkalosis
    Adrenergic stimuli or catecholamines
    Immediate postoperative period after heart surgery under cardiopulmonary bypass

talis without depressing myocardial contractility. Contraindications for the use of KCl include advanced heart block (second- and third-degree AV block), hyperkalemia, and anuria or oliguria. Dose: Oral KCl, 3–5 gm/day, diluted in chilled fruit juice. IV KCl, 0.5 mEq/kg/hour, IV drip until arrhythmias disappear or peaked T waves appear (maximum 3 mEq/kg/day).

(2) For tachyarrhythmias:
Lidocaine: 1 mg/kg IV bolus, followed by IV drip or 1–3 mg/kg/hour (maximum total dose = 5 mg/kg).
Phenytoin (Dilantin): 3–5 mg/kg show IV push, repeat in 10–15 min prn (maximum total dose = 500 mg in 4 hours).
Propranolol: 0.01 mg/kg, slow IV push q 2 min (maximum 0.1 mg/kg), followed by 1–4 mg/kg/day, PO, in 3–4 doses.
Cardioversion: Only if unresponsive to other measures. Start at 0.5 w-sec/kg, and increase by a small increment.

(3) For heart block:
Atropine: 0.01–0.03 mg/kg every 4–6 hours, prn (maximum 0.4 mg/kg).
Transvenous catheter pacing is usually indicated.

(4) Digoxin antibody (Digibind) has successfully been used in children.

c. Other Inotropic Agents
In infants with severe distress or those with renal dysfunction such as seen with infantile COA, rapidly acting catecholamines with short duration of action may be preferable to digoxin. Suggested dosages for IV drips are as follows:

1) Dopamine, 5–10 μg/kg/min.

2) Isoproterenol, 0.1–0.5 μg/kg/min.

3) Dobutamine, 5–8 μg/kg/min.

d. Afterload Reducing Agents
These agents reduce systemic vascular resistance and improve cardiac output, usually without changes in the contractile state of the myocardium. They are used in conjunction with digitalis and diuretics. Indications for vasodilator therapy include (a) cardiomyopathy, (b) myocardial ischemia, (c) postoperative cardiac patients, (d) severe MR or AR, and (e) systemic hypertension. Depending on the site of action, they may be divided into three groups: venodilator, arteriolar vasodilator, and mixed vasodilator. Dosages of these agents are presented in Table 27–6.

1) Venodilators (nitroglycerin, nitrates) act predominantly by dilating systemic veins. These agents are useful in patients with elevated ventricular filling pressure (such as seen with MS or AR); they reduce venous congestion, thereby improve pulmonary edema, but may not increase cardiac output.

2) Arteriolar vasodilators (hydralazine, captopril) act primarily by dilating the arteriolar bed. Hydralazine, the most commonly used arteriolar vasodilator, is often administered with propranolol because it activates the baroreceptor reflex with resulting tachycardia. Captopril (inhibitor of angiotensin-converting enzyme) reduces systemic vascular resistance by in-

TABLE 27–6.

Afterload Reducing Agents and Dosages

Drugs	Dosage and Route	Comments
Nitroglycerin	0.5–20 μg/kg/min IV drip (max 60 μg/kg/min IV)	Start with a small dose and titrate effects
Hydralazine (Apresoline)	0.5 mg/kg/day PO q6–8h (max 200 mg/day or 7.0 mg/kg/day PO) 1.5 μg/kg/min IV drip or 0.1–0.5 μg/kg IV q6h (max 2 mg/kg IV q 6h)	May cause tachycardia; may use with propranolol GI symptoms, neutropenia, lupus-like syndrome
Captopril (Capoten)	Neonates: 0.1–0.4 mg/kg/dose, PO q 6–24h Infants: 0.5–6.0 mg/kg/day PO q6–24h Children: 12.5 mg/dose PO q12–24h	May cause neutropenia, proteinuria Reduce dose in patients with impaired renal function
Nitroprusside (Nipride)	0.5–8 μg/kg/min IV drip	May cause thiocyanate or cyanide toxicity (fatigue, nausea, disorientation, etc.) Hepatic dysfunction Light sensitive
Prazosine (Minipress)	First dose: 5 μg/kg PO Increase up to 25 μg/kg/dose PO q6h	Fewer side effects (tachycardia) than hydralazine Orthostatic hypotension Tachyphylaxis may occur

hibition of angiotensin II generation and also by augmented production of bradykinin.

3) Mixed vasodilators (nitroprusside, prazosin) act on both arteriolar and venous beds. Nitroprusside is frequently used in postoperative cardiac patients, especially those who had pulmonary hypertension and those with postoperative rise in PA pressure. It is frequently used with dopamine or dobutamine. Continuous BP monitoring is necessary. Prazosin, a postsynaptic α-adrenergic blocking agent, produces far fewer side effects (tachycardia) than does hydralazine.

3. Surgical Management

If medical treatment with the above-mentioned regimen is not successful in treatment of CHF, specific palliative or corrective cardiac surgery for the underlying cardiac defect should be performed.

28 / Systemic Hypertension

Definition

Hypertension in children may be defined statistically as the presence of systolic and/or diastolic pressure levels greater than the 95th percentile for age and sex on at least three occasions. High normal blood pressure (BP) is defined as average systolic and/or diastolic BP between the 90th and 95th percentiles for age and sex. Values slightly above the 95th percentile may be considered significant hypertension, and values greater than the 95th percentile by 8–10 mm Hg may be considered severe hypertension. A prerequisite for these definitions is the availability of reliable normal BP values (see Tables 2–2 and 2–3). For adults, the World Health Organization has defined values of 140–150/90–95 mm Hg as borderline hypertension and values above 160/95 mm Hg as hypertension.

Etiology

Hypertension is classified into two general groups: essential (or primary) hypertension, in which a specific etiology cannot be identified, and secondary hypertension, in which a cause can be identified (Table 28–1). The incidence of essential hypertension in children is not known. However, over 90% of secondary hypertension in children is caused by three conditions: renal parenchymal disease, renal artery disease, and coarctation of the aorta (COA).

Table 28–2 lists the common causes of hypertension by age group in children. In general, the younger the child and the more severe the hypertension, the more likely one is to identify an underlying cause.

Diagnosis and Work-Up

Many children with mild hypertension are asymptomatic, and hypertension is diagnosed as the result of routine blood pressure measurement. Children with severe hypertension may be symptomatic (headache, dizziness, nausea and vomiting, irritability, personality changes). Occasionally, neurologic manifestations, CHF, renal dysfunction, and stroke may be the presenting symptoms.

Careful evaluation of history, physical findings, and simple laboratory tests usually point to the cause of hypertension.

1. History

Important past and present medical history and family history are as follows:

a. Past and current history:

1) Neonatal—use of umbilical artery catheters.

2) Cardiovascular—history of COA or surgery for it. History of palpitation, headache, and excessive sweating (excessive catecholamines).

3) Renal—history of obstructive uropathies, urinary tract infection, radiation, trauma, or surgery to the kidney area.

4) Endocrine—weakness and muscle cramp (hyperaldosteronism).

318

TABLE 28–1.

Causes of Hypertension

Primary (or essential) hypertension
Secondary hypertension
  Renal
    Renal parenchymal disease
      Glomerulonephritis, acute and chronic
      Pyelonephritis, acute and chronic
      Congenital anomalies (polycystic or dysplastic kidneys)
      Obstructive uropathies (hydronephrosis)
      Hemolytic-uremic syndrome
      Collagen disease (periarteritis, lupus)
      Renal damage from nephrotoxic medications, trauma, or radiation
    Renovascular diseases
      Renal artery disorders (stenosis, polyarteritis, thrombosis, etc.)
      Renal vein thrombosis
  Cardiovascular
    Coarctation of the aorta
    Conditions with large stroke volume (PDA, aortic insufficiency, systemic AV fistula, complete heart block) (these conditions cause only systolic hypertension)
  Endocrine
    Hyperthyroidism (systolic hypertension)
    Excessive catecholamines
      Pheochromocytoma
      Neuroblastoma
    Adrenal dysfunction
      Congenital adrenal hyperplasia
        11-β-hydroxylase deficiency
        17-hydroxylase deficiency
      Cushing's syndrome
      Hyperaldosteronism
        Primary
          Conn's syndrome
          Idiopathic nodular hyperplasia
          Dexamethasone-suppressible hyperaldosteronism
        Secondary
          Renovascular hypertension
          Renin-producing tumor (juxtaglomerular cell tumor)
    Hyperparathyroidism (and hypercalcemia)
  Neurogenic
    Increased intracranial pressure (any cause, especially tumors, infections, trauma)
    Poliomyelitis
    Guillain-Barré syndrome
    Dysautonomia (Riley-Day syndrome)
  Drugs and chemicals
    Sympathomimetic drugs (nose drops, cough medications, cold preparations)
    Amphetamines
    Steroids
    Oral contraceptives
    Heavy-metal poisoning (mercury, lead)
  Miscellaneous
    Hypervolemia and hypernatremia
    Stevens-Johnson syndrome

TABLE 28–2.

Most Common Causes by Age Group of Chronic Sustained Hypertension
in Pediatric Population*

Newborns:	Renal artery thrombosis, renal artery stenosis, congenital renal malformation, coarctation of the aorta, bronchopulmonary dysplasia
<6 yr:	Renal parenchymal disease, coarctation of the aorta, renal artery stenosis
6–10 yr:	Renal artery stenosis, renal parenchymal disease, primary hypertension
>10 yr:	Primary hypertension, renal parenchymal disease

*Adapted from the NIH Task Force (1987).

5) Medications—corticosteroids, amphetamines, antiasthmatic drugs, cold medications, oral contraceptives, nephrotoxic antibiotics.

6) Habits—smoking.

b. Family history:

1) Essential hypertension, atherosclerotic heart disease, and stroke.

2) Familial or hereditary renal disease (polycystic kidney, cystinuria, familial nephritis).

2. **Physical Examination**

a. Accurate measurement of blood pressure is essential.

b. Complete physical examination is also essential with emphasis on: delayed growth (renal disease), bounding peripheral pulse (PDA or aortic regurgitation), weak or absent femoral pulses (COA), abdominal bruits (renovascular), and tenderness of the kidney (renal infection).

3. **Routine Laboratory Tests**
Initial laboratory tests should be directed toward detecting renal parenchymal disease, renovascular disease, and COA, and therefore should include: urinalysis, urine culture, serum electrolytes, BUN, or creatinine, uric acid, ECG, chest x-rays, and possibly ECHO.

4. **More Extensive Studies**
More extensive studies may be indicated for detection of rare causes of secondary hypertension: excretory urography, plasma renin activity (PRA), aldosterone levels in serum and urine, 24-hour urine collection for catecholamines (norepinephrine, epinephrine) and their metabolites (vanillylmandelic acid [VMA]), renal vein renin, and abdominal aortogram.

Table 28–3 summarizes usefulness of the routine and more involved tests in identifying the cause of secondary hypertension. The decision to undertake special tests and procedures depends on the availability and familiarity with the procedure, severity of hypertension, the age of the patient, and history and physical findings suggestive of certain etiology. For example, children under 10 years of age with sustained hypertension require extensive evaluation, since identifiable and potentially curable causes are likely to be found. Adolescents with mild hypertension and positive family history of essential hypertension are more likely to have essential hypertension, and extensive studies are not indicated.

TABLE 28–3.

Routine and Special Laboratory Tests and Their Significance

Laboratory Tests	Significance of Abnormal Results
Urinalysis, urine culture, BUN, creatinine	Renal parenchymal disease
Serum electrolytes (hypokalemia)	Hyperaldosteronism, primary or secondary Adrenogenital syndrome Renin-producing tumors
ECG, chest x-rays	Cardiac cause of hypertension, also baseline function
Intravenous pyelography (or ultrasonography, radionuclide studies, CT of the kidneys)	Renal parenchymal diseases Renovascular hypertension Tumors (neuroblastoma, Wilms' tumor)

Plasma renin activity (PRA), peripheral	High-renin hypertension
	  Renovascular hypertension
	  Renin-producing tumors
	  Some Cushing's syndrome
	  Some essential hypertension
	Low-renin hypertension
	  Adrenogenital syndrome
	  Primary hyperaldosteronism

24-hr urine collection for 17-KS and 17-OHCS	Cushing's syndrome Adrenogenital syndrome
24-hr urine collection for catecholamines and VMA	Pheochromocytoma Neuroblastoma
Aldosterone	Hyperaldosteronism, primary or secondary Renovascular hypertension Renin-producing tumors
Renal vein PRA	Unilateral renal parenchymal disease Renovascular hypertension
Abdominal aortogram	Renovascular hypertension Abdominal coarctation of aorta Unilateral renal parenchymal diseases Pheochromocytoma

Management

1. Essential Hypertension

a. Nonpharmacologic intervention can be introduced as initial treatment. Counseling should be aimed at advice on weight reduction, if indicated, low-salt (and potassium-rich) foods, encouragement to be physically active and fit, and advice to avoid smoking and the use of oral contraceptives.

b. Drug Therapy:
Although there are no clear guidelines as to who should be treated with antihypertensive drugs, family history of early complications of hypertension, the presence of target organ damage (ocular, cardiac, renal, CNS, etc.), and the presence of other coronary artery risk factors favor drug therapy. However, possible adverse effects of long-term drug therapy on growing children have not been evaluated adequately.

The stepped-care approach is popular. Step 1 is initiated with a small dose of a single antihypertensive drug, either thiazide diuretic or an adrenergic inhibitor, and then proceeds to full dose, if necessary. In black, diabetic, or asthmatic patients, the diuretic is suggested as first-step therapy. (A β-adrenergic blocker may be contraindicated in diabetics and asthmatics; the diuretic works well in adult black patients.) In adolescents with a hyperdynamic-type hypertension (with a rapid pulse) or those associated with hyperthyroidism, a β-blocker is preferable. If the first drug is not effective, a second drug may be added to or substituted for the first drug, starting with a small dose and proceeding to full dose (step 2). If BP still remains elevated, a third drug, such as a vasodilator, may be added to the regimen (step 3). At this point, the possibility of a cause of secondary hypertension should be reconsidered. Table 28–4 shows the dosage of commonly used antihypertensive drugs for children.

1) Diuretics:

Diuretics are the cornerstone of antihypertensive drug therapy, except in patients with renal failure. Their action is related to a decrease in extracellular and plasma volume. The thiazide diuretics (hydrochlorothiazide and chlorothalidone) are most commonly used. The only important side effect of diuretic therapy in children is hypokalemia, occasionally requiring potassium supplementation in the diet or potassium salt.

2) Adrenergic Inhibitors:

If diuretics produce no clinical improvement at the maximum dose and over a sufficient length of time, a sympathetic inhibitor (propranolol, methyldopa, or reserpine) should be added to or substituted for the diuretic.

a) Propranolol (Inderal), a β-adrenergic blocker, acts at three important locations: on the juxtaglomerular apparatus of the kidney to suppress

TABLE 28–4.

Recommended Oral Dosages of Selected Antihypertensive Drugs for Children*

Drugs	Dose (mg/kg)	Times/day
Diuretics		
Hydrochlorothiazide	1–2	2
Chlorothiazide (Diuril)	0.5–2	1
Furosemide (Lasix)	0.5–2	2
Spironolactone (Aldactone)	1–2	2
Adrenergic inhibitors		
Propranolol (Inderal)	1–3	3
Methyldopa (Aldomet)	5–10	2
Vasodilators		
Hydralazine (Apresoline)	1–5	2–3
Minoxidil (Loniten)	0.1–1	2
Enzyme blockers		
Captopril (Capoten)		
<6 mo	0.05–0.5	3
>6 mo	0.5–2.0	3

*Modified from the NIH Task Force (1987).

the renin-angiotensin system, on the central vasomotor center to decrease systemic vascular resistance, and on the myocardium to suppress contractility. Adequacy of β-adrenergic blockade can be judged by suppression of the increase in heart rate when the patient stands up after a few minutes of recumbency. Propranolol is contraindicated in patients with CHF or asthma.

b) Methyldopa (Aldomet) appears to act by the reduction of systemic vascular resistance by direct action on the arterioles and its influence on the central vasomotor center rather than by forming a "false transmitter." The major adverse reaction is sedation occurring in the early stage of therapy. Other side effects include positive Coombs tests, lupus-like reaction, hepatitis, and colitis.

3) Vasodilators:

If a diuretic and/or a sympathetic inhibitor produce no clinical improvement, a vasodilator agent should be added. Vasodilators act directly on vascular smooth muscle to reduce vascular resistance.

Hydralazine (Apresoline) is the drug of choice in children. When used alone, it produces side effects related to increased cardiac output (flushing, headache, tachycardia, and palpitation) and salt and water retention. Therefore, the concomitant use of a β-adrenergic blocker and a diuretic is recommended. Minoxidil is a less commonly used vasodilator.

4) Specific Enzyme Blockers:

Captopril is an inhibitor of the angiotensin I-converting enzyme. An important side effect is postural hypotension.

2. Secondary Hypertension

Treatment of secondary hypertension should be aimed at removing the cause of hypertension whenever possible. Table 28–5 lists curable causes of systemic hypertension.

a. Renal parenchymal disease:

In nephritides, medical management should be instituted to lower blood pressure in the same manner as has been discussed for essential hypertension. Salt restriction, avoidance of excessive fluid intake, and antihypertensive drug therapy can control hypertension caused by most renal parenchymal diseases. Concomitant antibiotic therapy for infectious processes and

TABLE 28–5.

Curable Forms of Hypertension

Renal	Unilateral kidney disease (pyelonephritis, hydronephrosis, traumatic damage, radiation nephritis, hypoplastic kidney)
	Wilms' and other kidney tumors
Cardiovascular	Coarctation of the aorta
	Renal artery abnormalities (stenosis, aneurysm, fibromuscular dysplasia, thrombosis, etc.)
Adrenal	Pheochromocytoma and neuroblastoma
	Adrenogenital syndrome
	Cushing's syndrome
	Primary aldosteronism
Miscellaneous	Glucocorticoid therapy
	Oral contraceptives

general supportive measures may be indicated depending on the nature of renal disease. If hypertension is difficult to control and the disease is unilateral, unilateral nephrectomy may be considered.

  b. Surgical treatment:
  Renovascular disease may be cured by successful surgery, such as reconstruction of a stenotic renal artery, autotransplantation, or unilateral nephrectomy. Hypertension caused by tumors such as pheochromocytoma, neuroblastoma, and juxtaglomerular cell tumor that secrete vasoactive substances are treated primarily by surgery.

Hypertensive Crisis

A hypertensive emergency is present when a patient has any of the following features.

  a. Severe hypertension (greater than 180 mm Hg systolic or 110 mm Hg diastolic) or rapidly increasing blood pressures.

  b. Neurologic signs (hypertensive encephalopathy) with severe headache, vomiting, irritability, or apathy, seizures, papilledema, retinal hemorrhage, or exudate.

  c. Congestive heart failure or pulmonary edema.

Aggressive parenteral administration of antihypertensive drugs is indicated to lower blood pressure.

  a. Diazoxide (Hyperstat), 3–5 mg/kg as an IV bolus, or nitroprusside (Nipride), 1–3 µg/kg/min as an IV drip, is the treatment of choice.

  b. If hypertension is less severe, hydralazine (Apresoline), 0.15 mg/kg IV or IM, may be used. The onset of action is 10 minutes following an IV dose and 20–30 minutes following an IM dose. The dose may be repeated at a 4–6-hour interval.

  c. A rapid-acting diuretic, such as furosemide (1 mg/kg), is given IV to initiate diuresis.

  d. Fluid balance must be controlled carefully, so that intake is limited to urine output plus insensible loss.

  e. Seizures may be treated with slow IV infusion of diazepam (Valium), 0.2 mg/kg, or other anticonvulsant medication.

  f. When a hypertensive crisis is under control, oral medications will replace the parenteral medications (see Table 28–4 for oral dosages of antihypertensive drugs).

29 / Pulmonary Hypertension

Etiology

Pulmonary hypertension refers to a condition in which systolic and/or diastolic pressures in the pulmonary artery are increased. It is actually a group of conditions with multiple etiologies rather than a single entity. Therefore, pathogenesis and management are different among different entities. Table 29–1 lists conditions that give rise to pulmonary hypertension of either temporary or permanent nature, according to their pathogeneses. Four major causes of pulmonary hypertension are increased pulmonary blood flow, alveolar hypoxia, increased pulmonary venous pressure, and primary pulmonary vascular disease. Some oversimplification was inevitable in presenting this diverse group into four categories.

The term "cor pulmonale" is used to describe right ventricular hypertrophy and/or dilatation secondary to pulmonary hypertension caused by diseases of the lung parenchyma or pulmonary vasculature (including pulmonary veins). It does not include nonpulmonary causes of right ventricular dysfunction, such as mitral stenosis or LV failure.

Pathogenesis

Since pressure (P) is related to both flow (F) and vascular resistance (R), as shown in the formula:

$$P \propto F \times R$$

an increase in flow, an increase in vascular resistance, or a combination of both can result in pulmonary hypertension. Regardless of etiology, pulmonary hypertension eventually involves constriction of pulmonary arterioles with resulting increase in pulmonary vascular resistance (PVR).

Pulmonary hypertension associated with large left-to-right shunt lesions such as VSD and PDA (called "hyperkinetic" pulmonary hypertension) derives from a combination of an increase in flow, direct transmission of the systemic pressure into the pulmonary artery, and an increase in PVR by vasoconstriction. If there were no vasoconstriction, intractable CHF would result. Hyperkinetic pulmonary hypertension is usually reversible if the cause is eliminated before permanent changes take place in the pulmonary arterioles.

The lung is not just an organ of respiration; it is an active metabolic and endocrine organ. It synthesizes alveolar surfactant and selectively handles circulating vasoactive hormones. Certain vasoactive hormones (such as angiotensin I) are activated, and others (such as bradykinin, serotonin, and some prostaglandins) are inactivated by the lung. Synthesis and release of biologically active substances in the lung can be provoked by a number of physiologic and pathologic stimuli. It is well known that a reduction in PO_2 in the alveolar capillary region (alveolar hypoxia), either acute or chronic, elicits a pulmonary vasoconstrictor response. There is, however, a marked species and individual variation in the degree of response. Exact mechanism(s) of the pulmonary vasoconstrictor response is poorly understood. It may be caused by direct effects of reduced PO_2 on the

TABLE 29–1.

Causes of Pulmonary Hypertension

Large left-to-right shunt lesions ("hyperkinetic" pulmonary hypertension): VSD, PDA,
  ECD, etc.
Alveolar hypoxia
  Pulmonary parenchymal disease
    Extensive pneumonia
    Hypoplasia of lungs (primary or secondary such as seen in diaphragmatic hernia)
    Bronchopulmonary dysplasia (BPD)
    Interstitial lung disease (Hammon-Rich syndrome)
    Wilson-Mikity syndrome
  Airway obstruction
    Upper airway obstruction (large tonsils, macroglossia,
      micrognathia, laryngotracheomalacia)
    Lower airway obstruction (bronchial asthma, cystic fibrosis)
  Inadequate ventilatory drive (CNS diseases)
  Disorders of chest wall or respiratory muscles
    Kyphoscoliosis
    Weakening or paralysis of skeletal muscle
  High altitude (in certain hyperreactors)
Pulmonary venous hypertension
  Mitral stenosis, cor triatriatum, TAPVR with obstruction, chronic heart failure, left-
    sided obstructive lesions (AS, COA)
Primary pulmonary vascular disease
  Persistent pulmonary hypertension of the newborn
  Primary pulmonary hypertension—a rare, fatal form of pulmonary hypertension with
    obscure etiology
  Eisenmenger's physiology, secondary to long-standing "hyperkinetic" pulmonary
    hypertension
  Thromboembolism
    Ventriculovenous shunt for hydrocephalus, sickle cell anemia, thrombophlebitis,
      etc.
  Collagen disease
    Rheumatoid arthritis, scleroderma, mixed connective tissue disease

---

pulmonary arterioles, with resulting increase in plasma membrane permeability
to calcium, or indirectly by humoral agents which are either locally released or
activated in the lung. Vasoactive agents which have been implicated in the hy-
poxia-induced pulmonary vasoconstriction include histamine, prostaglandins and
related compounds (such as thromboxane and endoperoxides), angiotensin, catecholamines, and "slow releasing substances of anaphylaxis." The role of the autonomic nervous system is disputed. Alveolar hypoxia is the major clinical event,
not a low PO_2 in the pulmonary or systemic arterial blood, which stimulates the
pulmonary vasoconstrictor response.

Pulmonary venous hypertension produces reflex vasoconstriction of the pulmonary arterioles and possible alveolar hypoxia by pulmonary edema, resulting
in pulmonary arterial hypertension. Increased PVR seen with alveolar hypoxia
and increased pulmonary venous pressure is usually reversible when the cause is
eliminated.

Diverse conditions listed under primary pulmonary vascular disease appear to
be characterized by a decrease in the cross-sectional area of the pulmonary vascular bed by pathologic changes in vascular tissue itself, thromboembolism,
platelet aggregation, or a combination of these. In persistent pulmonary hyper-

tension of the newborn, the major pathology is a striking maldevelopment of the peripheral pulmonary arterial bed.

Eisenmenger's syndrome (pulmonary vascular obstructive disease, or PVOD) occurs in patients who have untreated large left-to-right shunt lesions such as VSD, PDA, or ECD. The time of onset of PVOD varies ranging from infancy to adult life, but the majority of the patients develop PVOD during late childhood or early adolescence. It may appear even later in patients with ASD. Many patients with TGA also develop PVOD within the first year of life, for reasons which are not entirely clear. Also, children with Down's syndrome with large left-to-right shunt lesions tend to develop PVOD much earlier than do normal children with similar lesions.

Etiology of primary pulmonary hypertension is not known; it is probably a heterogeneous disorder. It is characterized by progressive, irreversible vascular changes similar to those seen in Eisenmenger's syndrome, but without intracardiac lesions. The incidence of this condition in the pediatric age group is extremely low; it is a condition of adulthood and is more prevalent in females, with a poor prognosis.

Recurrent embolism may result in progressive hypertension secondary to a reduction in the total cross-sectional area of the pulmonary vascular bed. This may result from infective endocarditis, repeated thrombophlebitis, ventriculo-venous shunt for hydrocephalus, sickle cell anemia, etc. Some connective tissue disorders, especially lupus erythematosus, may be associated with arteritis of the small pulmonary arterioles, with resulting pulmonary hypertension. Pulmonary hypertension due to these disorders is usually progressive.

Regardless of the initial events that lead to pulmonary arterial hypertension, an elevated pressure in the pulmonary artery eventually induces anatomical changes in the pulmonary vessels. The changes are classified into six grades by Heath and Edwards. Grade 1 of the Heath-Edwards classification consists of hypertrophy of the medial wall of the small muscular arteries; grade 2, hyperplasia of the intima; and grade 3, hyperplasia and fibrosis of the intima with narrowing of the vascular lumen. Changes up to grade 3 are considered to be reversible if the cause is eliminated. Changes greater than grade 4 are considered to be irreversible; they consist of dilatation lesions with saccular formation and fibrinoid necrosis. These anatomical changes may augment the hypertension and sustain it even when the original stimulus is removed, especially when the condition is of long duration and the anatomical changes are far advanced. Chronic pulmonary hypertension leads to right ventricular hypertension and RVH on ECG.

Pathophysiology

1. If severe pulmonary hypertension develops suddenly in the presence of an unprepared (nonhypertrophied) RV, right heart failure develops. This is seen in infants with acute upper airway obstruction or in massive thromboembolism at any age.

2. With chronic pulmonary hypertension, gradual dilatation and hypertrophy of the RV develops. The RV pressure may exceed the level of systemic pressure.

3. Decrease in cardiac output may result from at least two mechanisms:

   a) Volume and pressure overload of the RV impairs cardiac function, primarily by (1) impairment of coronary perfusion of the hypertrophied and dilated RV, and (2) decreased LV function resulting from the dramatic leftward shift of the interventricular septum caused by the increasing RV volume. The latter alters LV geometry and decreases its compliance, resulting in increased LV end-diastolic pressure and an increase in LA pressure. This, in turn, results in low cardiac output and pulmonary venous congestion or edema.

   b) A sudden increase in PVR may decrease pulmonary venous return to the LA, with resulting circulatory shock in the absence of a right-to-left intracardiac shunt.

4. Pulmonary edema can occur without elevation of LA pressure. Direct disruption of the walls of small arterioles proximal to the hypoxically constricted arterioles in patients with hyperresponsive pulmonary vessels may be responsible, a mechanism similar to that proposed for high-altitude pulmonary edema. This is more likely if there is no hypertrophy of the muscles in the media of these vessels.

5. Deterioration of arterial blood gases: Hypoxemia, acidosis, and occasional hypercapnia may result from pulmonary venous congestion or edema, compression of small airways, or intracardiac shunts.

Clinical Manifestations
Regardless of the etiology, clinical manifestations of pulmonary hypertension are similar when a significant hypertension has been established.

History

   a) Dyspnea, fatigue, and syncope, related to exertion.

   b) History of heart defect or CHF in infancy in most cases of Eisenmenger's syndrome.

   c) Some patients may have history of headache or angina-like chest pain.

   d) Hemoptysis is a late and sometimes fatal development.

PE

   a) Cyanosis with or without clubbing may be present. Neck veins are distended with a prominent *a* wave.

   b) RV lift or tap on palpation.

   c) The S2 splits narrowly and usually not at all; the P2 is loud. An ejection click and an early diastolic decrescendo murmur of pulmonary regurgitation are usually present along the MLSB.

   d) A regurgitant systolic murmur of tricuspid regurgitation may be audible at the LRSB.

   e) Signs of right heart failure (such as hepatomegaly and ankle edema) may be present.

   f) Arrhythmias occur in the late stage.

ECG

   a) RAD and RVH with or without "strain" are seen with severe hypertension.

   b) RAH is frequently seen late.

X-Rays

   a) The heart size is normal or only slightly enlarged, unless CHF supervenes.

   b) A prominent MPA segment and dilated hilar vessels with clear lung fields.

   c) With acute exacerbation, pulmonary edema may be seen.

ECHO

Certain M-mode echocardiographic findings are frequently found in pulmonary hypertension, but one cannot rely on the ECHO to accurately estimate the PA pressure and PVR or to predict the reactivity of PVR.

a) Abnormal pulmonary valve motion (absent or diminished *a* wave, midsystolic closure, and flat e-f slope) has been suggested as an indicator of pulmonary hypertension, but no reliable correlation exists between these abnormalities and pulmonary artery pressures.

b) An increased ratio of RPEP/RVET is found, but it is not reliable in patients with VSD.

c) Hypertrophy of the RV free wall, and dilatation of the RV and PA.

d) Doppler ultrasound findings include short time to peak flow and increased peak velocity of tricuspid regurgitation jet.

Natural History, Complications, and Prognosis

a) Pulmonary hypertension secondary to airway obstruction is usually reversible when the etiology is eliminated.

b) Chronic conditions that produce alveolar hypoxia have a relatively poor prognosis. Pulmonary hypertension of variable degrees persists with right heart failure. Superimposed pulmonary infection may be an aggravating factor.

c) Pulmonary hypertension with large left-to-right shunt lesions ("hyperkinetic" type) or that associated with pulmonary venous hypertension improves or disappears after surgical repair of the cause, if done early.

d) Primary pulmonary hypertension is progressive, with fatal outcome, usually within 3–7 years after the diagnosis.

e) Pulmonary hypertension associated with Eisenmenger's syndrome, collagen disease, and chronic thromboembolism is usually irreversible, with poor prognosis, but may be stable for 2–3 decades.

f) Right heart failure is common at the late stage.

g) Chest pain, hemoptysis, and syncope are ominous signs.

h) Atrial and/or ventricular arrhythmias also occur late.

Diagnosis

1) History and physical findings suggestive of pulmonary hypertension.

2) Noninvasive tools (ECG, chest x-rays, and ECHO) are often useful in detecting pulmonary hypertension. Collectively, they are reasonably accurate in assessing the severity. Pulmonary artery pressures change rapidly in conditions in which alveolar hypoxia is the cause of pulmonary hypertension. Therefore, repeat ECHO studies are not very useful under these conditions; monitoring with a Swan-Ganz catheter may be more meaningful.

3) Cardiac catheterization demonstrates the presence and severity of pulmonary hypertension, as well as whether the elevated PA pressure is secondary to elevated PVR. Whether elevated PVR is due to active vasoconstriction or to permanent changes in the pulmonary arterioles may be assessed by the use of tolazoline (Priscoline) or other vasodilators or administration of oxygen during

cardiac catheterization. Characteristic angiographic findings have been described.

Management

1. Management of acute pulmonary hypertension:

   a) Improve arterial oxygen tension by intubation and respirator support with oxygen. Hyperventilation-induced respiratory alkalosis may produce pulmonary vasodilation.

   b) Inotropic agents: An ideal inotropic agent is one that does not increase PVR and that does not reduce systemic blood pressure (which is important for coronary perfusion to the RV).

      1) Digitalis and dopamine are often used, but may increase PVR.

      2) β-Adrenergic agents (dobutamine, isoproterenol) may lower systemic pressure and impair coronary perfusion to the RV. Additional intravascular volume may be needed to maintain systemic blood pressure.

      3) Occasionally, norepinephrine or phenylephrine may be used to provide adequate coronary perfusion.

   c) Diuretics for pulmonary edema.

   d) Avoid and eliminate factors that increase pulmonary vasoconstriction (alveolar hypoxia, acidosis, hypercapnia, vasoconstrictor drugs, fat emulsions, hypothermia, and high PEEP). High PEEP reduces intrapulmonary shunt, but increases edema and decreases cardiac output.

   e) Vasodilator drugs are not always salutary, as they may decrease SVR more than the PVR. Tolazoline, prazosin, nitroprusside, hydralazine, nifedipine, captopril, and corticosteroids have been tried with varying beneficial and deleterious effects.

2. Remove etiologies whenever possible.

   a) Tonsillectomy and adenoidectomy for upper airway obstruction.

   b) Open heart surgery for large-shunt VSD or PDA; banding MPA in early infancy may be necessary for large VSD.

3. Treat underlying diseases such as cystic fibrosis or asthma.

4. Only symptomatic treatment is available for irreversible forms of pulmonary hypertension.

   a. Plasmapheresis for polycythemia and severe headache.

   b. Treatment of CHF with chronic administration of digoxin, diuretics, and low-salt diet.

   c) Treatment of arrhythmias.

   d) Hemoptysis may be treated with bed rest and anticough medications.

   e) Avoid use of nitroglycerin for anginal pain; it may worsen the pain.

   f) Avoid strenuous exertion.

   g) Avoid trips to high altitudes and commercial aircraft flight.

   h) Oxygen supplement as needed.

30 / Hyperlipidemia in Childhood

A clear relationship has been established between elevated serum cholesterol levels (over 200 mg/dl) and an increased risk of coronary heart disease in the adult. Cholesterol appears to be the major blood lipid implicated in the pathogenesis of atherosclerotic heart disease.

It is widely believed that atherosclerotic lesions start to develop in childhood and progresses to irreversible lesions in adulthood. The following sequence of events in increasing order of severity is believed to occur in American population.

(1) Fatty streaks develop in the first and second decades, some of which may resolve.

(2) Fibrous plaque (2nd and 3rd decades).

(3) Complicated fibrotic and calcific lesions (4th and later decade).

(4) Clinical manifestations of atherosclerotic cardiovascular disease (myocardial infarction, gangrene of extremities, aortic aneurysm, etc.).

Since substantial and potentially irreversible atherosclerosis may already exist by the 4rd decade of life, efforts to lower serum cholesterol levels in children have been made in the hope of preventing or retarding the progress of atherosclerosis.

Reduction of elevated lipids is only one aspect of the total management plan. Other interrelated factors such as genetics, hypertension, diabetes mellitus, obesity, and smoking are important risk factors in the development of atherosclerotic cardiovascular disease. Physicians should play an increasing role not only in the detection of hyperlipidemia, but also in counseling for prevention of other risk factors.

Lipid Chemistry

The major lipids of plasma are cholesterol, triglycerides, phospholipids, and free fatty acids. Plasma lipids which are hydrophobic do not circulate freely but rather in the form of lipid-protein macromolecular complexes known as lipoproteins; free fatty acids are bound to albumin. Only cholesterol and triglyceride plasma levels are of diagnostic significance for familial hyperlipidemias.

By means of analytical ultracentrifugation, the serum lipoproteins are separated into four major groups based on differences in size and density: (a) chylomicron, (b) very low density lipoprotein (VLDL), (c) low density lipoprotein (LDL), and (d) α-lipoprotein (high density lipoprotein, or HDL). Electrophoretic techniques permit the separation of the serum lipoproteins based on differences in electrostatic charges; (a) chylomicrons (which remain at the origin), (b) β-lipoprotein (=LDL), (c) pre-β-lipoprotein (=VLDL), and (d) α-lipoproteins (=HDL). These fractions correlate well with those separated by the ultracentrifuge except for the order of β- and pre-β-bands.

Classification

Hyperlipidemia has been classified into five major groups according to the plasma lipoprotein patterns on paper electrophoresis or after ultracentrifugation. The types define the lipoprotein abnormality, whether the cause is genetic, environmental, or disease related. Brief outlines of each of the five groups are presented in Figure 30–1. In childhood, hypercholesterolemia is usually a manifestation of an increased amount of LDL cholesterol (type II hyperlipoproteinemia). In this type, the triglyceride levels are usually normal (type IIa), but are occasionally elevated (type IIb). About 20% of children with plasma cholesterol levels of 200–250 mg/dl have concentrations of LDL cholesterol below the 95th percentile with above average or high HDL cholesterol levels. High levels of HDL are thought to be protective against atherosclerosis. It is, therefore, important to determine HDL cholesterol levels in children with hypercholesterolemia to distinguish those with type II hyperlipoproteinemia from those with normal LDL levels.

Elevated plasma levels of lipids or lipoproteins may be primary or secondary. The primary form is genetically determined. The secondary form may result from diets high in cholesterol and saturated fat or from a variety of metabolic diseases. The possibility of secondary hyperlipoproteinemia should always be considered. Glycogen storage disease and congenital biliary atresia are the most common causes of hyperlipoproteinemia in infancy. Hypothyroidism, diabetes mellitus, and nephrotic syndrome are the most common causes later in childhood. Other causes include use of oral contraceptives, alcohol, and steroids.

Clinical Manifestations

Clinical manifestations will be presented according to the type of plasma lipids that are elevated (see Fig 30–1).

A. Hypercholesterolemia (Type II)

Hypercholesterolemia may occur without other lipoprotein abnormality (type IIa) or in association with a raised concentration of VLDL (type IIb) (see below and Fig 30–1).

a) Plasma total cholesterol levels are in the range of 250–500 mg/100 ml in the heterozygotes and 500–1,000 mg/100 ml in the homozygotes.

b) Heterozygotes are usually asymptomatic in the first decade. Tendon xanthomas develop during the 2nd decade, most commonly in the Achilles and extensor tendons of the hand (10%–15%). Rarely, angina pectoris is seen in the late teenage years.

c) Homozygotes present most commonly with xanthomas by the age of 5 years. Angina pectoris and myocardial infarction ordinarily occur before 20 years of age. Aortic stenosis may develop as the result of atherosclerosis of the valve.

B. Hypertriglyceridemia (Types I, IV, and V)

a) Life-threatening pancreatitis may develop.

b) Other clinical features include eruptive xanthomas, hepatosplenomegaly, and lipemia retinalis.

c) No predisposition for coronary heart disease exists in the adult.

d) *Familial combined hyperlipidemia* is a form of hypertriglyceridemia, which is characterized by increases of one or more lipoproteins in members of a single family (also called "multiple-type hyperlipoproteinemia"). Some fam-

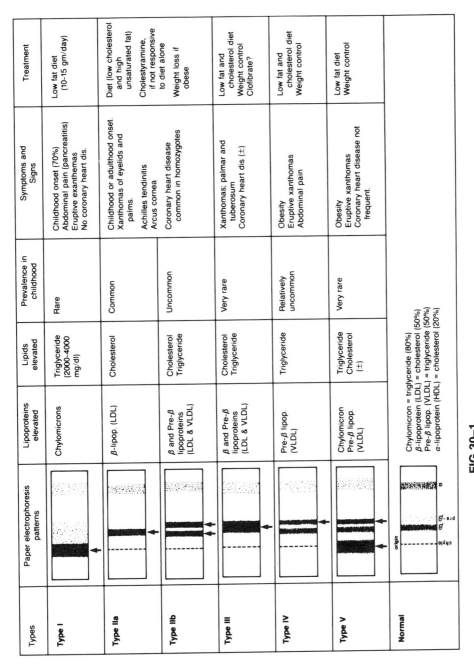

Types	Paper electrophoresis patterns	Lipoproteins elevated	Lipids elevated	Prevalence in childhood	Symptoms and Signs	Treatment
Type I		Chylomicrons	Triglyceride (2000–4000 mg/dl)	Rare	Childhood onset (70%) Abdominal pain (pancreatitis) Eruptive exanthemas No coronary heart dis.	Low fat diet (10–15 gm/day)
Type IIa		β-lipop. (LDL)	Cholesterol	Common	Childhood or adulthood onset. Xanthomas of eyelids and palms. Achilles tendinitis Arcus cornea	Diet (low cholesterol and high unsaturated fat) Cholestyramine, if not responsive to diet alone
Type IIb		β and Pre-β lipoproteins (LDL & VLDL)	Cholesterol Triglyceride	Uncommon	Coronary heart disease common in homozygotes	Weight loss if obese
Type III		β and Pre-β lipoproteins (LDL & VLDL)	Cholesterol Triglyceride	Very rare	Xanthomas; palmar and tuberosum Coronary heart dis (±)	Low fat and cholesterol diet Weight control Clofibrate?
Type IV		Pre-β lipop. (VLDL)	Triglyceride	Relatively uncommon	Obesity Eruptive xanthomas Abdominal pain	Low fat and cholesterol diet Weight control
Type V		Chylomicron Pre-β lipop. (VLDL)	Triglyceride Cholesterol (±)	Very rare	Obesity Eruptive xanthomas Coronary heart disease not frequent.	Low fat diet Weight control
Normal						

Chylomicron = triglyceride (80%)
β-lipoprotein (LDL) = cholesterol (50%)
Pre-β lipop. (VLDL) = triglyceride (50%)
α-lipoprotein (HDL) = cholesterol (20%)

FIG 30–1.
Summary of clinical features of hyperlipoproteinemia.

ily members have increases in VLDL alone (type IV), others have increases in LDL (type IIa), and still others have high levels of VLDL and LDL (type IIb). This rare form of hyperlipidemia may be found in childhood.

C. Familial Dysbetalipoproteinemia (Type III)

  a. The clinical hallmark of this rare form is unusual yellow deposits in the creases of the palms.

  b. Premature coronary heart disease may occur.

  c. Plasma cholesterol and triglyceride are both elevated.

Diagnosis

  1) Total cholesterol, total triglyceride, and HDL cholesterol levels should be measured after an overnight fast while the child is receiving *ad libitum* diet. The level of LDL cholesterol can be estimated using the following formula:

$$LDL\ cholesterol = total\ cholesterol - (triglycerides/5 + HDL\ cholesterol)$$

  Diagnosis of hypercholesterolemia or hypertriglyceridemia is made when levels of total cholesterol (or LDL cholesterol) or of triglycerides are above 95th percentile for the age and sex. The 95th percentile cholesterol is 200 mg/100 ml, that of LDL is 130 mg/100 ml, and that of triglyceride is 100–140 mg/100 ml.

  Electrophoresis is not useful as a diagnostic tool, since it is semiquantitative. Complete quantification of lipoproteins by ultracentrifugation is not usually accessible and is quite expensive.

  2) Secondary causes of hyperlipidemia must be ruled out, such as seen with hypothyroidism, diabetes mellitus, nephrotic syndrome, liver disease, lupus, etc.

  3) Turbid plasma may suggest hypertriglyceridemia (increases in chylomicron and pre-β bands).

  4) Indications for lipid studies:

  a) A family history of premature death or morbidity from atherosclerotic heart disease in either parent before age 50 years. (About 20% of children with such family history will have familial hypercholesterolemia.)

  b) All children with known family history of primary hypercholesterolemia and hypertriglyceridemia.

  c) Infants with unexplained postprandial irritability, or children with recurrent, unexplained abdominal pain, or children with obesity (above the ideal weight for height).

  d) Children from families with other risk factors (premature strokes, hypertension, diabetes, hyperuricemia, etc.).

Treatment

  1. For patients with all types of hyperlipidemia:

  a) Weight reduction to ideal weight for height.

  b) Maintenance of cardiovascular fitness by repetitive aerobic physical activity.

  c) Avoidance of excess calories, alcohol, and smoking.

2. Hypercholesterolemia (type II):

   a) Dietary management (with diet low in total fat, cholesterol, and polyunsaturated fat) is initially recommended; a knowledgeable dietician should be consulted.

   b. A bile acid sequestrant may be used if not responsive to diet alone.
      Cholestyramine, 4–16 gm of active resin/day, or
      Cholestepol resin, 5–10 mg/day.
      The bile acid sequestrants are ion exchange resins that form an insoluble resin-bile acid complex with the bile acid, which is excreted in the feces. Removal of the bile acids from the enterohepatic circulation accelerates the metabolism of cholesterol. The most common adverse effect is constipation; others include abdominal distention, belching, and nausea.

   c) Plasma exchange: The plasma of familial hypercholesterolemia homozygotes is exchanged for a cholesterol-free plasma fraction, and repeated every 2 weeks. This may result in marked reduction in total plasma and LDL cholesterol.

   d) Surgery: Partial ileal bypass or portacaval shunt may be needed if resistant to drug therapy.

   e) Liver transplantation is in experimental stage.

3. Hypertriglyceridemia (types I, IV, V):
   Hypertriglyceridemic patients respond quite well to dietary therapy (low in fat and cholesterol); the use of drugs is rarely, if ever, necessary.

4. Type III Hyperlipoproteinemia:

   a) Diet low in cholesterol and fat.

   b) Special drug (clofibrate) is always indicated.

31 / Child With Chest Pain or Syncope

I. CHEST PAIN

Chest pain is a frequently encountered complaint in children in office or emergency room practice. Although in the majority of pediatric patients chest pain does not indicate serious disease of the heart or other systems, in a society with a high prevalence of atherosclerotic cardiovascular disease, it is alarming to the child and his parents. In fact, chest pain means "heart disease" to the majority of these children and their parents. Making a referral to a cardiologist is not always a good idea; it may actually increase the family's concern. Physicians should be aware of the differential diagnosis of chest pain in children and should make every effort to find a specific cause of chest pain before reassuring the child and the parents.

Etiology

According to more recent studies, the most common cause of chest pain in children is costochondritis, occurring in 20%–75% of children. Two other common causes are trauma to the chest wall or muscle strain and respiratory disease, especially that associated with cough. In one study, no etiology could be found in 40% of the patients even after moderately extensive studies. Psychologic cause of chest pain should not be lightly assigned to these children without thorough history taking and follow-up evaluation. It is important to realize that cardiac disease rarely presents with chest pain in children. In more than 200 children presenting with chest pain as the chief complaint, only one was found to have abnormal cardiac findings, mitral valve prolapse (it may be coincidental rather than causal). Table 31–1 lists possible causes of chest pain in children.

Diagnostic Approach

Thorough history and physical examination are all that are required to make the diagnosis of the three most common causes of chest pain in children. If they fail to disclose the cause, and if abnormal cardiac findings are present, additional studies such as chest x-rays, ECG, and even ECHO may be indicated to rule out cardiac and certain respiratory or skeletal abnormalities. Cardiology consultation is occasionally indicated.

Costochondritis is diagnosed by the presence of tenderness to palpation of one or more costochondral or chondrosternal junctions. It is a benign condition that can be treated by reassurance and occasionally analgesics. History of vigorous exercise, weight lifting, or direct trauma and the presence of tenderness of chest wall or muscle are clear evidence of muscle strain or trauma.

A history of severe cough or bronchitis with tenderness of intercostal or abdominal muscles is an occasional cause of chest pain. Chest x-rays may confirm the diagnosis of pleural effusion, pneumonias, pneumothorax or abnormalities of the rib cage or the thoracic spine. Hyperventilation can produce chest discomfort and is often associated with paresthesia and lightheadedness. Gastrointestinal dis-

TABLE 31–1.

Causes of Chest Pain in Children

Cardiac
  Structural heart defects
    Severe obstructive lesions (severe AS, PS, HOCM)
    Pulmonary vascular obstructive disease
    Mitral valve prolapse (?)
    Anomalous origin of the coronary artery
  Inflammatory
    Pericarditis (viral, bacterial, rheumatic)
    Kawasaki's disease
  Arrhythmias
    Supraventricular tachycardia
    Frequent PVCs or ventricular tachycardia (?)
Thoracic cage
  Costochondritis
  Muscle strain or direct trauma to the chest wall
  Breast tenderness (mastalgia)
  Abnormalities of rib cage or thoracic spine
Respiratory
  Severe cough or bronchitis
  Pleural effusion
  Lobar pneumonia
  Spontaneous pneumothorax
  Pleurodynia or other viral infection
  Hyperventilation
Psychogenic
  Hyperventilation
  Conversion symptoms
  Somatization disorder
  Depression

orders may present as a cause of chest pain. The onset and relief of pain in relation to eating and diet may help to clarify the diagnosis.

Cardiac abnormalities that may result in chest pain can be divided into three categories: (1) structural abnormalities, (2) pericardial or myocardial inflammatory processes, and (3) arrhythmias. Chest pain of cardiac origin is usually the result of an imbalance of myocardial oxygen supply and demand or irritation of the pericardium. Severe obstructive lesions such as those of LV outflow tract (AS, subaortic stenosis, HOCM) or severe pulmonary stenosis may cause chest pain. It must be emphasized that mild stenotic lesions do not cause ischemic chest pain. Chest pain from severe obstructive lesions is usually exercise related and clearly the result of increased myocardial oxygen demands from tachycardia and increased blood pressure. Physical examination should reveal a loud heart murmur best heard at the upper right or left sternal border, usually with a thrill. ECGs may show ventricular hypertrophy with or without "strain" pattern. Exercise ECG may aid in the functional assessment of its severity. ECHO and Doppler studies will permit accurate determination of both the type and severity of the obstructive lesion. Patients with severe obstruction require relief of the obstruction.

Chest pain associated with mitral valve prolapse has been reported in about 20% of the patients. It is a vague, nonexertional pain. The pain is presumed to result from papillary muscle and/or LV endocardial ischemia, but there is increasing doubt as to the causal relationship between chest pain and mitral valve prolapse. Occasionally, supraventricular or ventricular arrhythmias seen in this syndrome may result in cardiac symptoms including chest discomfort. Thoracoskeletal deformities are common in these children. Nearly all patients with Marfan's syndrome have mitral valve prolapse. Cardiac examination should reveal a midsystolic click with or without late systolic murmur (see chap. 21 for detailed discussion of mitral valve prolapse). The ECG may show T wave abnormalities. ECHO confirms the diagnosis.

Coronary artery anomalies can rarely be the cause of chest pain. They include rare cases of anomalous origin of the left coronary artery from the pulmonary artery (usually symptomatic during early infancy), coronary artery fistula, aneurysm, or stenosis of coronary arteries as a result of clinical or subclinical Kawasaki's disease. Typical anginal pain is located in the precordial or subcostal region, radiating to the neck, upper extremities, or back, and is variously described as a pressure, choking, or squeezing sensation. Anginal pain is precipitated or worsened by exercise and ceases shortly after exercise stops. It is not exacerbated by deep breathing. Cardiac examination may be normal or may exhibit a heart murmur (systolic murmur of mitral regurgitation or continuous murmur of fistulas). ECGs may show evidence of myocardial ischemia or old myocardial infarction. Abnormal exercise ECG is a further indication of myocardial ischemia. Although ECHO can be helpful, coronary angiography is often indicated for a definitive diagnosis.

Irritation of the pericardium may result from inflammatory pericardial disease; it may be of viral, bacterial, or rheumatic origin. Acute myocarditis often involves the pericardium to a certain extent and can cause chest pain. Cardiomyopathy can cause chest pain either by ischemia, with or without exercise, or from rhythm disturbances. Chest x-ray and ECG may both suggest the correct diagnosis, with confirmation by ECHO.

Chest pain may result from a variety of arrhythmias, especially with sustained tachycardia resulting in myocardial ischemia. Even without ischemia, palpitation or forceful heartbeats may be expressed as chest pain by children. When chest pain is associated with dizziness and palpitation, a resting ECG and a 24-hour ambulatory ECG (Holter monitor) should be obtained. Alternatively, a telephone transmission device may be used to relay the ECG while the patient experiences symptoms.

In some children, a clear emotional origin of the pain may be demonstrated by careful history taking. Death or separation, stress from school or family, physical illness, or disability may be the cause of chest pain in children in whom other organic causes cannot be found. Psychologic or psychiatric consultation may bring out conversion symptoms, somatization disorder, or even depression.

II. SYNCOPE

Normal function of the brain depends on a constant supply of oxygen and glucose. Significant alterations in their supply may result in a transient loss or near-loss of consciousness, which is called syncope or fainting.

Etiology

Syncope may be due to circulatory, metabolic, or neuropsychologic causes. Table 31–2 lists possible causes of syncope.

TABLE 31–2.

Etiologic Classification of Syncope

Circulatory causes
  Extracardiac causes
    Common faint (or vasodepressor syncope)
    Orthostatic hypotension
    Failure of venous return (increased intrathoracic pressure, decreased venous return, hypovolemia, etc.)
    Cerebrovascular occlusive disease
  Intracardiac causes
    Severe obstructive lesions (AS, PS, HOCM, pulmonary hypertension, etc.)
    Arrhythmias (either extreme tachycardia or bradycardia)
Metabolic causes
  Hypoglycemia
  Hyperventilation syndrome
  Hypoxia
Neuropsychiatric causes
  Epilepsy
  Brain tumor
  Migraine
  Hysteria or nonconvulsive seizures

Clinical Manifestations

Only circulatory causes of syncope will be discussed in this chapter. Discussion of metabolic and neuropsychiatric causes of syncope is beyond the scope of this book.

1. Extracardiac Causes of Syncope

  a. Common faint (vasodepressor syncope):

    Common syncope is probably the most frequently encountered form. This is due to activation of the cholinergic vasodilator system, which leads to active dilatation of arterioles, a fall in blood pressure, and massive increase in blood flow to muscles. Initially, autonomic discharge of both sympathetic (tachycardia, pallor, hyperventilation, and pupillary dilatation) and parasympathetic (perspiration and nausea) systems is present. The initial tachycardia is transient and is replaced by bradycardia and persistent hypotension, leading to cerebral ischemia. It occurs with emotional stress or pain, in the fasting state, and in a hot, humid or crowded environment. Placing the patient in supine position until the circulatory crisis resolves may be all that is indicated. Inhalation of ammonia usually is effective.

  b. Orthostatic hypotension:

    Absence or inadequate response of normal vasoconstriction of arterioles and veins in the upright position results in hypotension without reflex increase in heart rate. It is due to failure of adrenergic vasoconstrictor activity. Too vigorous treatment of hypertension may result in orthostatic hypotension. The main differential point of this type of syncope from common faint is the absence of autonomic response, such as perspiration, pallor, or hyperventilation. The following have been used with varying degrees of success: elastic stocking, high-salt diet, sympathomimetic amines, and corticosteroids.

c. Decreased systemic venous return:

Normal return of venous blood to the heart is necessary to maintain normal left ventricular output and systemic pressures. Normally, the pressure in the RA is 5–10 mm Hg lower than in the venules and this makes blood flow toward the heart.

Decreased venous return may occur as a result of:

1. Increased intrathoracic pressure, such as seen in straining phase of Valsalva's maneuver, repetitive coughing, breath-holding, tracheal obstruction, etc.

2. Decrease in venous tone, which may be caused by pharmacologic agents that relax vascular smooth muscle (nitroglycerin) or that eliminate sympathetic tone (ganglionic blockers, guanethidine, etc.).

3. Decrease in intravascular volume secondary to hemorrhage or dehydration.

Treatment should be directed to the elimination or correction of identifiable causes.

d. Cerebrovascular occlusive disease:

Syncope from cerebrovascular occlusive disease is extremely rare in children. Adult patients with cerebrovascular occlusive disease may have syncope with a less significant fall in blood pressure than patients without it. It is often associated with short-term neurologic defects such as hemiparesis, transient blindness, diplopia, speech disturbance, confusion, and headache. Bruits over the carotid arteries may be present. Surgical therapy may be advisable.

2. **Cardiac Causes of Syncope**

a. Obstructive lesions:

Patients with AS, PS, HOCM, or pulmonary hypertension may have syncope. Syncope associated with these conditions is often precipitated by exercise. Peripheral vasodilation secondary to exercise is not accompanied by an adequate increase in cardiac output, thereby resulting in diminished perfusion to the brain.

These obstructive lesions and pulmonary hypertension can be diagnosed clinically by careful physical examination, ECG, chest x-ray, and echocardiography. Surgery is indicated for these conditions, with the exception of irreversible forms of pulmonary hypertension.

b. Arrhythmias:

Either extreme of ventricular rate, tachycardia or bradycardia, can depress cardiac output and lower the cerebral blood flow below the critical level. Commonly encountered arrhythmias include supraventricular tachycardia, ventricular tachycardia, sick sinus syndrome, and complete heart block. Arrhythmias that used to be rare in children are becoming increasingly frequent in the pediatric age group because of an increasing number of survivors of complex cardiac surgery. Those who require extensive surgery in the atria (such as the Mustard procedure for TGA) are prone to develop sick sinus syndrome (see chap. 23). Simple bradycardia is usually well tolerated in children, but the combination of tachycardia followed by bradycardia (overdrive suppression) is more likely to produce syncope. Long QT syndrome (see Table 1–2) is characterized by syncope owing to ventricular arrhythmias, prolongation of QT interval on the ECG, and occasional family history of sudden death. Congenital deafness is also a component of the syndrome in Jervell and Lange-Nielsen type but not in Romano-Ward type. Occasionally, mitral valve prolapse syndrome may present with syncope secondary to arrhythmias.

One must document causal relationships between arrhythmias and symptoms, by ECG recording, usually in the form of ambulatory monitoring (Holter monitoring) for 24 hours or longer. Some equivocal cases in which arrhythmias and symptoms are not causally related may require electrophysiologic studies.

Most arrhythmias respond to antiarrhythmic therapy. Patients with long QT syndrome respond well to propranolol. Propranolol or other antiarrhythmic drugs may be indicated in symptomatic patients with mitral valve prolapse syndrome. Occasionally, surgical treatment may be indicated (such as in WPW syndrome causing frequent supraventricular tachycardia). Implantation of a pacemaker with standby mode may be indicated in patients with sick sinus syndrome.

32 / Postoperative Syndromes

There are four well-recognized syndromes that are seen in the period following heart surgery in children.

I. POSTCOARCTECTOMY SYNDROME

This syndrome is believed to be caused by arteritis resulting from changes in pressure and flow dynamics following resection of the coarctation of the aorta, and the arteritis most often involves the superior mesenteric artery distribution.

Clinical Manifestations

a. Onset of the syndrome is 2–8 days following the surgery.

b. The syndrome is characterized by severe intermittent abdominal pain, fever, and leukocytosis, mimicking acute surgical abdomen.

c. In severe cases, abdominal distention, melena, and ascites associated with gangrenous bowel may develop.

d. Rebound systemic hypertension may be present

Management

a. Careful monitoring of blood pressure in the postoperative period to detect rebound hypertension. Make sure the hypertension in the arm is not due to residual coarctation of the aorta or to improper BP measuring techniques.

b. Delayed solid feeding postoperatively.

c. Prevention of rebound hypertension is important and may be accomplished by administration of (1) β-adrenergic blockers such as propranolol (0.01–0.05 mg/kg IV over 10 minutes, every 6–8 hours), (2) vasodilators such as hydralazine (0.15 mg/kg IM or IV, every 4–6 hours), or (3) sympatholytic drugs such as reserpine (0.07 mg/kg IM, every 6–8 hours).

d. Occasionally, exploratory laparotomy and resection of infarcted bowel may be necessary.

II. POSTPERICARDIOTOMY SYNDROME

This syndrome is believed to represent an immunologic phenomenon as a sequela of blood in the pericardial sac. A nonsurgical example of this syndrome is seen following myocardial infarction (Dressler's syndrome) and traumatic hemopericardium. A relationship to viral infection is implicated.

Clinical Manifestations

a. The onset of the syndrome is 2–3 weeks following a surgery that involves pericardiotomy. It is rare in infants less than 2 years.

  b. The syndrome is characterized by fever (sustained or spiking, up to 103° F), chest pain, pericardial friction rub, pericardial and pleural effusion, and hepatomegaly.

  c. Leukocytosis with shift to the left and elevated ESR are present.

  d. Chest x-rays show enlarged cardiac silhouette.

  e. The ECG shows persistent ST and T changes.

  f. Echocardiogram shows pericardial effusion.

Treatment

  a. Bed rest is all that is needed for a mild case (it subsides in 2–3 weeks).

  b. Aspirin may be used for chest pain.

  c. Moderate doses of corticosteroids for a few days may be indicated in severe cases.

  d. Pericardiocentesis for signs of cardiac tamponade (uncommon).

  e. Diuretics may be used for pleural effusion.

III. POSTPERFUSION SYNDROME

Postperfusion syndrome, which occurs following an open heart surgery using cardiopulmonary bypass, is believed to be due to cytomegalovirus infection.

Clinical Manifestations

  a. The onset occurs 3–6 weeks following an open heart surgery.

  b. It is characterized by the triad of fever (up to 103°F), splenomegaly (lasting for 8 weeks), and atypical lymphocytosis (lasting 2–3 weeks).

Management

  a. No specific treatment is available.

  b. The syndrome is self-limited, lasting for a few weeks to a few months.

IV. HEMOLYTIC ANEMIA SYNDROME

Hemolytic anemia may occur following a cardiac surgery, especially following repair of endocardial cushion defect or aortic or mitral valve replacement. It is caused by trauma of red blood cells or by autoimmune reaction.

Clinical Manifestations

  a. The onset occurs 1–2 weeks following the surgery.

  b. It is characterized by low-grade fever, jaundice, hepatomegaly, and reticulocytosis.

Management

  a. Medical treatment of the anemia, either by iron replacement therapy or blood transfusion.

  b. Surgical correction of turbulence if the anemia is severe and the correction is technically possible.

Appendix

Appendix

Pediatric Drug Dosage

Drug	Route and Dosage	Toxicity or Side Effects
	CARDIAC GLYCOSIDES	
Digoxin (Lanoxin)	Total digitalizing dose (TDD): (PO): Prematures 0.02 mg/kg Full-term newborn 0.03 mg/kg 1 mo.–2 yr 0.04–0.05 mg/kg Over 2 yr 0.03–0.04 mg/kg (IV): 75% of the PO dose Maintenance dose: (PO, IV): 25% of TDD/day in 2 doses	AV conduction disturbances, arrhythmias, nausea and vomiting (see Table 26–4 for ECG signs)
Digitoxin	Total digitalizing dose (TDD): (PO): Prematures and Full-term newborn 0.02 mg/kg 1 mo.–2 yr 0.03 mg/kg Over 2 yr 0.02 mg/kg Maintenance dose: (PO): 15% (10%–20%) of TDD once a day	Same as above
	DIURETICS	
Chlorothiazide (Diuril)	(PO): 20–40 mg/kg/day in 2 doses	Hypokalemia, hyponatremia
Furosemide (Lasix)	(IV): 0.5–2.0 mg/kg/dose (PO): 1–2 mg/kg/dose, 2–3 × a day, if necessary	Same as above
Hydrochlorothiazide (HydroDiuril)	(PO): 2.0–4.0 mg/kg/day in 2 doses	Same as above
Spironolactone (Aldactone)	(PO): 2.0–3.0 mg/kg/day in 2–3 doses	Hyperkalemia, hyponatremia
	ANTIHYPERTENSIVES	
Hydrochlorothiazide	(PO): 1–2 mg/kg, 2 × a day	Hypokalemia
Chlorthalidone	(PO): 1 mg/kg, once a day (max 2 mg/kg/day)	Hypokalemia
Propranolol (Inderal)	(PO): 1–3 mg/kg, 2–3 × a day	Cardiac depression
Methyldopa (Aldomet)	(PO): 5–10 mg/kg, 2 × a day (max 40 mg/kg/day)	Sedation, hypotension, lupus-like syndrome, hepatitis, colitis
Prazosine (Minipress)	(PO): 0.5–7 mg/kg, 3 × a day	Orthostatic hypotension
Hydralazine (Apresoline)	(PO): 1–5 mg/kg, 2–3 × a day (IV, IM): 0.15–0.2 mg/kg for emergency	Hypotension, tachycardia, and palpitation
Minoxidil (Loniten)	(PO): 0.1–1.0 mg/kg, 2 × a day	Hypotension
Diazoxide (Hyperstat)	(IV): 5 mg/kg, IV push for emergency	Hypotension, hyperglycemia
Nitroprusside (Nipride)	(IV): 0.5–0.8 μg/kg/min (usually 2–3 μg/kg/min) for emergency (with careful BP monitoring)	Hypotension
Captopril (Capoten)	(PO): <6 mo.: 0.05–0.5 mg/kg, 3 × a day > 6 mo.: 0.5–2.0 mg/kg, 3 × a day	Neutropenia, proteinuria
	ANTIARRHYTHMICS	
Quinidine sulfate	(PO): Start with 3–6 mg/kg, every 2–3 hr × 5 May increase to 12 mg/kg every 2–3 hr × 5 Maintain minimum effective dose every 4–6 hr	Intraventricular conduction disturbance (prolonged QRS), ventricular arrhythmias, nausea, and vomiting

(Continued.)

Pediatric Drug Dosage   (cont.).

Drug	Route and Dosage	Toxicity or Side Effects
Quinidine gluconate	(PO): 10–30 mg/kg/day, in 2–3 doses	Same as above
Procainamide HCl (Pronestyl)	(IV): 10–100 mg, slow IV drip over 5 min every 10–30 min if necessary (PO): 40–60 mg/kg/day in 4 doses	Hypotension, ventricular arrhythmias, lupus-like syndrome, blood dyscrasias
Lidocaine (Xylocaine)	(IV): See *Drugs Used in CPR* (this table)	Myocardial depression, hypotension, seizures, ataxia
Diphenylhydantoin (Dilantin)	(IV): 3–5 mg/kg over 5 min (PO): 2–6 mg/kg/day in 2–3 doses	Myocardial depression, hypotension, lupus-like syndrome, gingival hyperplasia, blood dyscrasias
Propranolol HCl (Inderal)	(IV): 0.01 mg/kg, every 2 min (max 0.1 mg/kg) (PO): 1–4 mg/kg/day in 3–4 doses	Myocardial depression (heart failure), AV block, bronchospasm
Amiodarone*	(PO): 3–12 mg/day, once a day	Skin discoloration, photosensitivity
Verapamil*	(IV): 0.15 mg/kg, every 60 sec (PO): 3–5 mg/kg/day in 3–4 doses	Cardiac depression

MISCELLANEOUS DRUGS

K-triplex or K chloride (20%)	(PO): 0.5 ml/kg, 2–3 × daily will supply half of the maintenance (K supplementation for diuretic therapy)	
Bishydroxycoumarin (Dicumarol)	(PO): Initial, 50–100 mg; Maintenance, 10–50 mg/day	Bleeding
Warfarin (Coumadin)	(PO): Initial, 50–100 mg/day; Maintenance, 1–5 mg/day; Maintain prothrombin time 1.5–2 × normal for Dicumarol and Coumadin	Same as above (vitamin D is antidote for Coumadin and Dicumarol)
Heparin	(IV): 100 units/kg, every 4 hr, Keep clotting time 2–3 times normal	Hemorrhage (protamine sulfate is antidote for heparin)

DRUGS USED IN CARDIOPULMONARY RESUSCITATION

Epinephrine	(IV): 0.01 mg/kg/dose (IV drip): Start at 0.5 μg/kg/min up to 1.0–1.5 μg/kg/min	Tachycardia, hypertension, arrhythmias
Sodium bicarbonate	(IV): 2 mEq/kg, stat, 1 mEq/kg every 15 min if necessary	
Atropine	(IV): 0.02 mg/kg (range 0.01–0.03 mg/kg)	Tachycardia, dry mouth, blurred vision
Calcium 10% solution of	(IV): 5–10 mg ionized calcium/kg	Bradycardia or sinus arrest, slough if extravasated, sinus arrest
Ca chloride	0.3 ml/kg	
Ca gluceptate	0.5 ml/kg	
Ca gluconate	1.0 ml/kg	
Dopamine (Intropin)	(IV): 2–5 μg/kg/min up to max of 50 μg/kg/min, Titrate to desired effect	Tachycardia, arrhythmias
Isoproterenol (Isuprel)	(IV): 0.1 μg/kg/min, Titrate to desired effect	Tachycardia, arrhythmias
Lidocaine (Xylocaine)	(IV): 1 mg/kg loading dose, followed by 1–3 mg/kg/hr IV drip	Myocardial depression, hypotension, seizures
Defibrillation	2 w-sec/kg	Myocardial damage
Cardioversion	0.5 w-sec/kg	Ventricular fibrillation

*Investigative drugs for children.

Suggested Readings

General

Adams FH, Emmanouilides GC: *Moss' Heart Disease in Infants, Children, and Adolescents*, ed 3. Baltimore, Williams & Wilkins Co, 1983.

Anthony CL, Arnon RG: *Pediatric Cardiology*, revised ed. New Hyde Park, Medical Examination Publishing Co, Inc, 1983.

Feigenbaum H: *Echocardiography*, ed 4. Philadelphia, Lea & Febiger, 1986.

Goldberg SJ, Allen HD, Sahn DJ: *Pediatric and Adolescent Echocardiography*, ed 2. Chicago, Year Book Medical Publishers, 1980.

Keith JD, Rowe RD, Vlad P: *Heart Disease in Infancy and Childhood*, ed 3. New York, MacMillan Publishing Co, 1978.

Kirklin JW, Barratt-Boyes BG: *Cardiac Surgery*. New York, John Wiley & Sons, 1986.

Park MK, Guntheroth WG: *How to Read Pediatric ECGs*, ed 2. Chicago, Year Book Medical Publishers, 1987.

Rudolph AM: *Congenital Diseases of the Heart*. Chicago, Year Book Medical Publishers, 1974.

Chapter 1. History Taking

Nadas AS, Fyler DC: *Pediatric Cardiology*, ed 3. Philadelphia, WB Saunders Co, 1972, pp 3–20.

Noonan JA: Syndromes associated with cardiac defects. *Cardiovasc Clin* 1980; 11/2:97–116.

Nora JJ: Etiologic aspects of heart disease, in Adams FH, Emmanouilides GC (eds): *Moss' Heart Disease in Infants, Children, and Adolescents*, ed 3. Baltimore, Williams & Wilkins Co, 1983, pp 2–10.

Chapter 2. Physical Examination

Guntheroth WG: Initial evaluation of the child for heart disease. *Pediatr Clin North Am* 1978; 25:657–675.

Leon DF, Shaver JA: *Physiologic Principles of Heart Sounds and Murmur*. New York, American Heart Association, 1975.

Nadas AS, Fyler DC: *Pediatric Cardiology*, ed 3. Philadelphia, WB Saunders Co, 1972, pp 3–20.

Park MK, Menard SM: Accuracy of blood pressure measurement by the Dinamap monitor in infants and children. *Pediatrics* 1987; 79:907–914.

Rosenthal A: How to distinguish between innocent and pathologic murmurs in childhood. *Pediatr Clin North Am* 1984; 31:1229–1240.

Chapter 3. Electrocardiography I.

Park MK, Guntheroth WG: *How to Read Pediatric ECGs*, ed 2. Chicago, Year Book Medical Publishers, 1987.

Chapter 4. Chest Roentgenography

Elliott LP, Schiebler GL: A roentgenologic-electrocardiographic approach to cyanotic forms of heart disease. *Pediatr Clin North Am* 1971; 18:1133–1161.

Gedgaudas E, Knight L: Plain-film diagnosis of heart disease: A physiologic approach. *JAMA* 1975; 232:63–67.

Nadas AS, Fyler DC: *Pediatric Cardiology*, ed 3. Philadelphia, WB Saunders Co, 1972, pp 21–35.

Chapter 5. Flow Diagram

Kawabori I: Cyanotic congenital heart defects with decreased pulmonary blood flow. *Pediatr Clin North Am* 1978; 25:759–776.

Kawabori I: Cyanotic congenital heart defects with increased pulmonary blood flow. *Pediatr Clin North Am* 1978; 25:777–795.

Stevenson JG: Acyanotic lesions with normal pulmonary blood flow. *Pediatr Clin North Am* 1978; 25:725–742.

Stevenson JG: Acyanotic lesions with increased pulmonary blood flow. *Pediatr Clin North Am* 1978; 26:743–758.

Chapter 6. Noninvasive Techniques of Cardiac Evaluation

Cumming GR, Everatt D, Hartman L: Bruce treadmill test in children: Normal values in a clinic population. *Am J Cardiol* 1978; 41:69–75.

Murphy DJ, Meyer RA, Kaplan S: Non-invasive evaluation of newborns with suspected congenital heart disease. *Am J Dis Child* 1985; 139:589–594.

Porter CJ, Gillette PC, McNamara DG: Twenty-four hour ambulatory ECGs in the detection and management of cardiac arrhythmias in infants and children. *Pediatr Cardiol* 1980; 1:203–208.

Reeder GS, Currie PJ, Hagler DJ, et al: Use of Doppler techniques (continuous-wave, pulsed-wave, and color flow imaging) in the non-invasive hemodynamic assessment of congenital heart disease. *Mayo Clin Proc* 1986; 61:725–744.

Sherman FS, Sahn DJ: Pediatric Doppler echocardiography, 1987: Major advances for technology. *J Pediatr* 1987; 110:333–342.

Tajik AJ, Seward JB, Hagler DJ, et al: Two-dimensional real-time ultrasonic imaging of the heart and great vessels: Technique, image orientation, structure identification, and validation. *Mayo Clin Proc* 1978; 53:271–303.

Chapter 7. Invasive Studies

Elliott LP, Bargeron LM, Bream PR, et al: Axial cineangiography in congenital heart disease. *Circulation* 1977; 56:1084–1093.

Hoffer FA, Fellows KE, Wyly JB, et al: Therapeutic catheter procedures in pediatrics. *Pediatr Clin North Am* 1985; 32:1461–1476.

Jarmakani JM: Catheterization and angiocardiography, in Adams FH, Emmanouilides GC (eds): *Moss' Heart Disease in Infants, Children and Adolescents*, ed 3. Baltimore, Williams & Wilkins Co, 1983, pp 83–100.

Park SC, Neches WH, Mullins CE, et al: Blade atrial septostomy: Collaborative study. *Circulation* 1982; 66:258–266.

Chapter 8. Fetal and Perinatal Circulation

Guntheroth WG, Kawabori I, Stevenson JG: Physiology of the circulation: Fetus, neonate, and child, in Kelley VC (ed): *Practice of Pediatrics*. Philadelphia, Harper & Row, 1982-83, vol 8, chap 23.

Rudolph AM: *Congenital Disease of the Heart*. Chicago, Year Book Medical Publishers, 1974.

Chapter 9. Pathophysiology of Left-to-Right Shunt Lesions

Heath D, Edwards JE: The pathology of hypertensive pulmonary vascular disease. *Circulation* 1958; 18:533–547.

Moller JH, Amplatz K, Edwards JE: *Congenital Heart Disease*. Kalamazoo, Mich, The Upjohn Co, 1971.

Rudolph AM: *Congenital Diseases of the Heart*. Chicago, Year Book Medical Publishers, 1974.

Rudolph AM: The changes in the circulation after birth: Their importance in congenital heart disease. *Circulation* 1970; 41:343–359.

Chapter 10. Pathophysiology of Obstructive and Valvular Regurgitant Lesions

Moller JH, Amplatz K, Edwards JE: *Congenital Heart Disease*. Kalamazoo, Mich, The Upjohn Co, 1971.

Chapter 11. Pathophysiology of Cyanotic Congenital Heart Defects

Fischbein CA, Rosenthal A, Fischer EG, et al: Risk factors for brain abscess in patients with congenital heart disease. *Am J Cardiol* 1974; 34:97–102.

Guntheroth WG, Morgan BC, Mullins GL: Physiologic studies of paroxysmal hyperpnea in cyanotic congenital heart disease. *Circulation* 1965; 31:70–76.

Moller JH, Amplatz K, Edwards JE: *Congenital Heart Disease.* Kalamazoo, Mich, The Upjohn Co, 1971.

Rudolph AM: *Congenital Disease of the Heart.* Chicago, Year Book Medical Publishers, 1974.

Chapter 12. Left-to-Right Shunt Lesions

Capelli H, Andrade JL, Somerville J: Classification of the site of ventricular septal defect by 2-dimensional echocardiography. *Am J Cardiol* 1983; 51:1474–1480.

Feldt RH, Edwards WD, Puga FJ, et al: Atrial septal defects and atrioventricular canal, in Adams FH, Emmanouilides GC (eds): *Moss' Heart Disease in Infants, Children and Adolescents,* ed 3. Baltimore, Williams & Wilkins Co, 1983, pp 118–134.

Graham TP Jr: When to operate on the child with congenital heart disease. *Pediatr Clin North Am* 1984; 31:1275–1291.

Heymann MA: Patent ductus arteriosus, in Adams FH, Emmanouilides GC (eds): *Moss' Heart Disease in Infants, Children and Adolescents,* ed 3. Baltimore, Williams & Wilkins, 1983, pp 158–171.

Keith JD: Ventricular septal defect, in Keith JD, Rowe RD, Vlad P (eds): *Heart Disease in Infancy and Childhood,* ed 3. New York, MacMillan Publishing Co, 1978, pp 320–379.

Chapter 13. Obstructive Lesions

Beekman RH, Rocchini AP, Behrendt DM, et al: Re-operation for coarctation of the aorta. *Am J Cardiol* 1981; 48:1108–1114.

Friedman WF, Benson LB: Congenital aortic stenosis, in Adams FH, Emmanouilides GC (eds): *Moss' Heart Disease in Infants, Children and Adolescents,* ed 3. Baltimore, Williams & Wilkins, 1983, pp 171–188.

Graham TP Jr: When to operate on the child with congenital heart disease. *Pediatr Clin North Am* 1984; 31:1275–1291.

Hoffman JIE: The natural history of congenital isolated pulmonic and aortic stenosis. *Annu Rev Med* 1969; 20:15–28.

Chapter 14. Cyanotic Congenital Heart Defects

Allwork SP, Bentall HH, Becker AE, et al: Congenitally corrected transposition of the great arteries: Morphologic study of 32 cases. *Am J Cardiol* 1976; 38:910–923.

Danielson GK, Fuster V: Surgical repair of Ebstein's anomaly. *Ann Surg* 1982; 196:499–504.

Elliott LP, Anderson RH, Bargeron LM Jr, et al: Single or univentricular heart, in Adams FH, Emmanouilides GC (eds): *Moss' Heart Disease in Infants, Children and Adolescents,* ed 3. Baltimore, Williams & Wilkins Co, 1983, pp 386–400.

Emmanouilides GC, Baylen BG, Nelson RJ: Pulmonary atresia with intact ventricular septum, in Adams FH, Emmanouilides GC (eds): *Moss' Heart Disease in Infants, Children and Adolescents,* ed 3. Baltimore, Williams & Wilkins Co, 1983, pp 263–271.

Engle MA: Cyanotic congenital heart disease. *Am J Cardiol* 1976; 37:283–308.

Fontan F, Deville C, Quaegebeur J, et al: Repair of tricuspid atresia in 100 patients. *J Thorac Cardiovasc Surg* 1983; 85:647–660.

Gillette PC, Kugler JD, Gutgesell HP, et al: Mechanisms of cardiac arrhythmias after the Mustard operation for transposition of the great arteries. *Am J Cardiol* 1980; 45:1225–1230.

Graham TP Jr: When to operate on the child with congenital heart disease. *Pediatr Clin North Am* 1984; 31:1275–1291.

Guntheroth WG, Kawabori I, Baum D: Tetralogy of Fallot, in Adams FH, Emmanouilides GC (eds): *Moss' Heart Disease in Infants, Children and Adolescents,* ed 3. Baltimore, Williams & Wilkins Co, 1983, pp 215–228.

Hagler DJ, Ritter DG, Puga FJ: Double-outlet right ventricle, in Adams FH, Emmanouilides GC (eds): *Moss' Heart Disease in Infants, Children and Adolescents*, ed 3. Baltimore,
Williams & Wilkins Co, 1983, pp 215–228.

Kirklin JW, Blackstone EH, Kirklin JK, et al: Surgical results and protocols in the spectrum
of tetralogy of Fallot. *Ann Surg* 1983; 198:251–265.

Kirklin JK, Blackstone EH, Kirklin JW, et al: The Fontan operation: Ventricular hypertrophy, age and date of operation as risk factors. *J Thorac Cardiovasc Surg* 1986; 92:1049–
1064.

Lucas RV Jr: Anomalous venous connections, pulmonary and systemic, in Adams FH, Emmanouilides GC (eds): *Moss' Heart Disease in Infants, Children and Adolescents*, ed 3.
Baltimore, Williams & Wilkins Co, 1983, pp 458–491.

Mair DD, Edwards WD, Fluster V, et al: Truncus arteriosus, in Adams FH, Emmanouilides GC (eds): *Moss' Heart Disease in Infants, Children and Adolescents*, ed 3. Baltimore,
Williams & Wilkins Co, 1983, pp 400–410.

Paul MH: Transposition of the great arteries, in Adams FH, Emmanouilides GC (eds): *Moss'
Heart Disease in Infants, Children and Adolescents*, ed 3. Baltimore, Williams & Wilkins
Co, 1983, pp 296–333.

Quaegebeur JM, Rohmer J, Ottenkamp J, et al: The atrial switch operation: An eight-year
experience. *J Thorac Cardiovasc Surg* 1986; 92:361–384.

Turley K, Tucker WY, Ullyot DJ, et al: Total anomalous pulmonary venous connection in
infancy: Influence of age and type of lesions. *Am J Cardiol* 1980; 45:92–97.

Chapter 15. Vascular Ring
Shuford WH, Sybers RG: *The Aortic Arch and Its Malformations*. Springfield, Ill, Charles
C Thomas Publisher, 1973.

Chapter 16. Chamber Localization and Cardiac Malposition
Huhta JC, Hagler DJ, Seward JB, et al: Two-dimensional echocardiographic assessment of
dextrocardia: A segmental approach. *Am J Cardiol* 1982; 50:1351–1360.

Van Praagh R, Vlad P: Dextrocardia, mesocardia and levocardia: The segmental approach
to diagnosis in congenital heart disease, in Keith JD, Rowe RD, Vlad P (eds): *Heart Disease in Infancy and Childhood*, ed 3. New York, MacMillan Publishing Co, 1978, pp 638–
695.

Chapter 17. Miscellaneous Congenital Cardiac Conditions
Sapire DW, Ho SY, Anderson RH, et al: Diagnosis and significance of atrial isomerism. *Am
J Cardiol* 1986; 58:342–346.

Chapter 18. Primary Myocardial Disease
Edwards JE: Cardiac tumors, in Adams FH, Emmanouilides GC (eds): *Moss' Heart Disease
in Infants, Children and Adolescents*, ed 3. Baltimore, Williams & Wilkins Co, 1983, pp
741–748.

Keith JD, Rose V, Manning JA: Endocardial fibroelastosis, in Keith JD, Rowe RD, Vlad P
(eds): *Heart Disease in Infancy and Childhood*, ed 3. New York, MacMillan Publishing
Co, 1978, pp 941–957.

Maron BJ: Cardiomyopathies, in Adams FH, Emmanouilides GC (eds): *Moss' Heart Disease
in Infants, Children and Adolescents*, ed 3. Baltimore, Williams & Wilkins Co, 1983, pp
757–780.

Chapter 19. Cardiovascular Infections
Crowley DC: Cardiovascular complications of mucocutaneous lymph node syndrome. *Pediatr
Clin North Am* 1984; 31:1321–1329.

Johnson DH, Rosenthal A, Nadas AS: A 40-year review of bacterial endocarditis in infancy
and childhood. *Circulation* 1975; 51:581–588.

Kavey RW, Frank DM, Byrum CJ, et al: Two-dimensional echocardiographic assessment of
infective endocarditis in children. *Am J Dis Child* 1983; 137:851–856.

Melish ME, Hicks RV, Reddy V: Kawasaki syndrome: An update. *Hosp Pract* 1982; 17:99–
106.

Newburger JW, Takahashi M, Burns JC, et al: The treatment of Kawasaki syndrome with
intravenous gamma globulin. *N Engl J Med* 1986; 315:341–347.

Noren GR, Kaplan EL, Staley NA: Non-rheumatic inflammatory disease, in Adams FH, Emmanouilides GC (eds): *Moss' Heart Disease in Infants, Children and Adolescents*, ed 3. Baltimore, Williams & Wilkins Co, 1983.

Shulman ST, Amren DP, Bino AL, et al: Prevention of bacterial endocarditis. *Circulation* 1984; 70:1123A–1127A.

Weinstein L, Schlesinger JJ: Pathoanatomic, pathophysiologic and clinical coorelation in endocarditis. *N Engl J Med* 1974; 291:832–837, 1122–1126.

Chapter 20. Acute Rheumatic Fever

Ayoub EM, Schiebler GL: Acute rheumatic fever, in Kelley VC (ed): *Practice of Pediatrics*, Philadelphia, Harper & Row, 1987, vol 8, chap 27.

Markowitz M, Gordis L: *Rheumatic Fever*. Philadelphia, WB Saunders Co, 1972.

Shulman ST, Amren DP, Bisno AL, et al: Prevention of rheumatic fever. *Circulation* 1984; 70:1118A–1122A.

Chapter 21. Valvular Heart Disease

Bisset GS III, Schwartz DC, Meyer RA, et al: Clinical spectrum and long term follow-up of isolated mitral valve prolapse in 119 children. *Circulation* 1980; 62:423–429.

Levine RA, Triulzi MO, Harrigan P, et al: The relationship of mitral annular shape to the diagnosis of mitral valve prolapse. *Circulation* 1987; 75:756–767.

Park MK: Acquired valvular heart disease, in Kelley VC-(ed): *Practice of Pediatrics*. Philadelphia, Harper & Row, 1987, vol 8, chap 28.

Chapter 22. Cardiac Involvement in Systemic Diseases

Caddell JL: Metabolic and nutritional diseases, in Adams FH, Emmanouilides GC (eds): *Moss' Heart Disease in Infants, Children and Adolescents*, ed 3. Baltimore, Williams & Wilkins Co, 1983, pp 596–626.

Child JS, Perloff JK, Bach PM, et al: Cardiac involvement in Friedreich's ataxia: A clinical study of 75 patients. *J Am Coll Cardiol* 1986; 7:1370–1378.

Freedom RM, Keith JD: Cardiac involvement in the Callagen disease, in Keith JD, Rowe RD, Vlad P (eds): *Heart Disease in Infancy and Childhood*, ed 3. New York, MacMillan Publishing Co, 1978, pp 970–977.

Friedli B, Rowe RD: Marfan's syndrome: Arachnodactyly, in Keith JD, Rowe RD, Vlad P (eds): *Heart Disease in Infancy and Childhood,* ed 3. New York, MacMillan Publishing Co, 1978, pp 1004–1012.

Perloff JK, DeLeon AC Jr, O'Doherty D: The cardiomyopathy of progressive muscular dystrophy. *Circulation* 1966; 33:625–648.

Rowe RD, Freedom RM: The heart in neuromuscular disorders, in Keith JD, Rowe RD, Vlad P (eds): *Heart Disease in Infancy and Childhood*, ed 3. New York, MacMillan Publishing Co, 1978, pp 978–986.

Chapter 23. Arrhythmias and Disturbances of Atrioventricular Conduction

Dick M II, Campbell RM: Advances in the management of cardiac arrhythmias in children. *Pediatr Clin North Am* 1984; 31:1175–1195.

Garson A, Gillette PC, McNamara DG: Supraventricular tachycardia in children: Clinical features, response to treatment and long-term follow-up in 217 patients. *J Pediatr* 1981; 98:875–882.

Guntheroth WG, Park MK, Kawabori I, et al: Disorders of heart rate and rhythm, in Kelley VC (ed): *Practice of Pediatrics*. Philadelphia, Harper & Row, 1982–83, vol 8, chap 28.

Chapter 24. ST Segment and T Wave Changes

Park MK, Guntheroth WG: *How to Read Pediatric ECGs*, ed 2. Chicago, Year Book Medical Publishers, 1987.

Chapter 25. Special Features in Cardiac Evaluation of the Newborn

Lees MH, Sunderland CO: Heart disease in the newborn, in Adams FH, Emmanouilides GC (eds): *Moss' Heart Disease in Infants, Children and Adolescents*, ed 3. Baltimore, Williams & Wilkins Co, 1983, pp 658–669.

Taybi H: Roentgen evaluation of cardiomegaly in the newborn period and early infancy. *Pediatr Clin North Am* 1971; 18:1031–1058.

Chapter 26. Cardiac Problems of the Newborn

Dooley KJ: Management of the premature infant with a patent ductus arteriosus. *Pediatr Clin North Am* 1984; 31:159–174.

Fox WW, Duara S: Persistent pulmonary hypertension in the neonate: Diagnosis and management. J Pediatr 1983; 103:505–514.

Freed MD, Heymann MA, Lewis AB, et al: Prostaglandin E in infants with ductus-dependent congenital heart disease. *Circulation* 1981; 64:899–905.

Gutgesell HP, Speer ME, Rosenberg HS: Characterization of the cardiomyopathy in infants of diabetic mothers. *Circulation* 1980; 61:441–450.

Huhta JC, Cohen M, Gutgesell HP: Patency of the ductus arteriosus in normal neonates: Two-dimensional echocardiography versus Doppler assessment. *J Am Coll Cardiol* 1984; 4:561–564.

McCue CM, Mantakas ME, Tingelstad JB, et al: Congenital heart block in newborns of mothers with connective tissue disease. *Circulation* 1977; 56:82–90.

Norwood WI, Lang P, Hansen D: Physiologic repair of aortic atresia-hypoplastic left heart syndrome. *N Engl J Med* 1983; 308:23–26.

Ramsay JM, Murphy DJ Jr, Vick GW III, et al: Response of the patent ductus arteriosus to indomethacin treatment. *Am J Dis Child* 1987; 141:294–297.

Rowe RD, Freedom MR, Mehrizi A: *The Neonate With Congenital Heart Disease*. Philadelphia, WB Saunders Co, 1981.

Rowe RD, Hoffman T: Transient myocardial ischemia of the newborn infant: A form of severe cardiopulmonary distress in full term infants. *J Pediatr* 1972; 81:243–250.

Stevens DC, Schreiner RL, Hurwitz RA, et al: Fetal and neonatal ventricular arrhythmias. *Pediatrics* 1979; 63:771–777.

Talner HS, Berman MA: Postnatal development of obstruction in coarctation of the aorta: Role of the ductus arteriosus. *Pediatrics* 1975; 56:562–569.

Chapter 27. Congestive Heart Failure

Artman M, Parrish MD, Graham TP Jr: Congestive heart failure in childhood and adolescents: Recognition and management. *Am Heart J* 1983; 105:471–480.

Berman W Jr, Yabek SM, Dillon T, et al: Effects of digoxin in infants with a congested circulatory state due to a ventricular septal defect. *N Engl J Med* 1983; 308:363–366.

Friedman WF, George BL: New concepts and drugs in the treatment of congestive heart failure. *Pediatr Clin North Am* 1984; 31:1197–1227.

Park MK: The use of digoxin in infants and children with specific emphasis on dosage. *J Pediatr* 1986; 108:871–877.

Talner NS: Heart failure, in Adams FH, Emmanouilides GC (eds): *Moss' Heart Disease in Infants, Children and Adolescents*, ed 3. Baltimore, Williams & Wilkins Co, 1983.

Chapter 28. Systemic Hypertension

Berenson GS, Cresanta JL, Webber LS: High blood pressure in the young. *Annu Rev Med* 1984; 35:535–560.

Park MK, Guntheroth WG: Systemic hypertension, in Kelly VC (ed): *Practice of Pediatrics*. Philadelphia, Harper & Row, 1982–83, vol 8, chap 35.

Report of the Second Task Force on Blood Pressure Control in Children—1987. *Pediatrics* 1987; 79:1–25.

Chapter 29. Pulmonary Hypertension

Heath D, Edwards JE: The pathology of hypertensive pulmonary vascular disease: A description of 6 grades of structural changes in the pulmonary arteries with special reference to congenital cardiac septal defects. *Circulation* 1958; 18:533–547.

Hoffman JIE, Rudolph AM, Heymann MA: Pulmonary vascular disease with congenital heart lesions: Pathologic features and causes. *Circulation* 1981; 64:873–877.

Perkin RM, Anas NG: Pulmonary hypertension in pediatric patients. *J Pediatr* 1984; 105:511–522.

Chapter 30. Hyperlipidemia in Children

Diagnosis and treatment of primary hyperlipidemia in childhood: A joint statement for physicians by the committee on atherosclerosis and hypertension in childhood of the Council of Cardiovascular Disease in the Young and Nutrition Committee, American Heart Association. *Circulation* 1986; 74:1181A–1188A.

Strong WB: *Atherosclerosis: Its Pediatric Aspects*. New York, Grune & Stratton, 1978.

Chapter 31. Child With Chest Pain or Syncope

Brenner JI, Ringel RE, Berman MA: Cardiologic perspectives of chest pain in childhood: A referral problem? To whom? *Pediatr Clin North Am* 1984; 31:1241–1258.

Diehl AM: Chest pain in children: Tip-offs to cause. *Postgrad Educ* 1983; 73:335–342.

Driscole DJ, Glicklich LB, Gallen WJ: Chest pain in children: A prospective study. *Pediatrics* 1976; 57:648–651.

Pantell RH, Goodman BW Jr: Adolescent chest pain: A prospective study. *Pediatrics* 1983; 71:881–887.

Chapter 32. Postoperative Syndromes

Engle MA: Postoperative problems, in Adams FH, Emmanouilides GC (eds): *Moss' Heart Disease in Infants, Children and Adolescents*. Baltimore, Williams & Wilkins Co, 1983, pp 748–757.

Index